# ARTHROPLASTY:
## An Atlas of Surgical Technique

MICHAEL J. BRONSON, M.D.
Lenox Hill Hospital *and*
Columbia University College
of Physicians and Surgeons
New York, New York

EDWARD V. CRAIG, M.D.
University of Minnesota
Minneapolis, Minnesota

SUSAN M. CRAIG, M.D.
St. Luke's—Roosevelt Hospital *and*
Columbia University College
of Physicians and Surgeons
New York, New York

PETER GEAREN, M.D.
University of Florida College
of Medicine *and*
Shands Teaching Hospital and Clinics
Gainesville, Florida

RICHARD D. SCOTT, M.D.
Harvard Medical School *and*
Brigham and Women's Hospital *and*
Northeast Baptist Hospital
Boston, Massachusetts

ROBERT G. VOLZ, M.D.
Arizona Health Sciences Center
Tucson, Arizona

# ARTHROPLASTY: An Atlas of Surgical Technique

Edited by

**W. Norman Scott, M.D.**

Lenox Hill Hospital
New York, New York

**William Thomas Stillwell, M.D.**

St. John's Episcopal Hospital
Smithtown, New York
and
State University of New York
Stony Brook, New York
and
Columbia University
New York, New York

AN ASPEN PUBLICATION®
Aspen Publishers, Inc.

1987

Rockville, Maryland
Royal Tunbridge Wells

Library of Congress Cataloging-in-Publication Data

Arthroplasty : an atlas of surgical technique.

Includes bibliographies and index.
1. Arthroplasty. 2. Arthroplasty—Atlases. I. Scott, W. Norman. Stillwell, Williams Thomas. [DNLM: 1. Arthroplasty—atlases. WE 17 A787]
RD686.A75 1986 617'.58 86-28686
ISBN: 0-87189-390-8



Editorial Services: Lisa J. McCullough

Library of Congress Catalog Card Number: 86-28686
ISBN: 0-87189-390-8

*Printed in the United States of America*

1 2 3 4 5

# TABLE OF CONTENTS

# Preface

In the rapidly evolving sphere of joint arthroplasty, progress seems to be directly proportional to biomechanical advances and improved surgical technique. Material properties, geometric configurations, and modes of fixation represent the primary investigative areas of biomechanical research. Developing the ideal material necessitates an evaluation of its strength, ductility, and durability in a bone-prosthetic-interface composite. In vitro geometric considerations, e.g., collar versus collarless hip prosthesis, do not always have the same in vivo characteristics; thus the interaction between laboratory and clinical investigations has been the cornerstone of success. The biomechanical failure of joint replacements has usually occurred at the interface and readily explains the perpetual interest in evaluating all methods of fixation. Until recently, cemented prostheses were felt to be doomed for failure, as evidenced by the abundant research into noncemented fixation. Recent data, however, suggests that in hip arthroplasty utilizing modern cement techniques, the 10 year results are better than previous experience and, indeed, cement might not be "so bad."[1] Although the issue will only be resolved with continued analysis, there is no controversy as to the interaction of good surgical technique and biomechanical design. In the 67 cemented Total Condylar knee replacements evaluated at least 10 years postoperatively with "decent" alignment of 0–10° valgus, there was only one failure.[2]

The development of this book originates from the belief that surgical technique is at least as important for a successful arthroplasty as the biomechanical considerations. All too often, however, in promoting a "new" design or set of instrumentation, the principles of insertion are ignored. Although details of surgical technique can usually be found, they have never been pictorially contrasted using artistic representation and operative pictures in the same volume.

It is not our intent to champion any specific prostheses but rather in an atlas fashion to allow the surgeon the opportunity of analyzing any significant differences in surgical technique. It would be impossible to delineate every detail of all primary arthroplasties, and for this information we refer the reader to the original articles. It is our hope that medical students, residents, and orthopedists will be able to use this volume as a pictorial reference before observing their "first" joint arthroplasty or as a "refresher" prior to undertaking new techniques. In developing this theme, we felt it best to use recognized experts for each chapter. The written introduction is cursory since, in this rapidly evolving field, the perpetual lag between textbook information and periodicals puts the former at a distinct disadvantage. The operative pictures are from the individual authors and interspersed to allow the reader the chance to compare differences. The artwork, for the most part, has been contributed by an orthopedist, and a professional artist, William Thomas Stillwell, who has elaborated on the differences between schematics and "what it really looks like."

The individual contributors are to be congratulated and, from the editors' perspective, applauded for their tireless effort in developing this novel approach of disseminating information for the good of the surgeon's understanding and, ultimately, the patient's benefit.

## References

1. Lachiewicz, P. Ten to 12 year follow-up of Harris total hip replacement: Don't throw away the cement. Paper No. 245, AAOS Meeting, February 24, 1986.
2. Insall, J. Participant panel discussion. The Knee Society, February 20, 1986, New Orleans.

# Shoulder Arthroplasty

# 1

Edward V. Craig

## Introduction

Under normal nonpathologic conditions the glenohumeral joint achieves its unique capacity for range of motion by a stable, painless articulation between the glenoid and humeral head and the integrated action of the acromioclavicular, sternoclavicular, and scapulothoracic articulations. The critical contribution of the surrounding capsule and musculotendinous units cannot be overemphasized. The glenoid shape is only slightly curved and has a surface area of 25% of the humeral head. Thus, the humeral head "rests" against the glenoid and relies on the associated soft tissue for stability as well as mobility. Scarring or contracture of these soft tissues, excessive laxity or capsular incompetence, deltoid or rotator cuff weakness from neurological disease, or loss of the function of the rotator cuff through degeneration or wear will severely compromise normal shoulder function.

Any discussion of the role, indications, and technique of shoulder replacement arthroplasty must take into consideration the multiple variables that can affect these surrounding soft tissue and bony structures. The technique of component insertion is but a small part of a process that must include proper patient selection; evaluation of sternoclavicular, acromioclavicular, and scapulothoracic relations; evaluation of the integrity and function of the rotator cuff, the laxity or contracture of the capsule and glenohumeral ligaments, and the power of the deltoid muscle; and the ability of surgeon and patient to cooperate in the critical rehabilitation necessary for successful arthroplasty. Pain relief following arthroplasty is quite predictable if these many variables can be handled successfully. Although passive motion may be established with meticulous attention to soft tissue and bony technique, active motion will depend almost entirely on the rehabilitation and strength of the muscles powering the shoulder girdle. Implant stability will be possible only with competent soft tissue around an unconstrained implant or the reliance on an implant with more inherent constraint.

In no other arthroplasty is it as important to understand the disease process leading to the joint degeneration, because the particular features of each arthropathy will present unique problems of bone and soft tissue reconstruction. In primary osteoarthritis it is the circumferential osteophyte (Fig. 1-38) and uneven wear of the glenoid (Fig. 1-39). In rheumatoid arthritis it is the associated acromioclavicular joint disease, lower extremity pathology, elbow and wrist disability, associated rotator cuff pathology, severe bone wear, and osteopenia (Figs. 1-41 and 1-42). Old trauma presents the problem of extensive scarring, contracted soft tissue, malunited tuberosities, and the frequency of associated nerve injuries (Fig. 1-46). In cuff tear arthropathy, the excessive wear into the AC joint, acromion, and glenoid, and the associated massive cuff deficiency is particularly challenging (Fig. 1-43). In arthroplasty of dislocations, technical difficulties can be produced by scarred tendon, shortened subscapularis, and the presence of hardware (Fig. 1-44). Revision arthroplasty with its bone deficits, dense adhesions, and patient disappointment at failure of the primary procedure is as troublesome in the shoulder as it is in other joints.

Thus, a single operative technique that will be applicable in all situations is unrealistic. This chapter is only a guide to some of the techniques of implant arthroplasty of the shoulder. This is in no way an attempt to provide a cookbook approach to total shoulder replacement and should not be thought of as such.

Because the need for total shoulder replacement does not arise as frequently as for total hip or total knee replacements, because each case is often unique in its particular bony or soft tissue anatomy, because the operation is invariably technically difficult, and because of the unique role of patient motivation in rehabilitation of the shoulder, few surgeons obtain enough experience to handle comfortably the multiple variables in total shoulder replacement. As with other areas where experience of any one orthopaedic surgeon is limited, consideration should be given to observing several shoulder replacements at any one of a number of centers experienced in this technique and to performing implantation and dissection in a cadaver model before attempting total shoulder replacement.

## Prosthetic Selection

A number of prosthetic designs have been developed in the evolving history of shoulder replacement. By far the most popular has been the nonconstrained implant designed by Neer. The popularity of this prosthesis stems from the fact that its insertion requires the removal of only that part of the humeral head and glenoid normally covered with articular cartilage. This minimal removal of bone allows for the duplication of normal anatomy, and the nonconstrained implant also allows some bone stock for salvage through arthrodesis should this become necessary. In the Neer design the proximal humeral component comes in two thicknesses of head (15 and 23 mm), each with the same radius of curvature. There are three different diameters of stem (6.3, 9.5, and 12.7 mm) for each thickness of head. The extra long stem (252 mm) is used in tumor resection or for associated humeral shaft fractures, whereas the extra short stem (63 mm) is used in special situations such as in juvenile rheumatoid arthritis or where there is epiphyseal dysplasia. The proximal humerus can be used with or without bone cement, and since its radius of curvature approximates the normal humeral head, it can be used without a glenoid component if the situation warrants it, such as in fractures or if there is no associated glenoid disease (Fig. 1-1).

The standard glenoid component approximates the surface of the average adult glenoid and is made of a high density polyethylene. It has a keel that must be inserted into the neck of the scapula and a radiographic marker wire (Fig. 1-2). Its radius of curvature matches that of the proximal humerus (Fig. 1-3). More recently, a metal-backed glenoid has been utilized to minimize the possibility of keel breakage of the standard polyethylene glenoid (Fig. 1-4).

Other nonconstrained designs have included the Bechtol and O'Leary-Walker models. A bit more constraint has been built into the prosthetic design of the UCLA and MacNab-English prostheses. Since the nonconstrained implant duplicates the normal anatomy, it has a critial reliance on the soft tissue integrity around the shoulder to both stabilize and move the implant. The surgeon must thus have the tools to treat capsular laxity or contracture should this be present and must be able to reconstruct the rotator cuff should there be a significant defect.

In an effort to avoid the pitfalls of this difficult soft tissue reconstruction, efforts have been made to design prostheses with more inherent stability. The trispherical prosthesis of Gristina, the "floating socket" of Buechel, the prostheses designed by Fenlin, Post, and Stanmore, and the Zippel models are the most constrained. These more constrained prostheses do not allow the stresses in the shoulder to be dissipated by the surrounding soft tissues, and complications in some series have been high.[1,2] These designs may be considered when there is no functioning rotator cuff.[3] The amount of necessary bone resection is sometimes great, making salvage difficult, and loosening may still be considered the greatest problem. Most surgeons would still prefer a nonconstrained implant with meticulous reconstruction of soft tissues for coverage or stability. For this reason, the technique of insertion of the nonconstrained implant will be the technique outlined.

## Indications and Contraindications

The main indication for implant arthroplasty of the shoulder is pain from an incongruous glenohumeral joint unresponsive to other forms of conservative treatment such as rest, antiinflammatory medication, or an occasional intraarticular injection. It is critical that the surgeon identify that the pain is coming from the glenohumeral joint itself. Some patients may have mild radiographic arthritic changes, while their predominant pain is coming from associated acromioclavicular joint disease, cervical spine pathology, or impingement syndrome. A radiographic finding of mild arthritis in a patient with recurrent dislocation may suggest that dislocation arthropathy is the source of pain, while the pain may be coming from continued instability or hardware protrusion into the joint. A patient with rheumatoid arthritis may benefit from AC joint resection or bursectomy if the radiographic changes are not severe. In addition, there is a precollapse phase before the development of cuff tear arthropathy when acromioplasty and cuff repair, rather than shoulder replacement, is better advised.

Improved range of motion is a less common indication for prosthetic replacement, because in general the gain in active range of motion is less predictable than pain improvement. Range of motion will depend to a great degree on the ability to reconstruct and rehabilitate the musculotendinous units moving the implant. Rheumatoid patients may in fact have a limited active range of motion because of associated rotator cuff weakness or rheumatoid myopathy, and implant insertion will not correct this. A patient with cuff tear arthropathy may have pain relief without a necessarily improved active range of motion, since the cuff may be irreversibly weakened because of the length of time before treatment. Nevertheless, there are some patients, notably those with ankylosing spondylitis or other rheumatic disease, in whom a restricted range of motion may affect the activities of daily living or put undue stress on more distal joints. In this situation it is probably reasonable to attempt to gain range of motion with prosthetic replacement.

Indications for prosthetic replacement are also identified by the disease process. Humeral head replacement alone is indicated in the following situations:

1. Some forms of primary osteoarthritis where the glenoid still has some cartilage remaining, although this is not common
2. Avascular necrosis, where the disease process has caused collapse and deformity of the humeral head but has not yet caused disease of the glenoid
3. Four-part fractures where it is anticipated that the articular segment is completely devoid of soft tissue attachments and blood supply, making avascular necrosis likely
4. A head-splitting fracture where the articular segment is destroyed
5. Recurrent, acute, or chronic dislocations where the impression fracture (Hill-Sachs) lesion is 40% of the articular surface or more
6. Those severe disease processes where there is not glenoid bone stock available for insertion of the implant, such as in some forms of rheumatoid arthritis
7. Elderly patients with nonunion of the surgical neck of the humerus and an osteoporotic humeral head
8. Resectable tumors of the proximal humerus
9. Very young patients when, perhaps, consideration should be given for an uncemented humeral head prosthesis alone if there is not severe destruction of the glenoid

Unconstrained total shoulder replacement has been utilized for approximately 15 years. However, reports of long-term results have been limited. Preliminary results have suggested, however, that the arthroplasty is an excellent solution to most shoulder arthropathies if attention is paid to the details of surgery and rehabilitation. The most common indications for total shoulder replacement are as follows:

1. Primary osteoarthritis with destruction of both humeral head and glenoid (Figs. 1-38 and 1-39)
2. Avascular necrosis where the incongruity of the humeral head has also destroyed the glenoid
3. Rheumatoid arthritis, which usually affects both glenoid and humeral head (Figs. 1-41 and 1-42)
4. Posttraumatic arthritis, where joint incongruity or malunion has destroyed the glenoid (Fig. 1-46)
5. Cuff tear arthropathy, the arthropathy of long-standing, untreated rotator cuff tears (Fig. 1-43A)
6. Severe arthritis of dislocations, the result of repeated instability of the humeral head. (Fig. 1-44)
7. Old infection, which is quiescent or treated
8. Failed prosthetic replacement, humeral head resection, or arthrodesis

Contraindications at present include those patients whose symptoms or disease process are not severe enough to warrant arthroplasty, active or recent infection, and paralysis of anterior deltoid and rotator cuff muscles. Since the nonconstrained implants rely so much on the reconstructed rotator cuff tendon and deltoid for power, nerve injury to axillary and suprascapular nerves or other extensive paralytic processes will so weaken and destabilize the replacement that arthrodesis may be preferable. A Charcot joint is usually a contraindication, although in some neuropathic joints stiffness and pain predominate, and implantation could probably be considered. A massive rotator cuff tear can usually be reconstructed using a remnant of a tendon, tendon transfers, and grafting and does not usually present a contraindication to a nonconstrained implant. If the cuff is totally nonreconstructable, consideration should probably be given to a more constrained implant. In the rare patient with cuff tear arthropathy and paraplegia, since most of the strength is required below shoulder level for transfers, consideration may well be given to an arthrodesis rather than total shoulder replacement. Bone loss that is reconstructable by grafting techniques is not at present a contraindication to a nonconstrained implant, although some patients have such severe erosion and bone loss of glenoid that insertion of a glenoid component may be impossible, and the humeral head alone can be used. A final relative contraindication to unconstrained arthroplasty is the patient who is unable or unwilling to cooperate with the extensive rehabilitation necessary for adequate functioning of the implant.

## Present and Future Research

Large series of total shoulder replacements have noted the presence of lucent lines around the glenoid component. In the Neer series[4] there was a 30% incidence of radiolucent lines appearing around the glenoid component, although none of these were progressive and were thought to be related to cementing techniques. In Cofield's series,[1] there were 80% lucent lines surrounding the glenoid, and 33% were progressive. Thus, recent research has centered on the area of glenoid fixation, with studies currently underway utilizing ingrowth material for the glenoid component. Several designs are now being tested, and the results are promising.[5] It remains to be seen whether the early motion so necessary for a normal return of shoulder function will be compatible with bone ingrowth designs of the glenoid.

A still unsolved problem is the patient with incapacitating glenohumeral arthritis and a massive rotator cuff defect. Attempts have been made to circumvent this by building more constraint into the prosthesis, although the complications with constrained implants may be higher than with unconstrained implants. Nevertheless, investigation into new prosthetic designs continues. It is likely that the problem of a severely deficient rotator cuff will be better solved by innovative tendon transfers and, perhaps, tendon substitution materials so that this most difficult problem will still be able to be solved with an unconstrained implant.

Another area of potential development centers around the attempts to simplify the complicated and lengthy rehabilitation of the patient following nonconstrained implant arthroplasty. At present a knowledgeable surgeon and physical therapist, a motivated patient, and careful supervision of the rehabilitation process are critical elements of successful arthroplasty. It has recently been observed that the patient need not wait 5–6 days after a shoulder replacement to begin rehabilitation, and some patients may begin their range of motion the day of surgery either with therapist-monitored passive range of motion or the use of a continuous passive motion device.[6] Early initiation of range of motion seems to simplify the rehabilitation, allowing earlier achievement of range of motion and hospital discharge and making the early postoperative period less painful. However, the rehabilitation following total shoulder replacement will continue to need to be individualized.

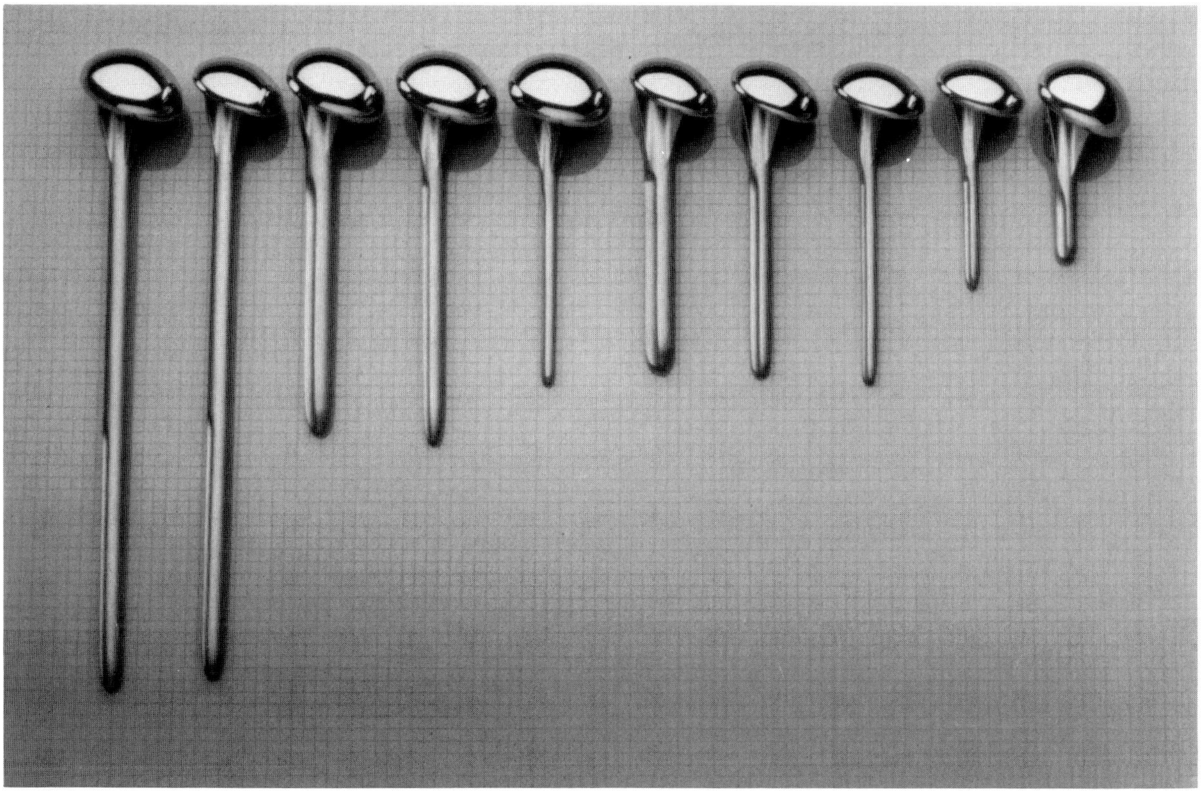

**Fig. 1-1** Neer II proximal humerus. There are two thicknesses of head (15 and 23 mm), three different stem diameters (6.3, 9.5, and 12.7 mm), and different stem lengths.

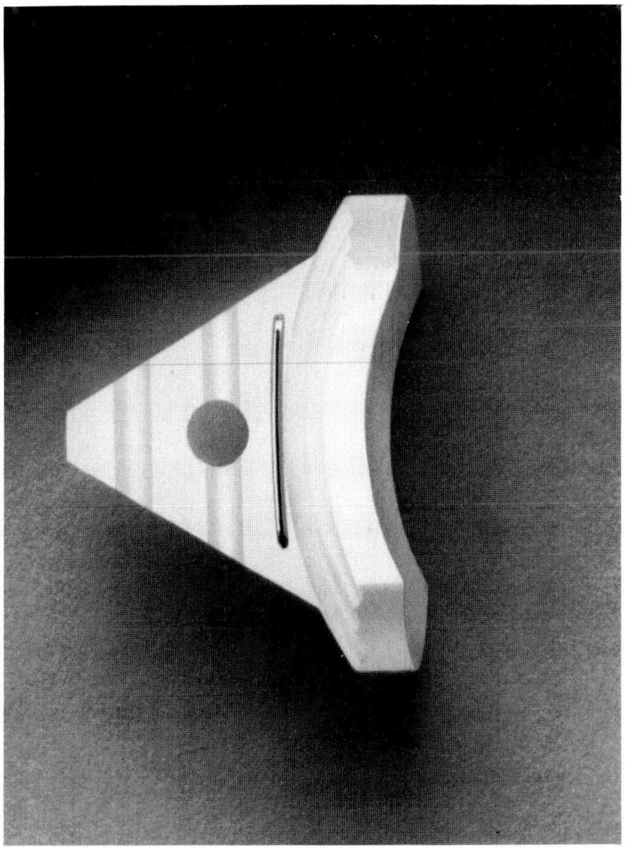

**Fig. 1-2** The standard polyethylene glenoid.

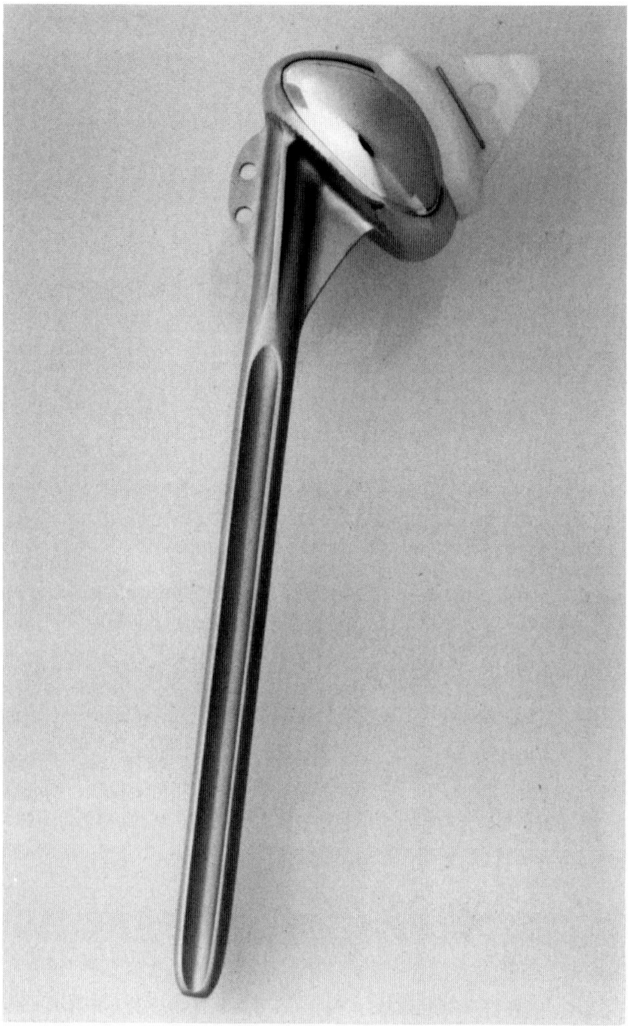

**Fig. 1-3** The total shoulder replacement, unconstrained.

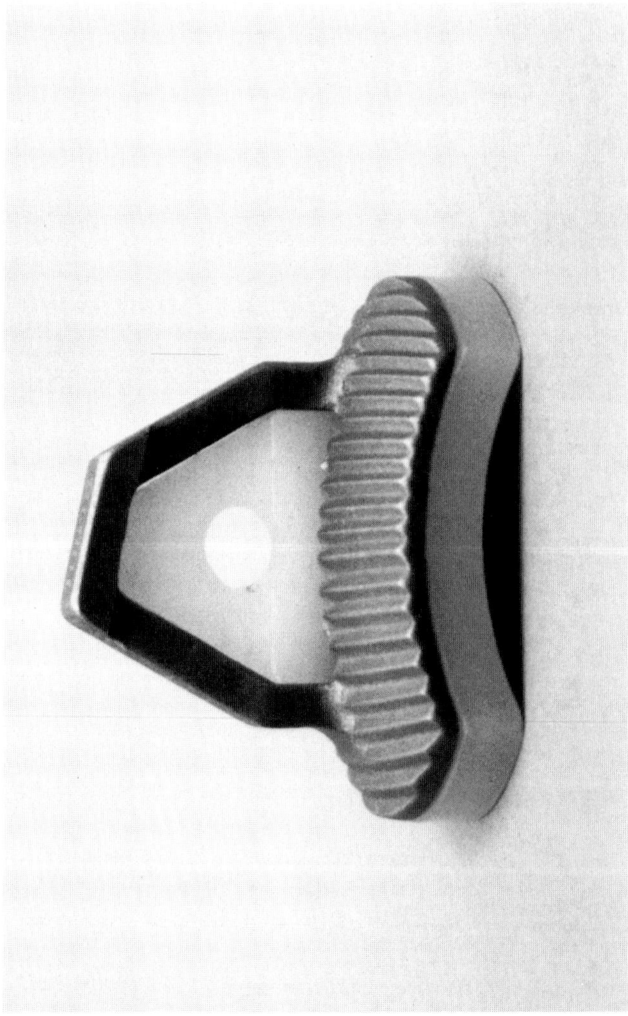

**Fig. 1-4** The metal-backed polyethylene glenoid.

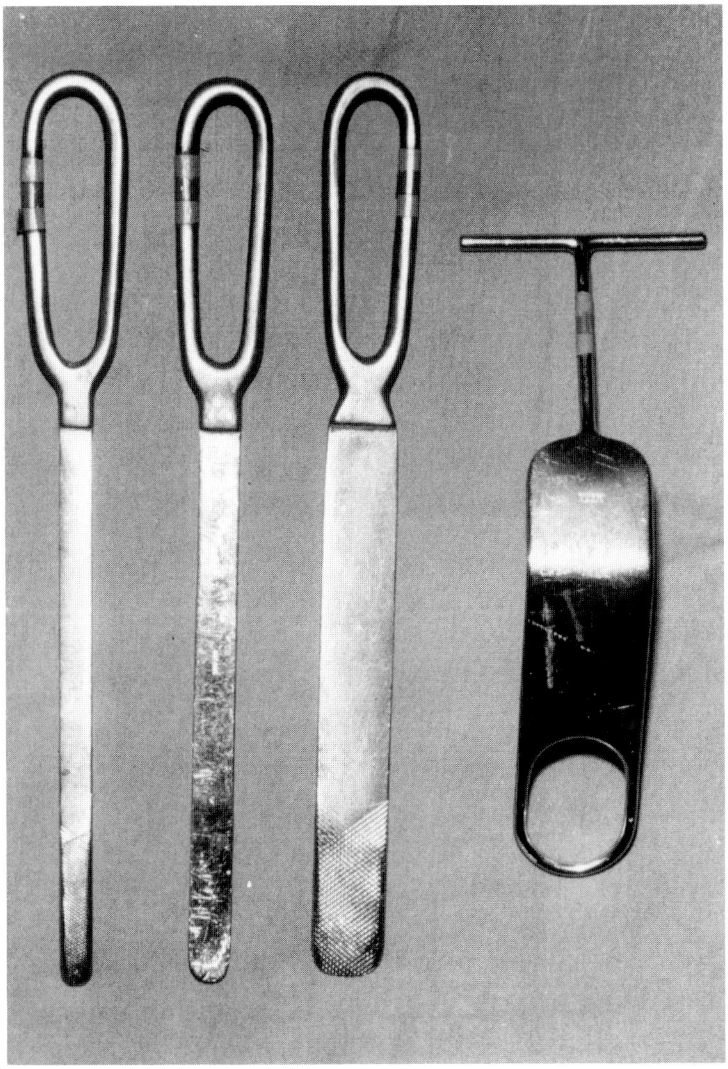

**Fig. 1-5** The Darrach and Fukuda (ring) retractors.

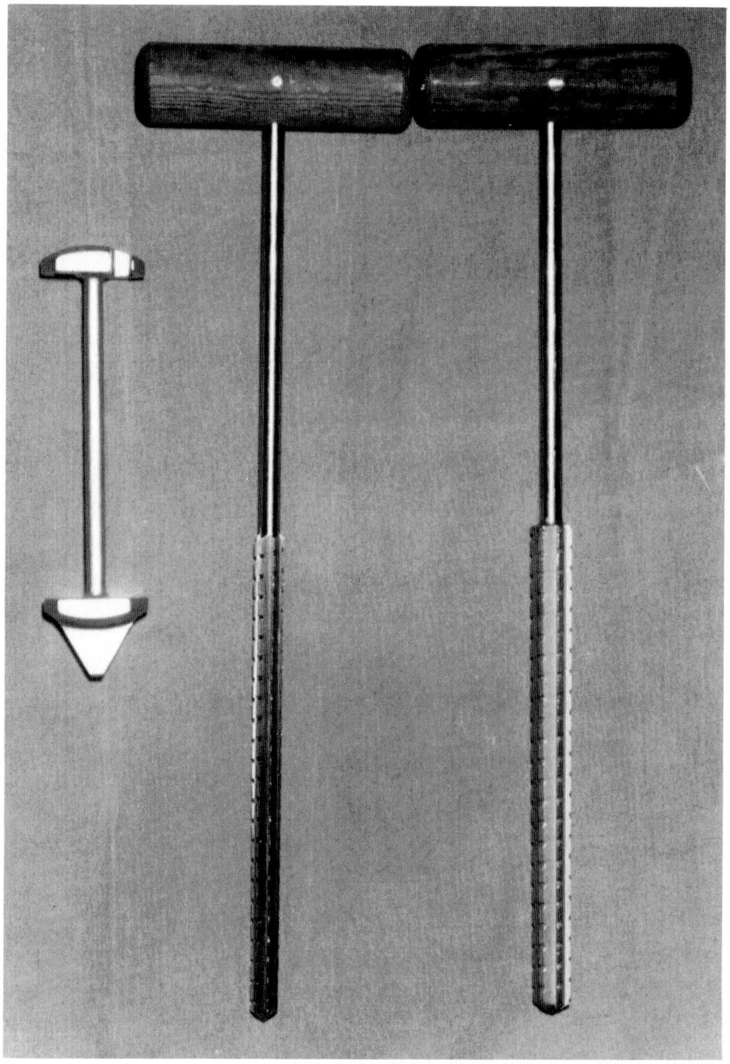

**Fig. 1-6** The T-handled reamers and glenoid guide.

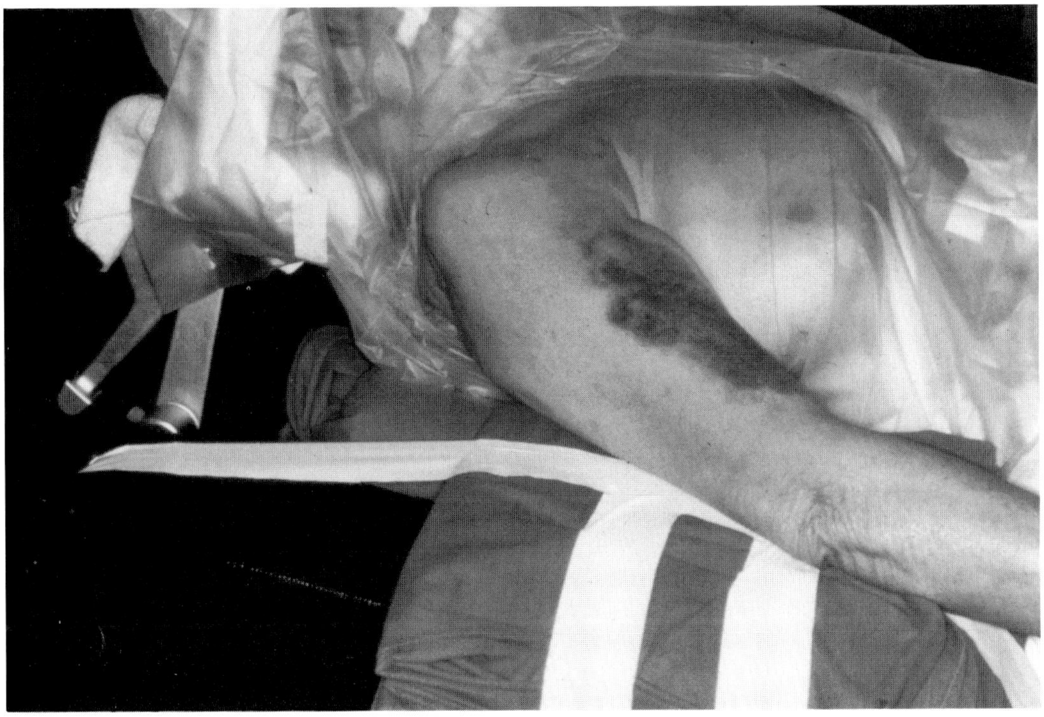

**Fig. 1-7** The arm board is useful for support of the humerus at the glenoid insertion.

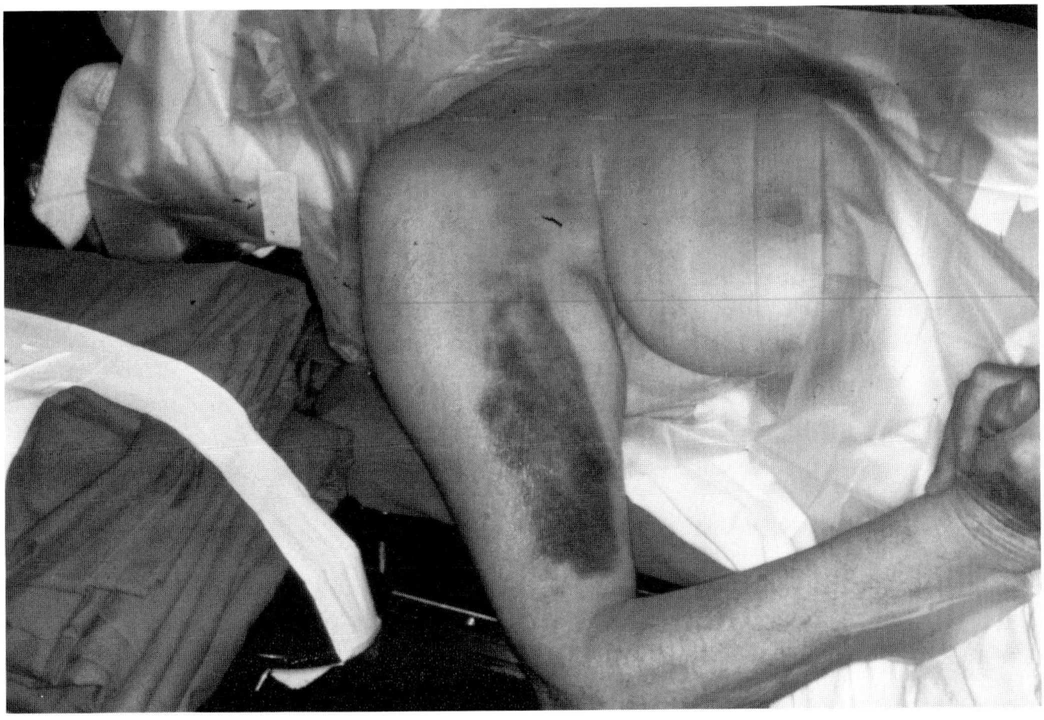

**Fig. 1-8** The arm board must be able to be moved away for insertion of the humeral component since hyperextension is necessary.

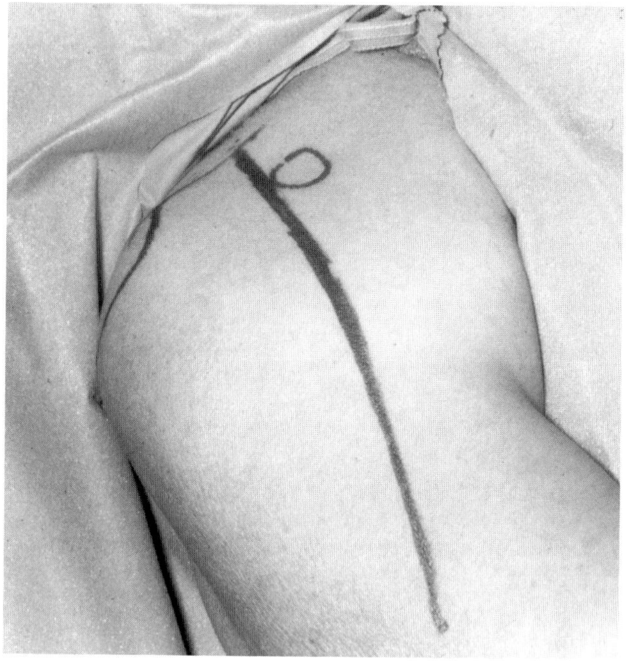

**Fig. 1-9** A long deltopectoral incision. The coracoid process is outlined.

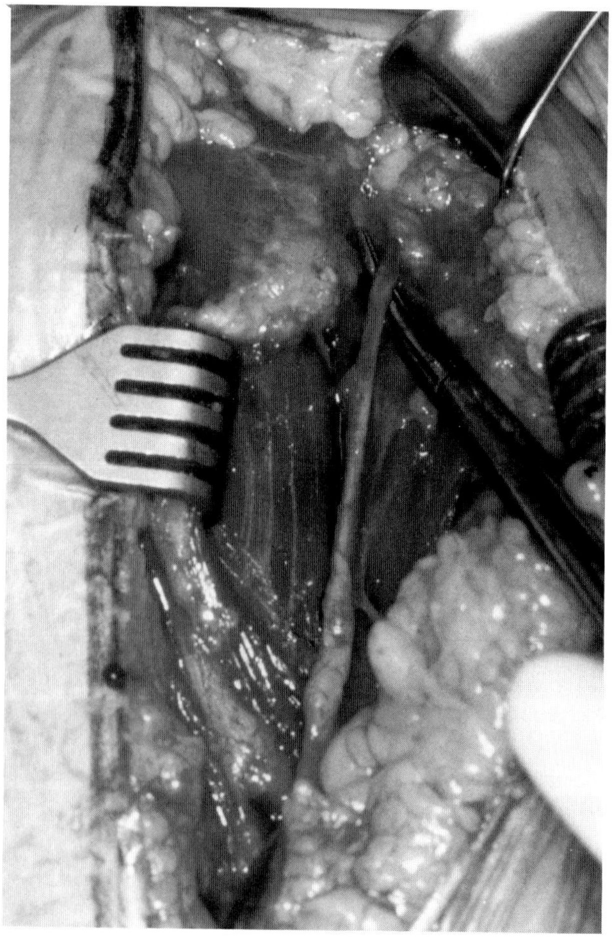

**Fig. 1-10** Ligation and excision of the cephalic vein.

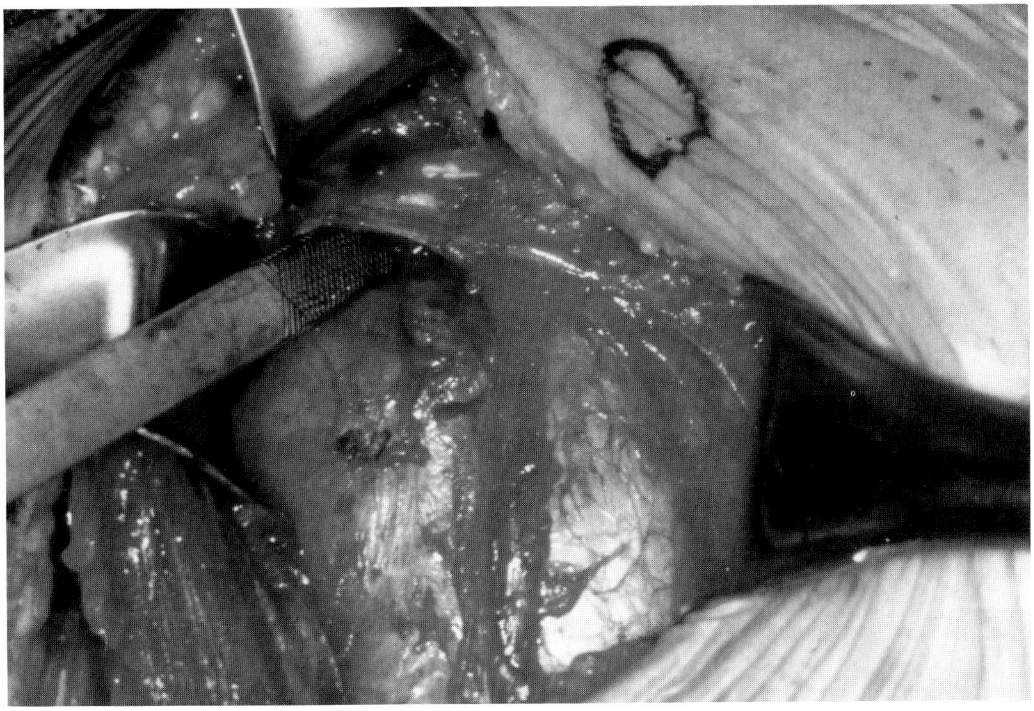

**Fig. 1-11A** The deltoid and pectoralis retracted. A Darrach retractor is under the coracoacromial ligament.

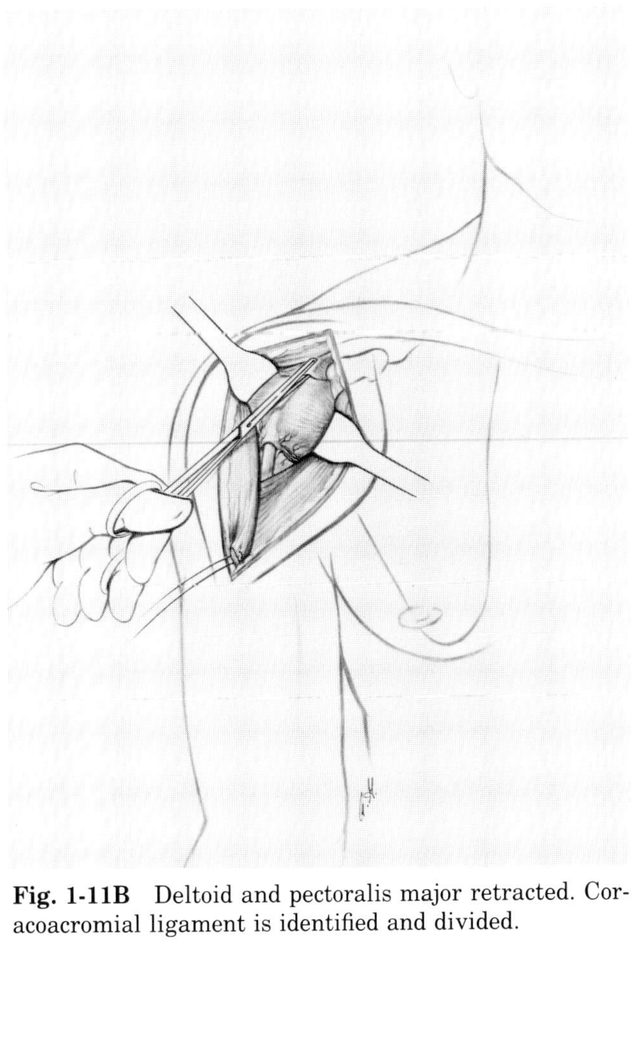

**Fig. 1-11B** Deltoid and pectoralis major retracted. Coracoacromial ligament is identified and divided.

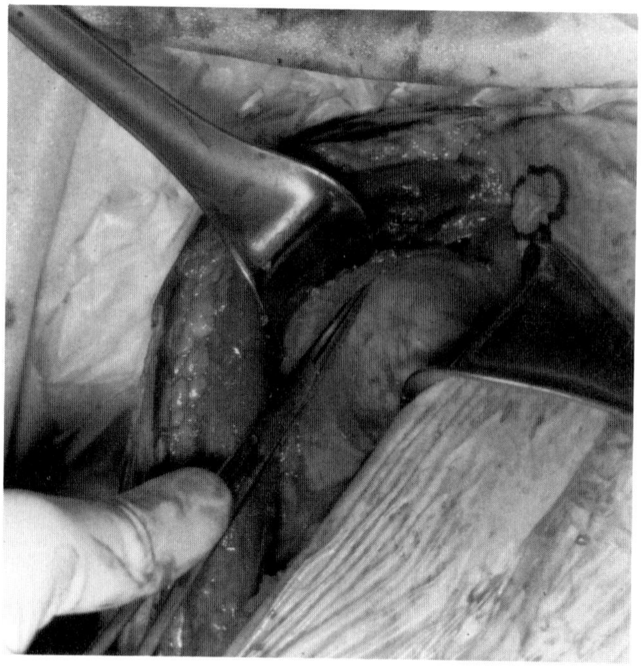

**Fig. 1-12A** Clamp marks the edge of the subscapularis to be divided.

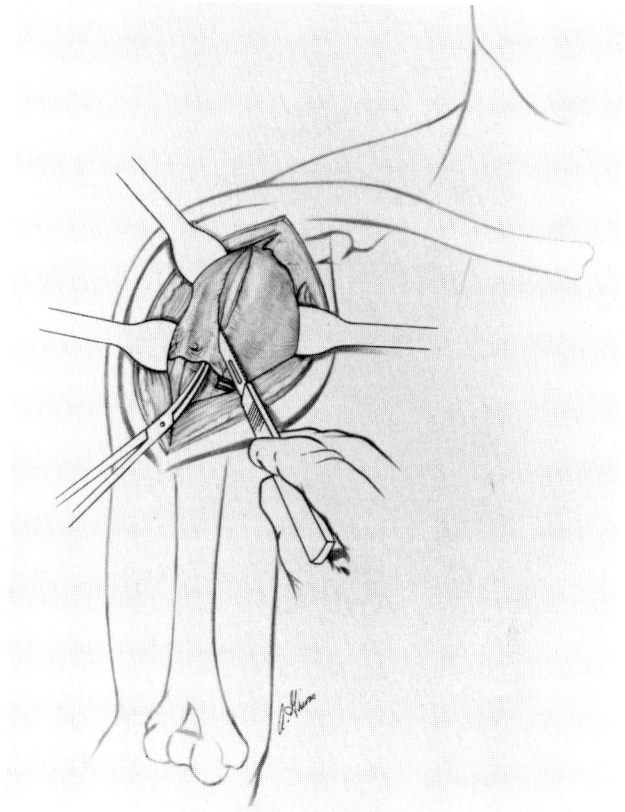

**Fig. 1-12B** Anterior-humeral circumflex vessels identify the lower border of the subscapularis.

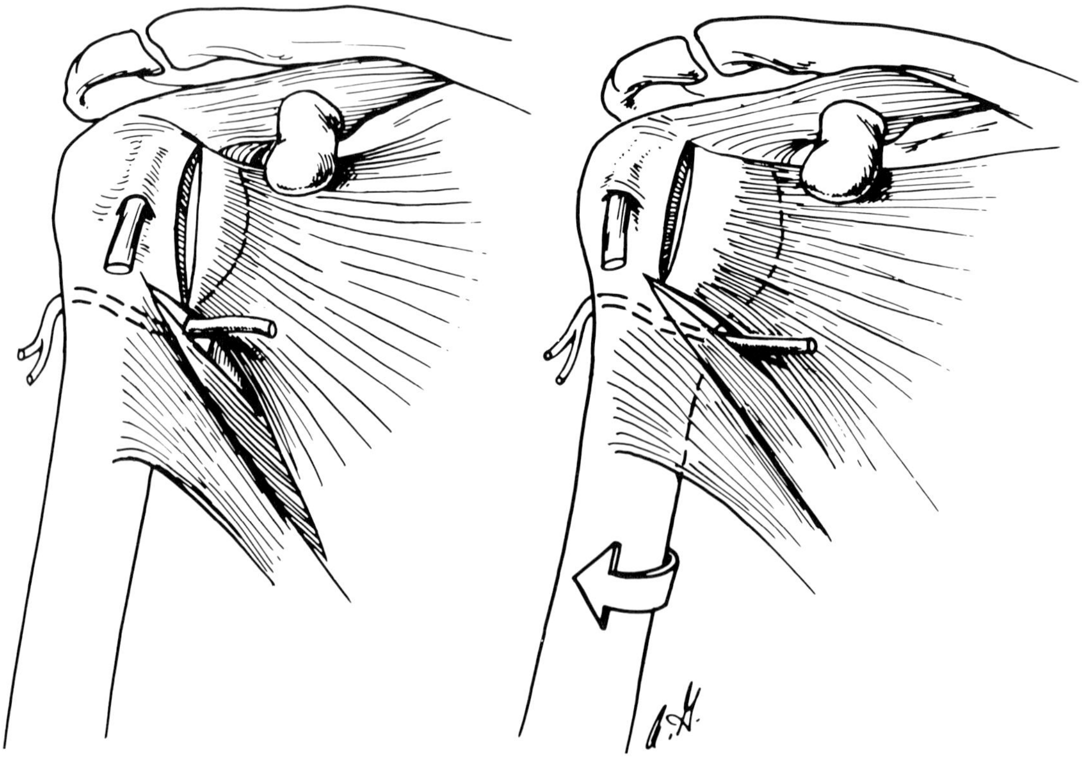

**Fig. 1-12C** Externally rotating arm during division of subscapularis tendon keeps the axillary nerve away from dissection.

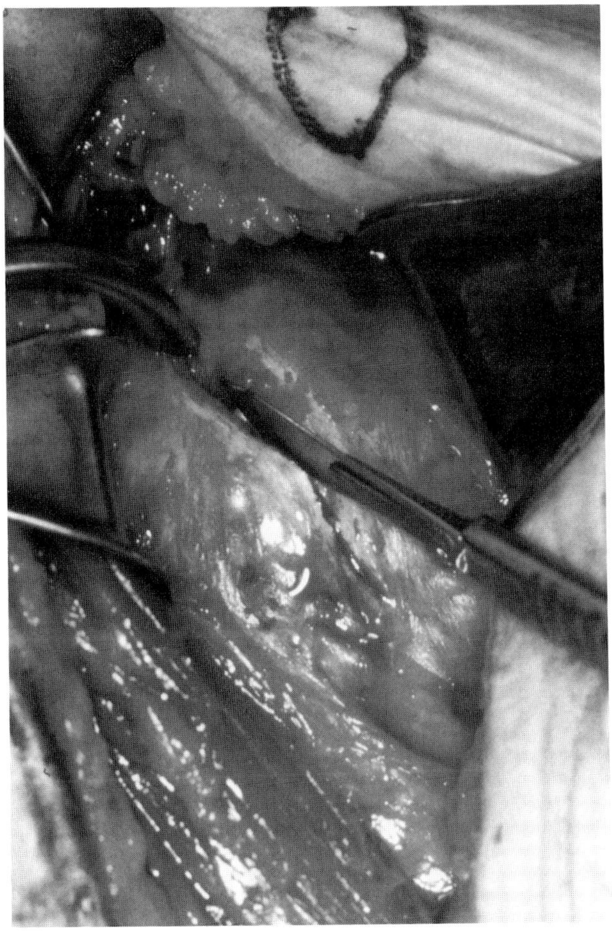

**Fig. 1-13** Subscapularis is divided 1½ cm medial to the bicipital groove.

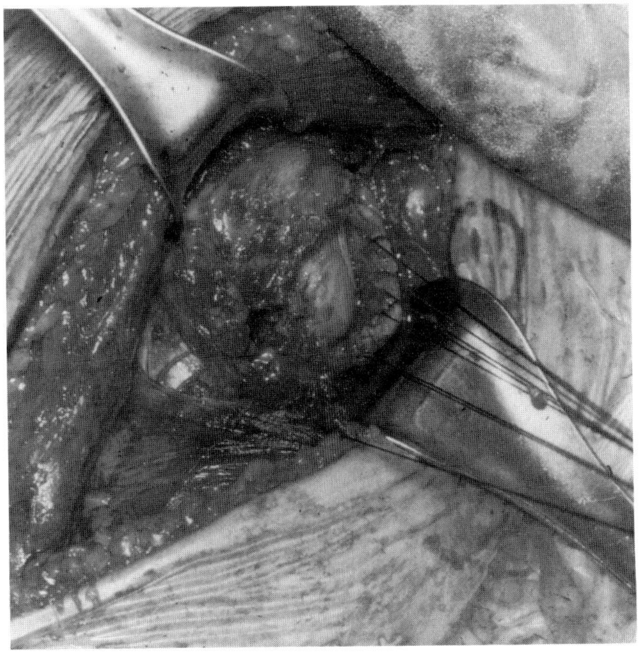

**Fig. 1-14A** Stay sutures placed in the subscapularis for retraction. This is the only muscle divided during the procedure. It allows the head to be dislocated for osteotomy.

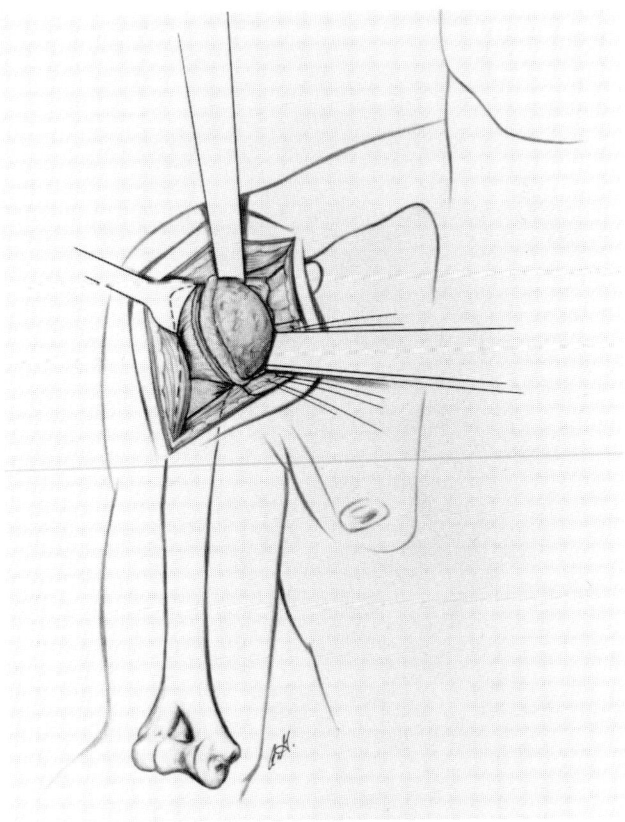

**Fig. 1-14B** Humeral head is dislocated. The osteophyte is identified and removed. The retractor protects the biceps tendon and supraspinatus superiorly and subscapularis medially.

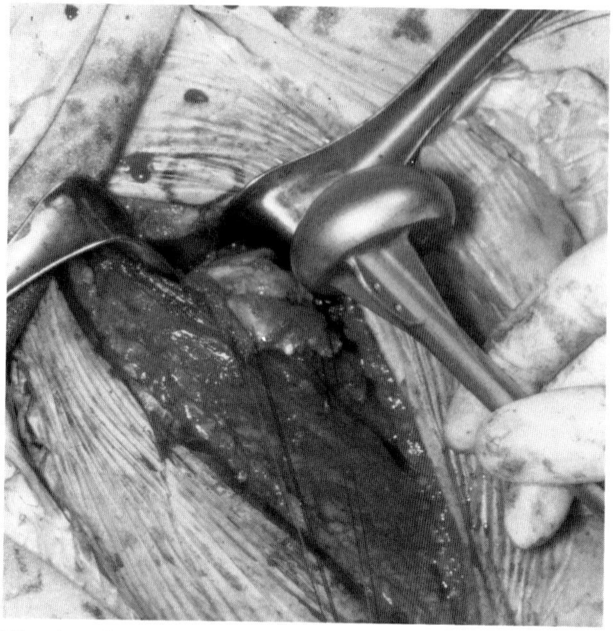

**Fig. 1-15A** Trial humeral component for orientation of the head osteotomy site.

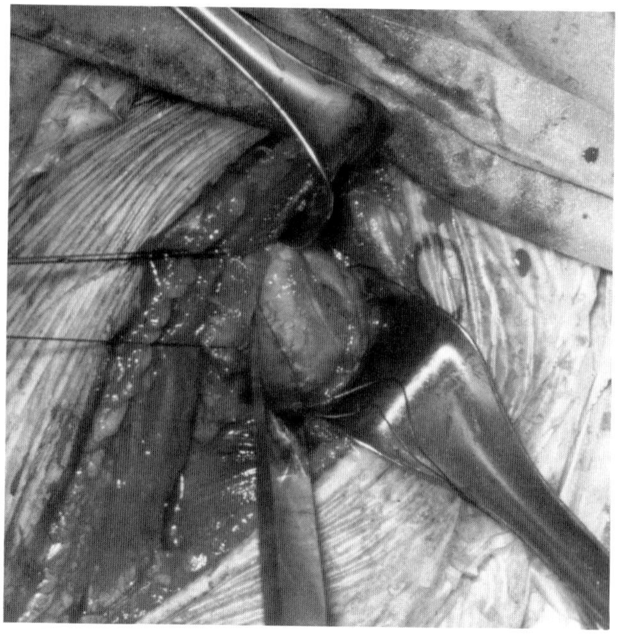

**Fig. 1-16A** The head is osteotomized using a broad osteotome at an angle of 45° to the humeral shaft.

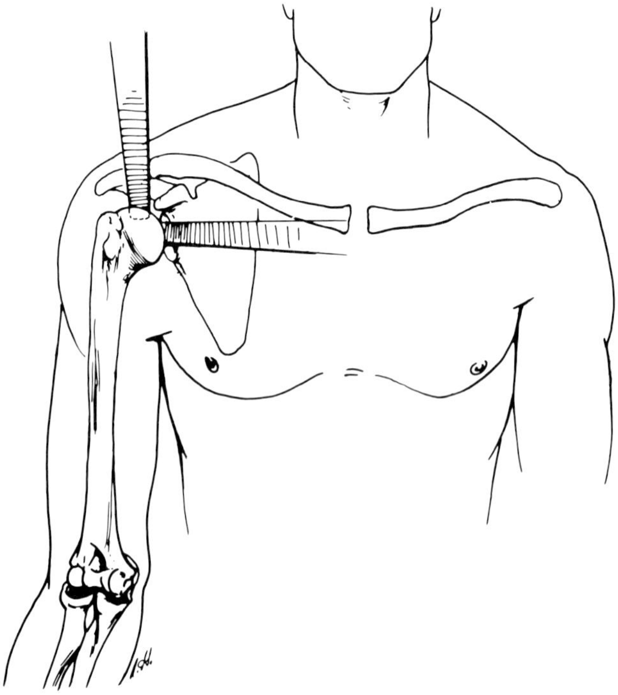

**Fig. 1-15B** Retractors behind humeral head aid exposure.

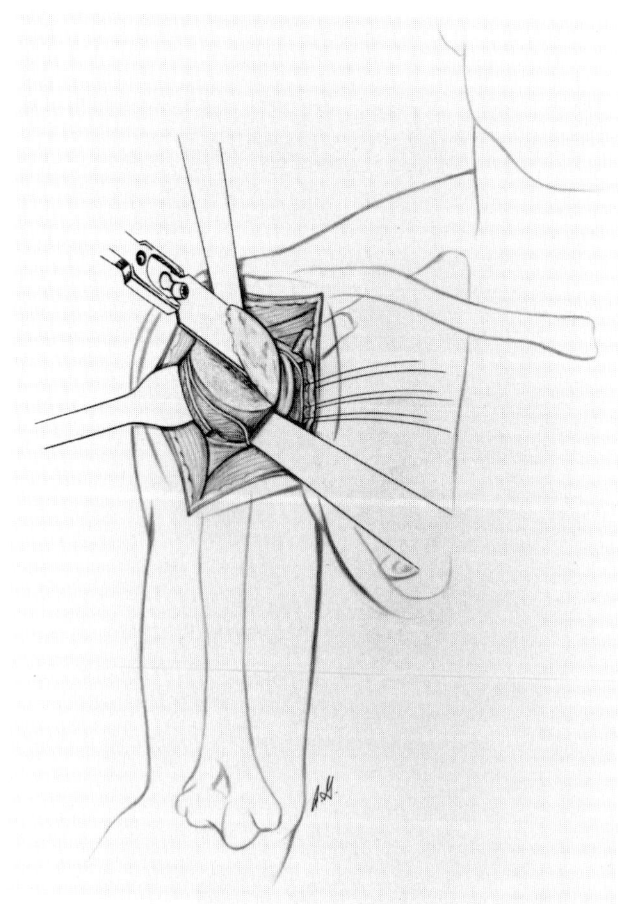

**Fig. 1-16B** The humeral head is osteotomized using a sharp osteotome. Only that amount of humeral head normally covered by articular cartilage is removed.

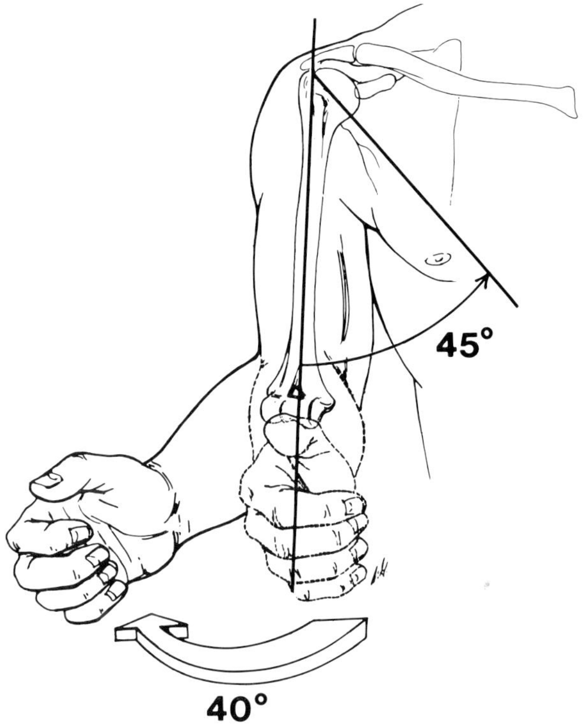


**Fig. 1-16C** The arm is externally rotated 40° during osteotomy for the correct amount of retroversion.

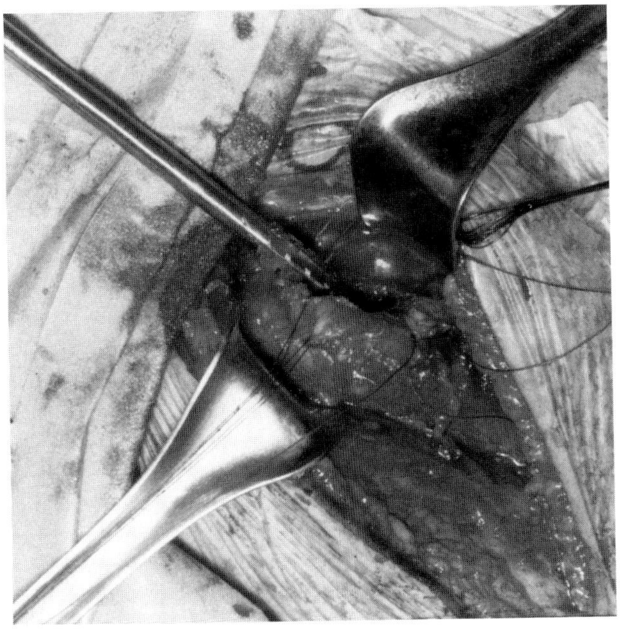

**Fig. 1-18** The T-handled reamers are used to prepare the humeral shaft.

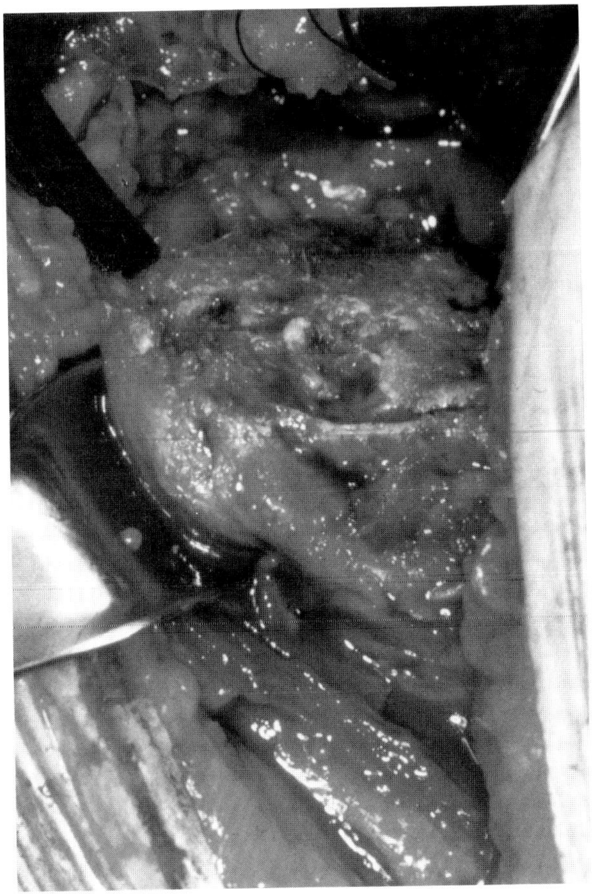

**Fig. 1-17** The osteotomized head is prepared for reaming.

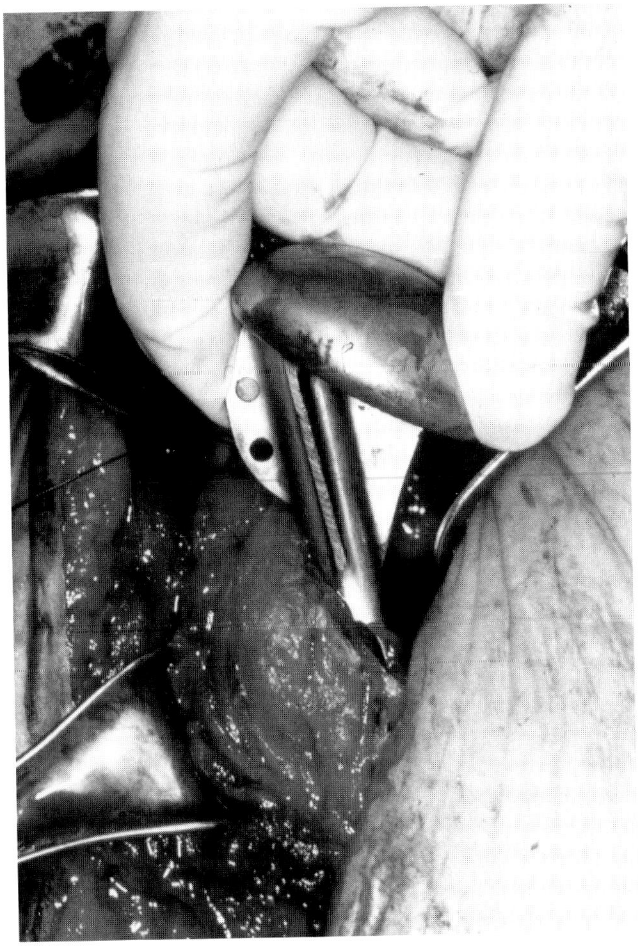

**Fig. 1-19** The correct trial humeral head is inserted.

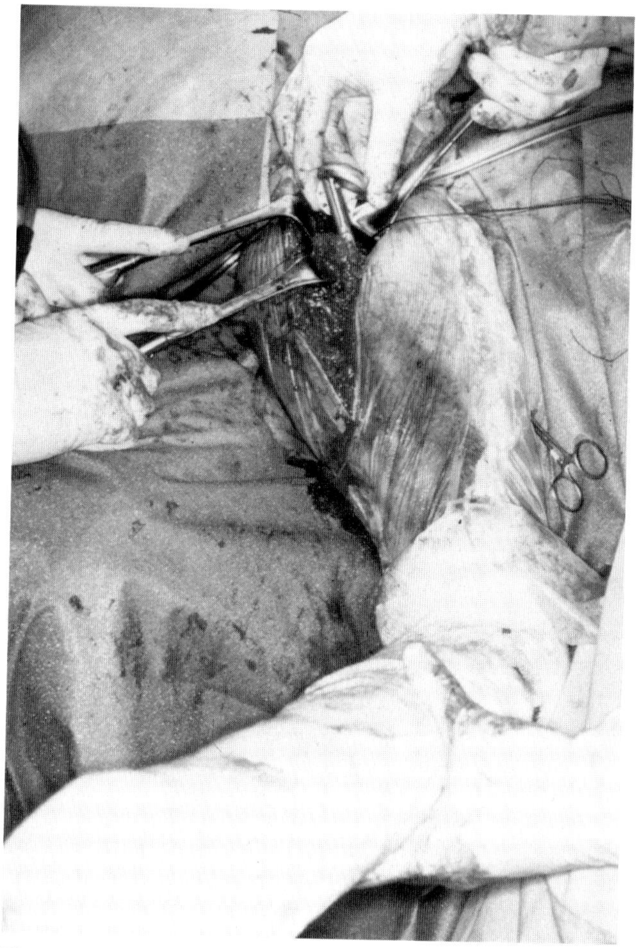

Fig. 1-20 The trial humerus is inserted in approximately 40° of retroversion to the transverse axis of the elbow. It is then removed so that the glenoid can be prepared.

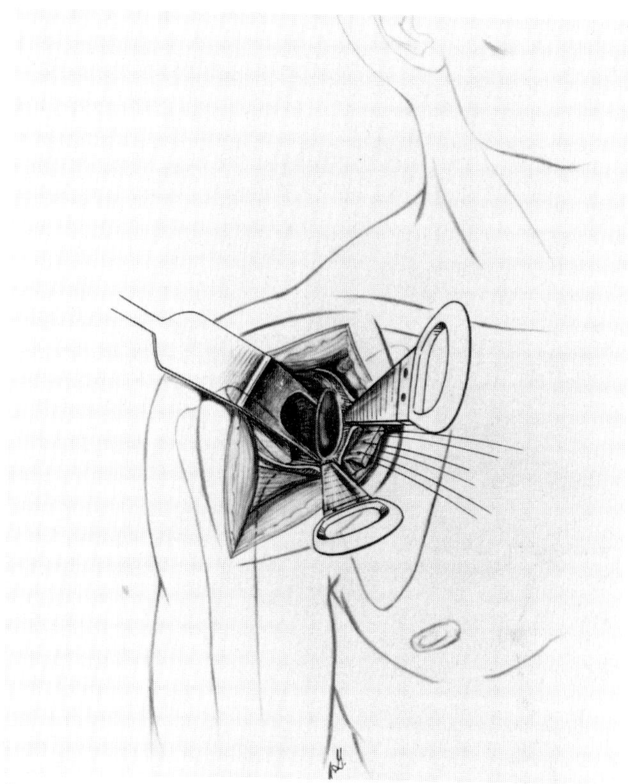

A

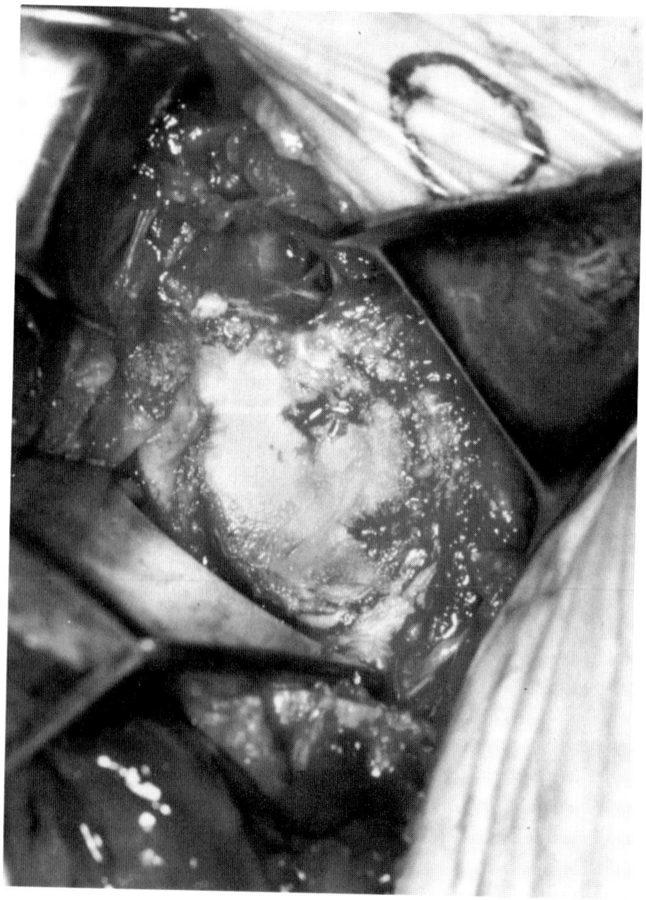

B

Fig. 1-21A & B The humerus, resting on the armboard, is retracted posteriorly for glenoid exposure. Anterior and posterior labrum are excised. The inferior retractor aids exposure and protects the axillary nerve. The anterior retractor aids the identification of glenoid neck angle for the slot in the glenoid. The Fukuda retractor is exposing the glenoid and retracting the humeral head.

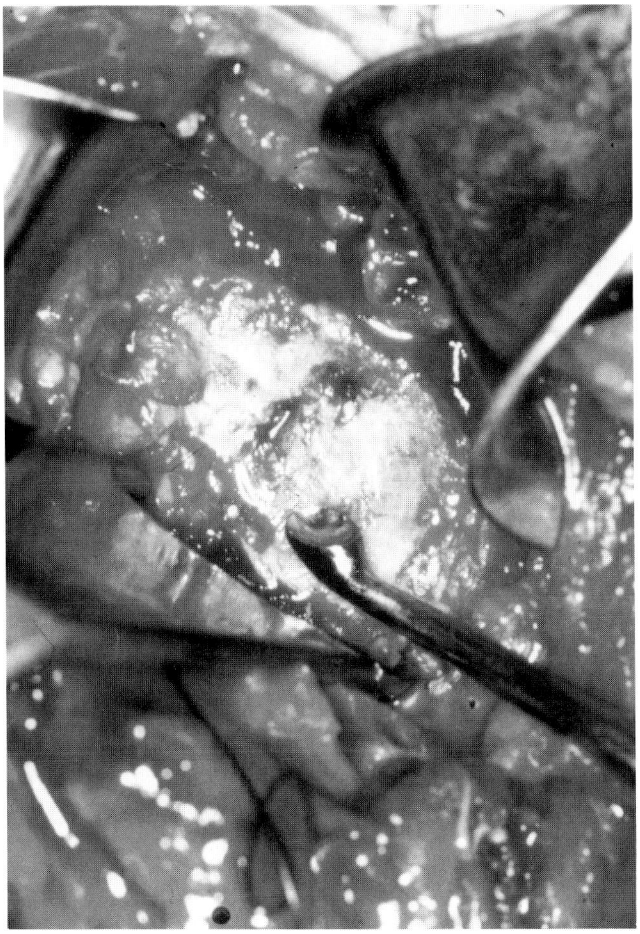

Fig. 1-21C The remaining articular cartilage is curetted from the glenoid surface.

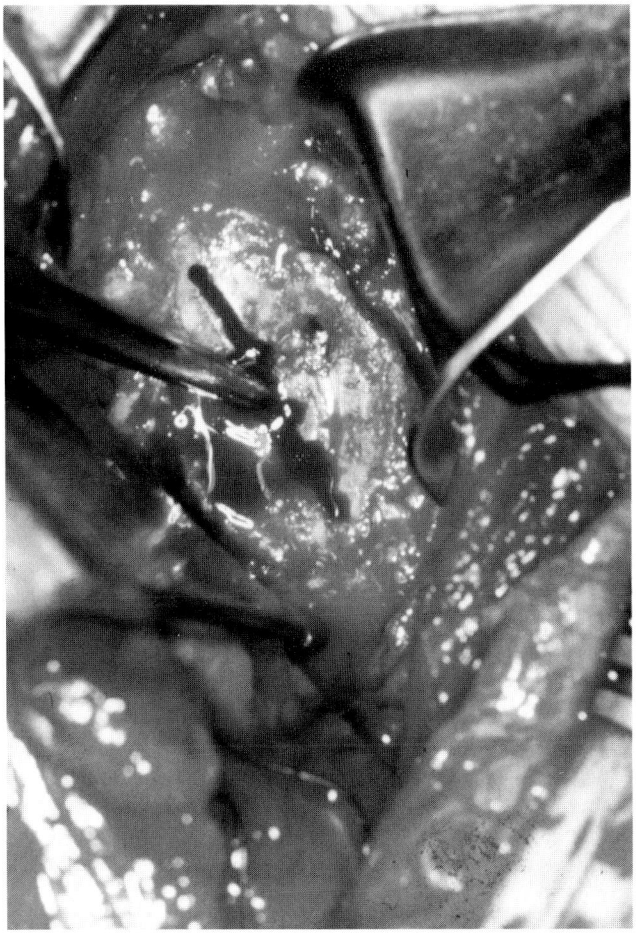

Fig. 1-22 The glenoid slot is made with a drill and enlarged and deepened with a curette.

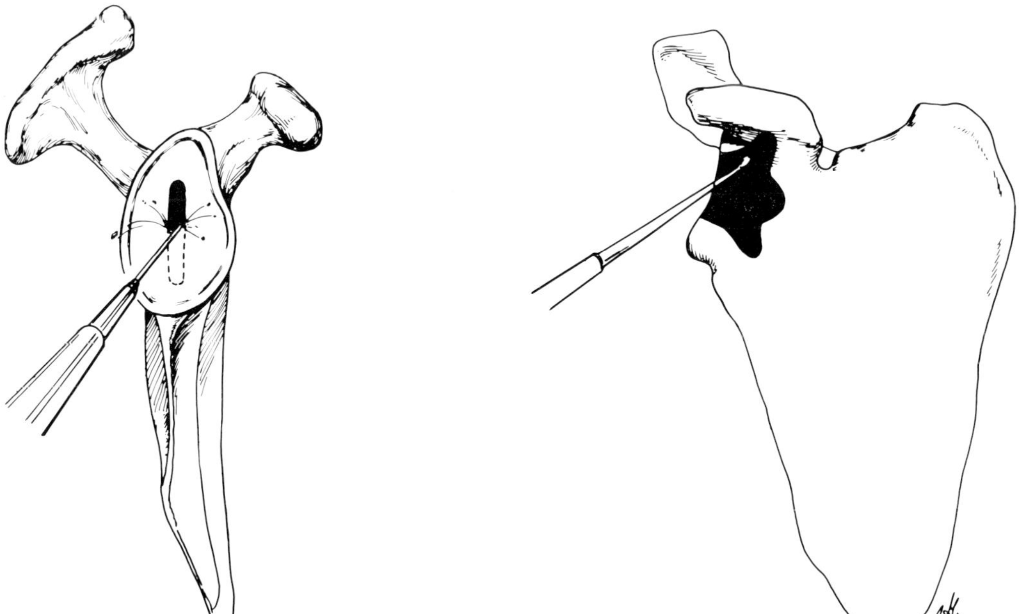

Fig. 1-23 The glenoid slot is made along the exact axis of the glenoid neck. The slot is undermined into the cancellous bone at base of coracoid superiorly and the cancellous portion of the neck inferiorly.

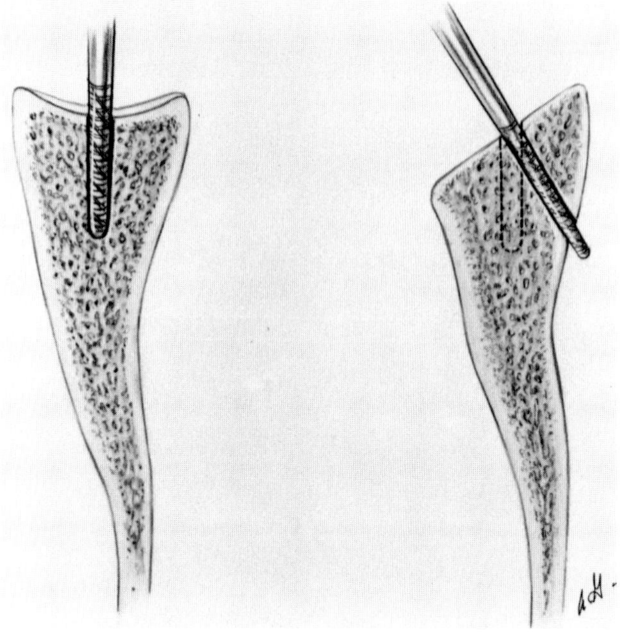

**Fig. 1-24** Slot in the glenoid is made along the exact axis of the glenoid. With excessive wear anteriorly or posteriorly, there is danger of perforating the cortex if the drill bit is oriented perpendicular to the exposed glenoid rather than perpendicular to the glenoid neck.

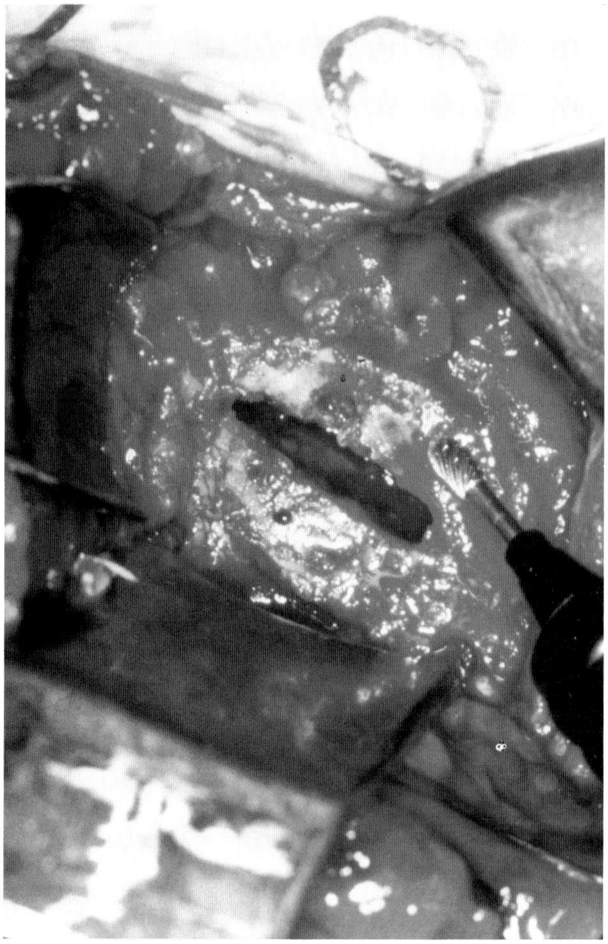

**Fig. 1-26A** A burr is used to remove any uneven buildup of the glenoid surface for the final preparation of the glenoid.

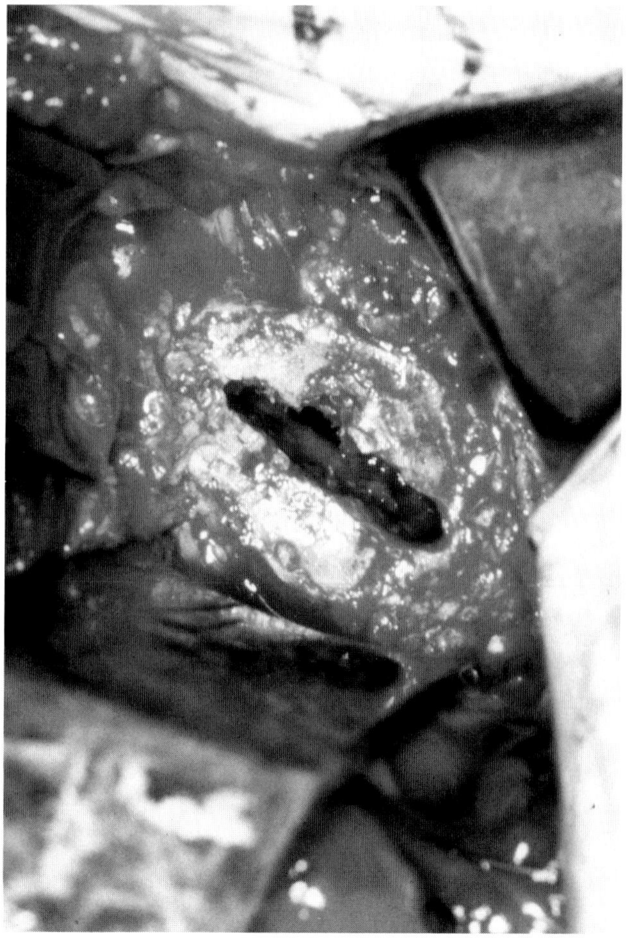

**Fig. 1-25** The completed glenoid slot.

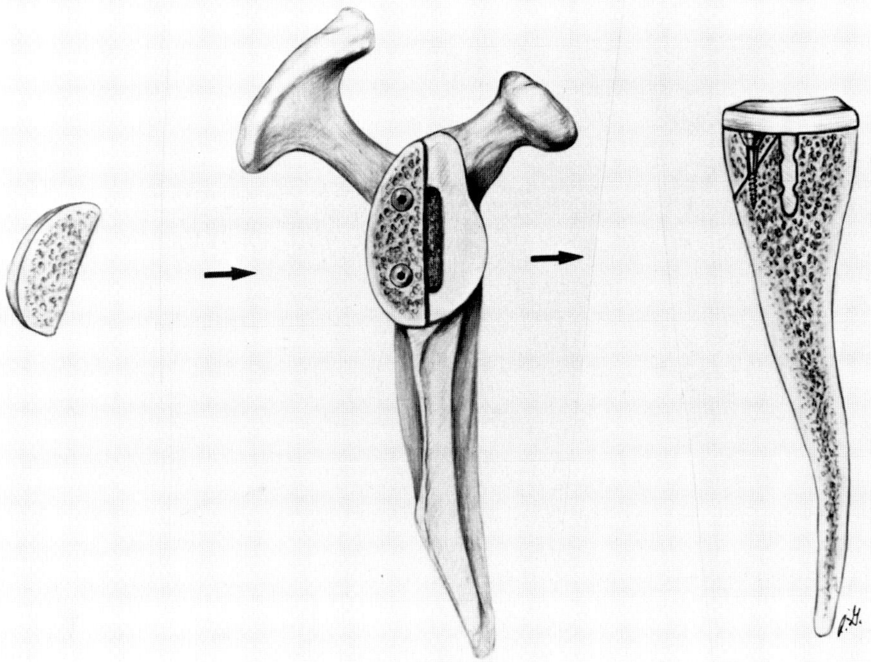

**Fig. 1-26B** The technique of using bone graft for proper seating of glenoid if significant asymmetric wear is present.

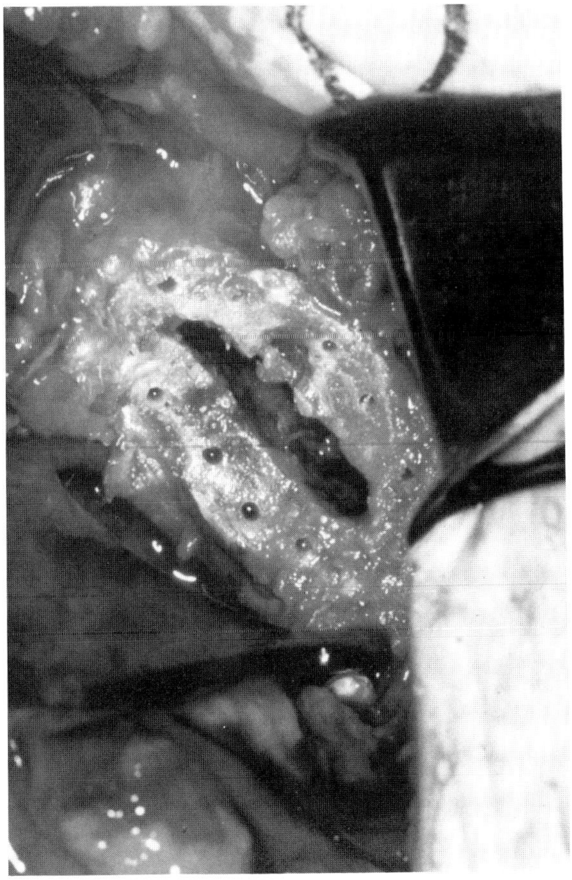

**Fig. 1-27** Several drill holes into the subchondral bone of the glenoid.

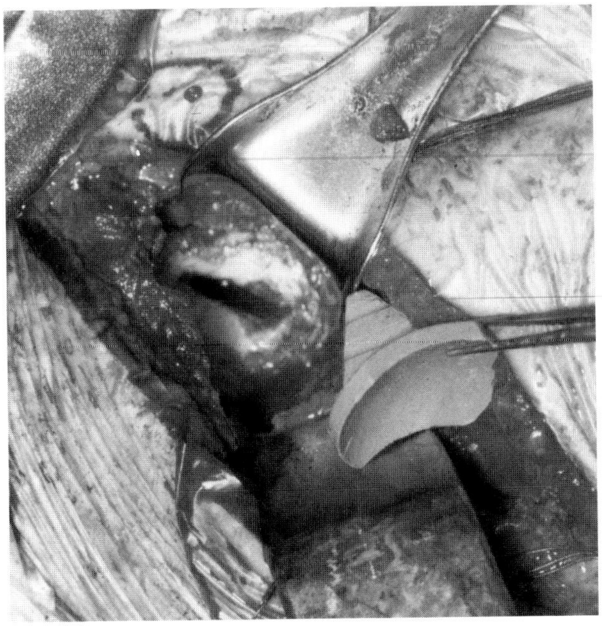

**Fig. 1-28** The trial glenoid being prepared to be inserted.

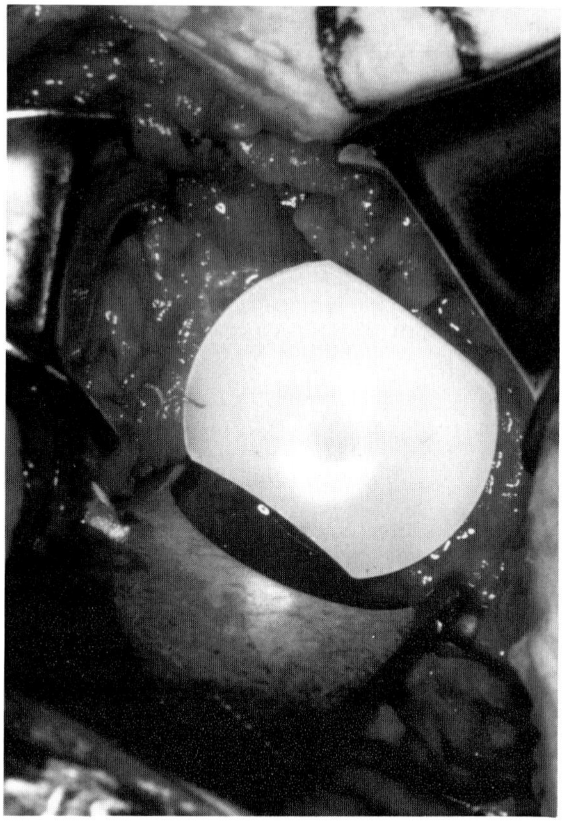

Fig. 1-29 The standard polyethylene glenoid inserted.

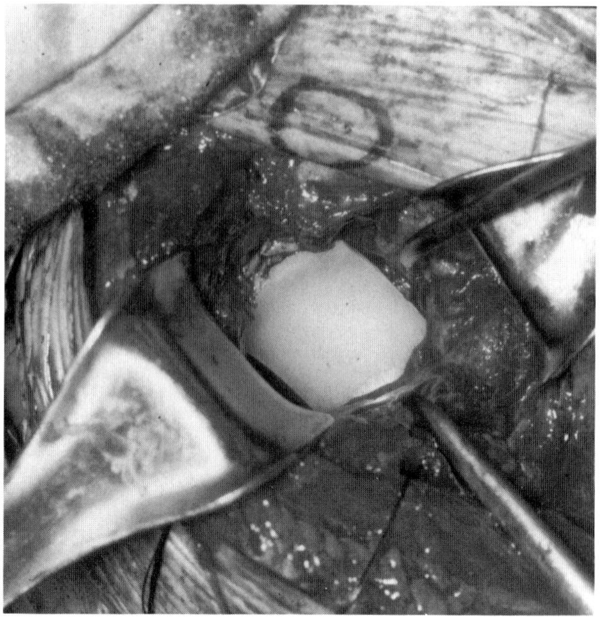

Fig. 1-30 Excess cement is removed. A bone hook is placed around the proximal humerus as the humerus is gently externally rotated to clear the glenoid so that the humeral implant can be inserted.

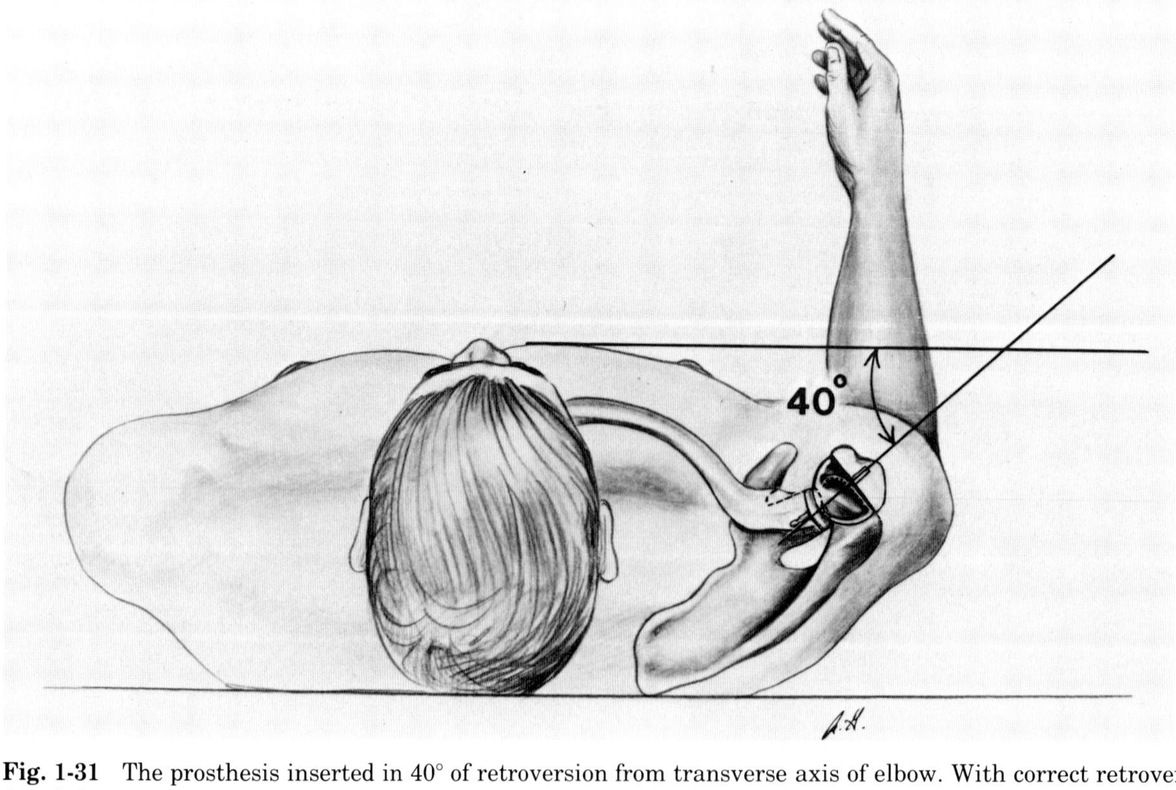


Fig. 1-31 The prosthesis inserted in 40° of retroversion from transverse axis of elbow. With correct retroversion, the fin of the prosthesis is usually lateral to the bicipital groove, and, with the arm in neutral rotation, the humeral component faces directly toward the glenoid.

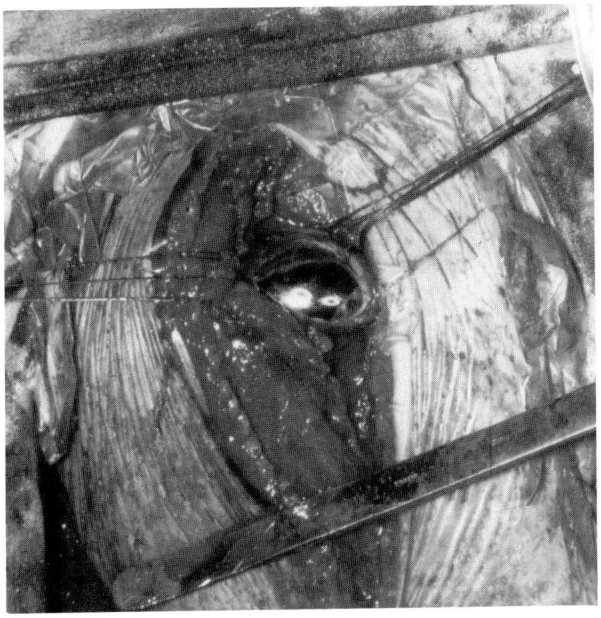

**Fig. 1-32** The previously sized proximal humerus is inserted in 40° of retroversion.

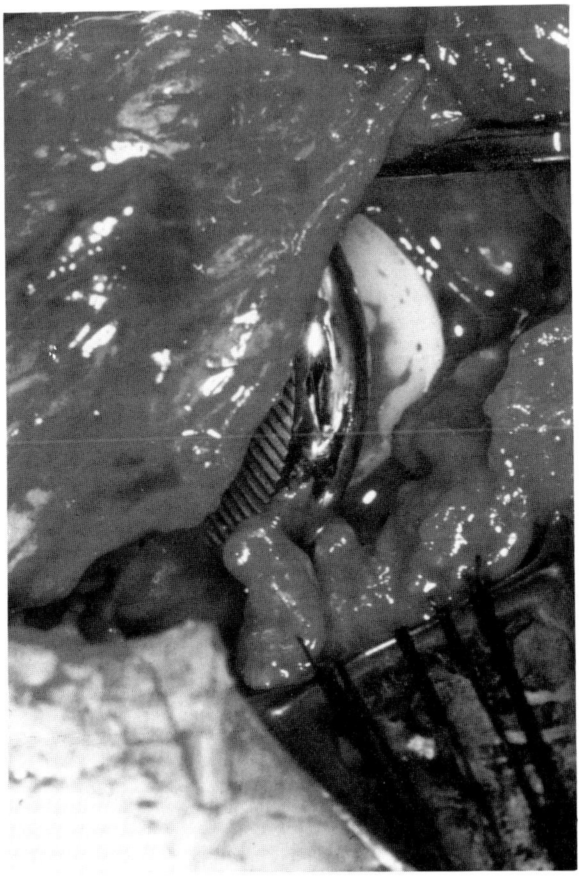

**Fig. 1-33** In the correct amount of retroversion, the humeral component should face directly toward the glenoid. The subscapularis is ready to be closed around the humeral implant.

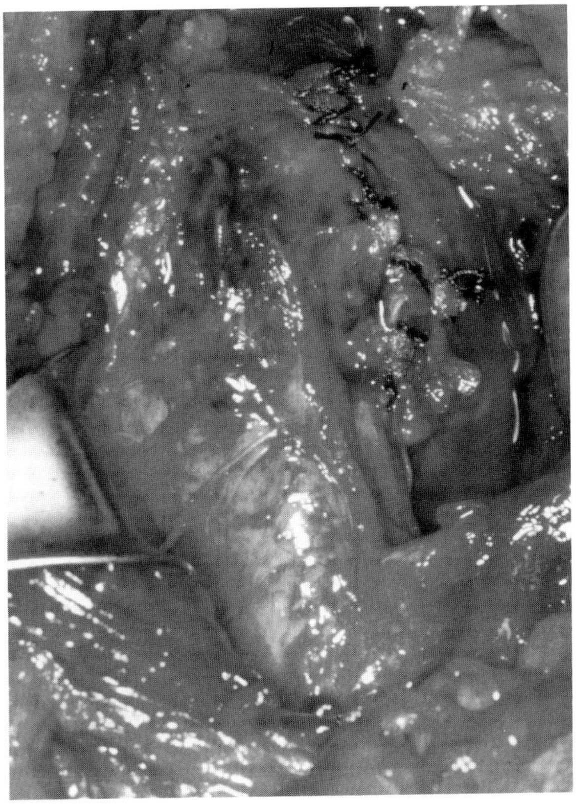

**Fig. 1-34** The only detached muscle, the subscapularis, is resutured to the site of its detachment.

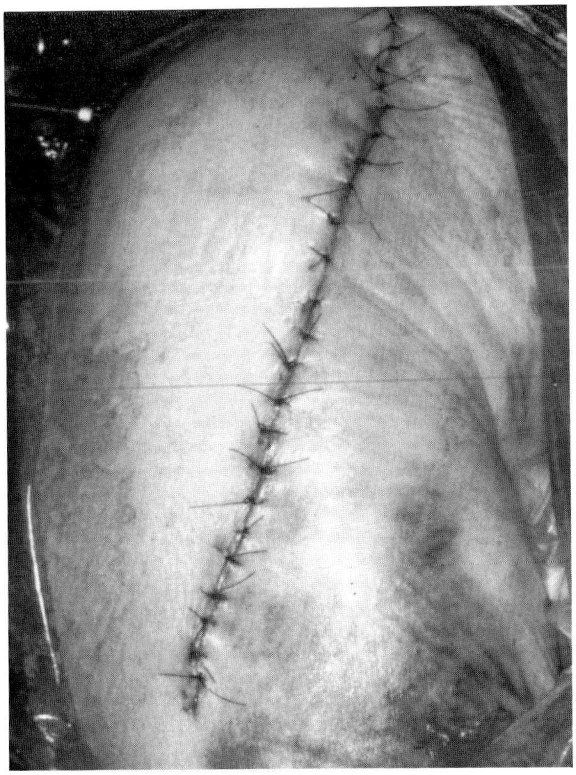

**Fig. 1-35** The wound is closed with an interrupted suture.

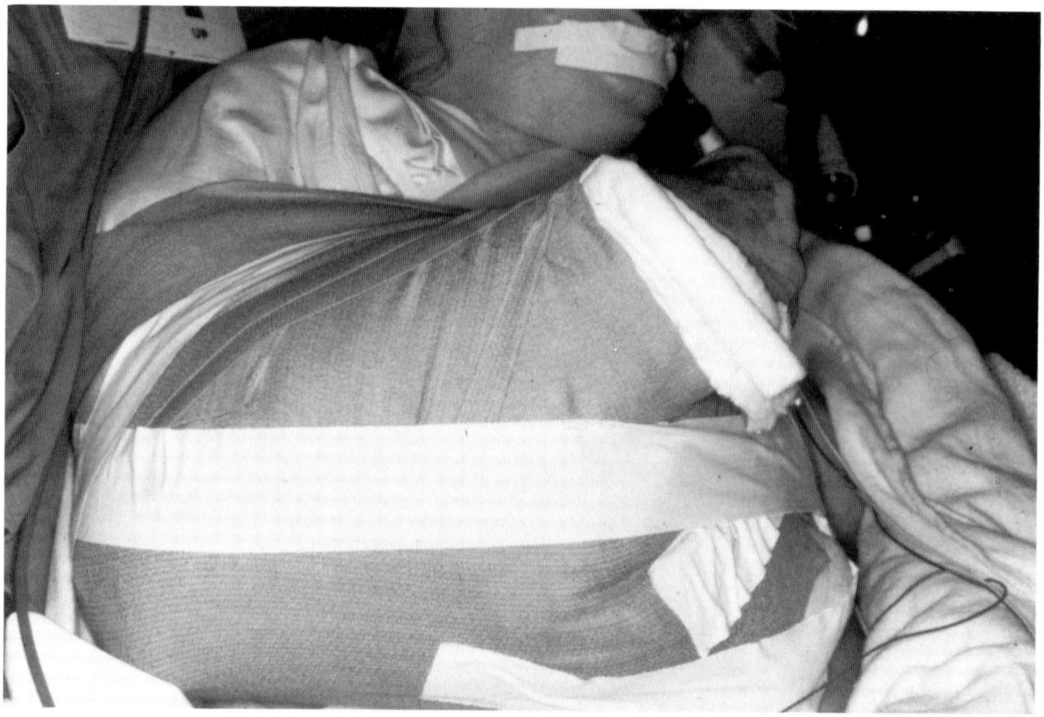

**Fig. 1-36A** The arm is placed in a sling and elastic bandage with the arm in a neutral rotation.

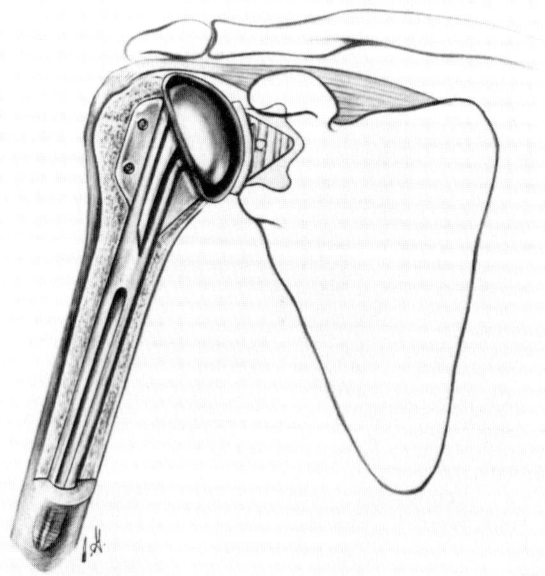

**Fig. 1-36B** The completed total shoulder arthroplasty.

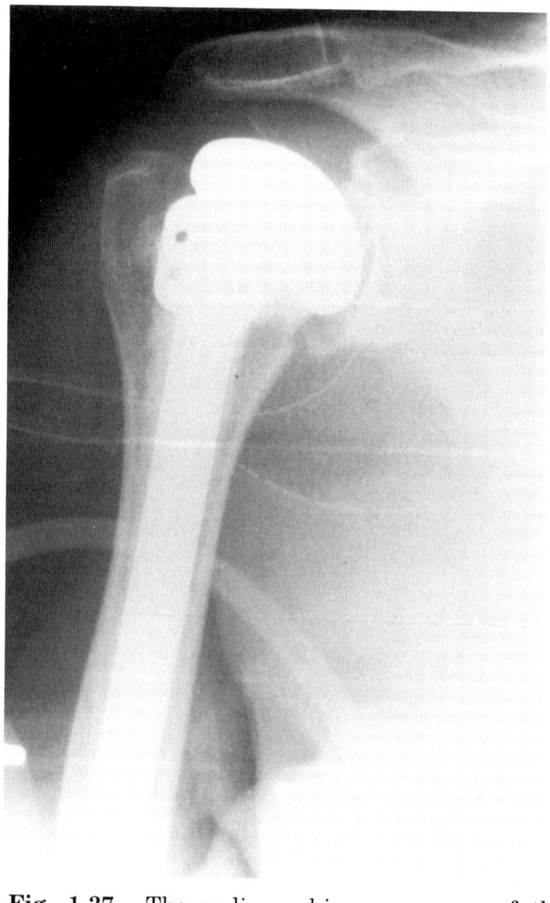

**Fig. 1-37** The radiographic appearance of the total shoulder replacement. The top of the humeral head should sit just superior to the greater tuberosity.

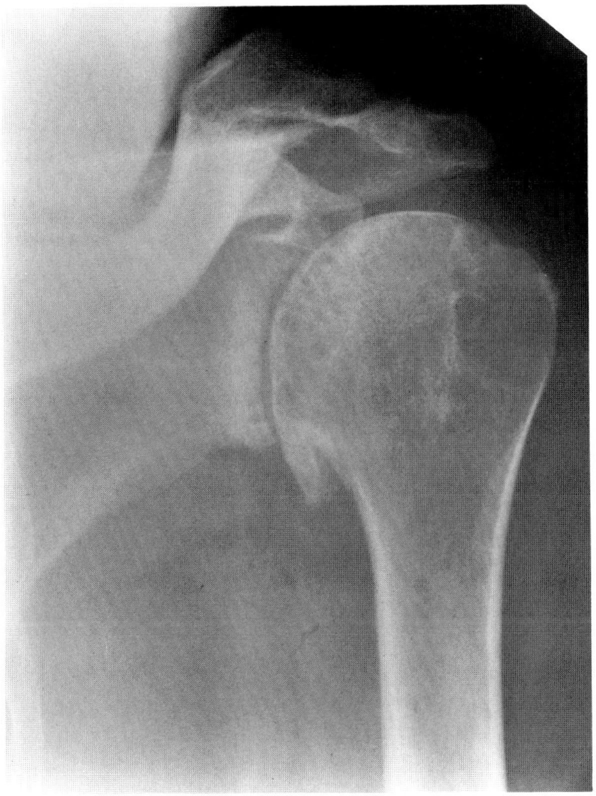

**Fig. 1-38** Primary osteoarthritis of the shoulder with radiographically inferiorly protruding osteophyte.

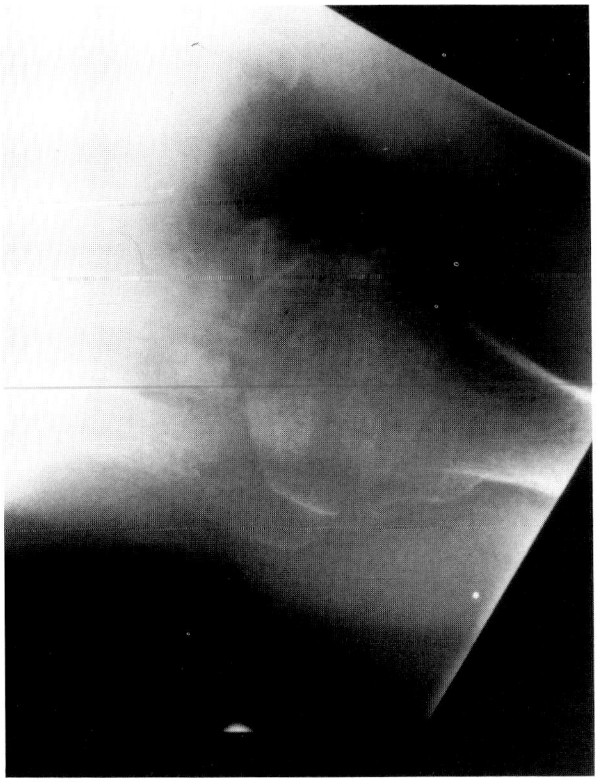

**Fig. 1-39** An axillary X-ray of primary osteoarthritis. Posterior subluxation and asymmetric erosion of the glenoid, showing more posterior glenoid wear than anterior wear, are evident.

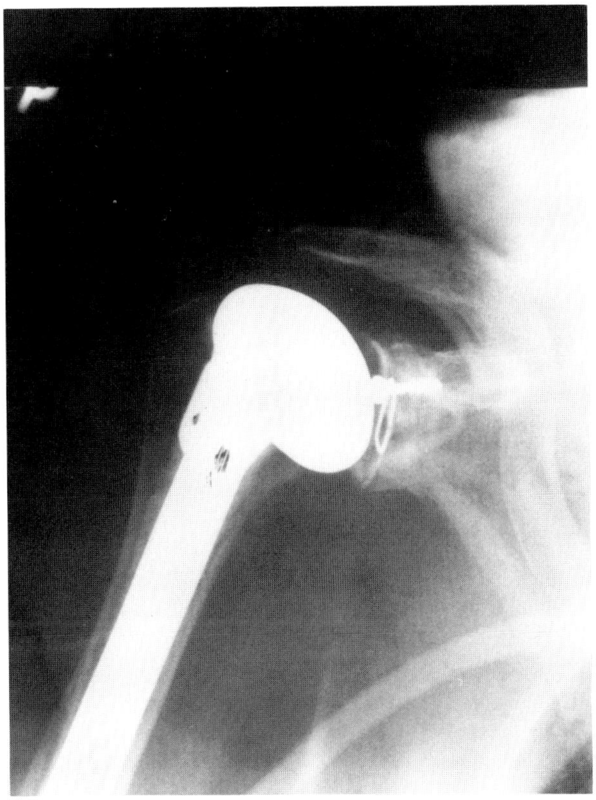

**Fig. 1-40** Total shoulder replacement with glenoid bone grafting for asymmetric glenoid wear. The graft is fixed with a navicular screw.

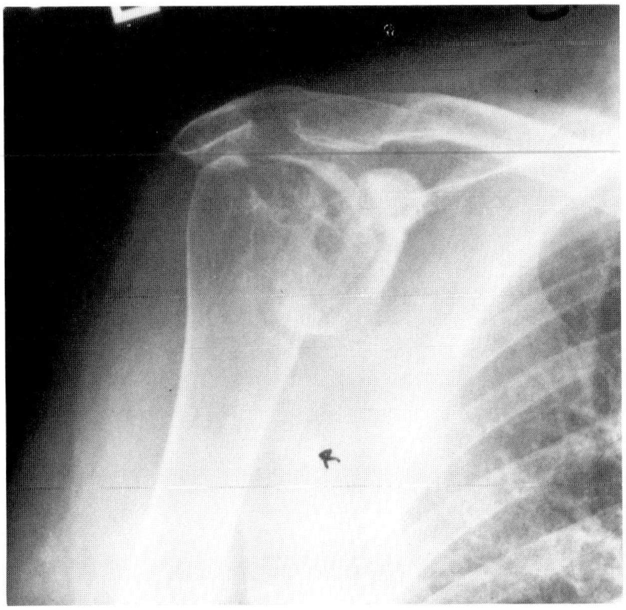

**Fig. 1-41** Rheumatoid arthritis with superior migration of the humeral head.

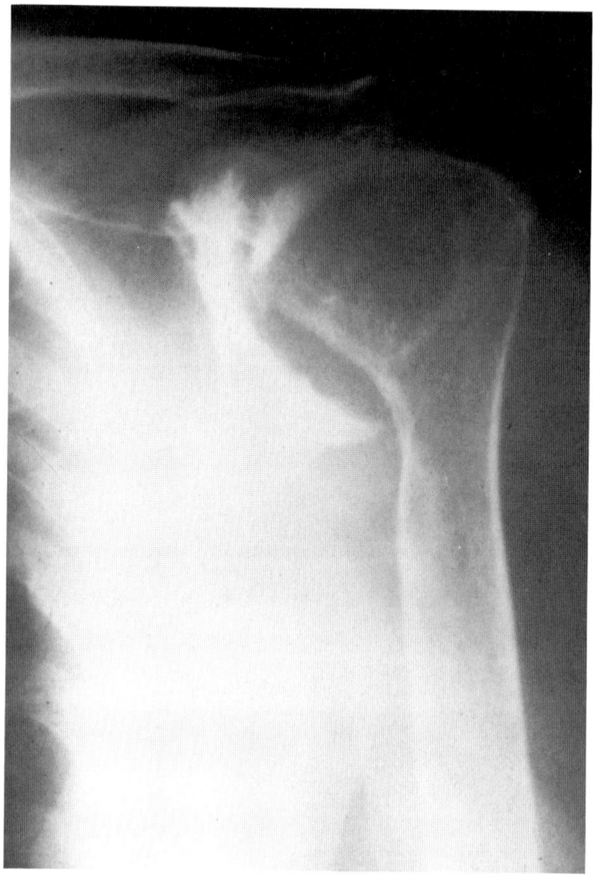

**Fig. 1-42** Rheumatoid arthritis with severe glenoid bone destruction.

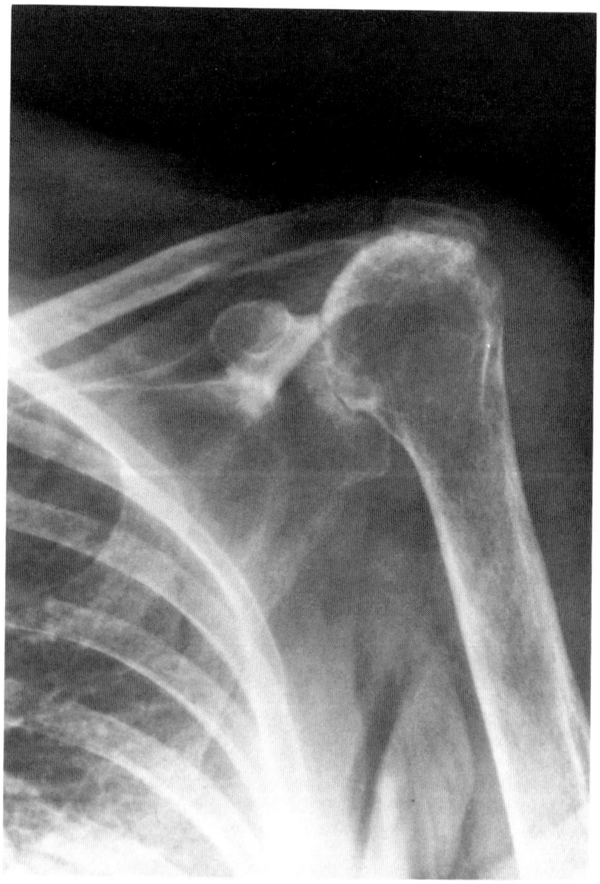

**Fig. 1-43A** Cuff tear arthropathy with severe wear into the glenoid and coracoid process and superior migration of the humeral head.

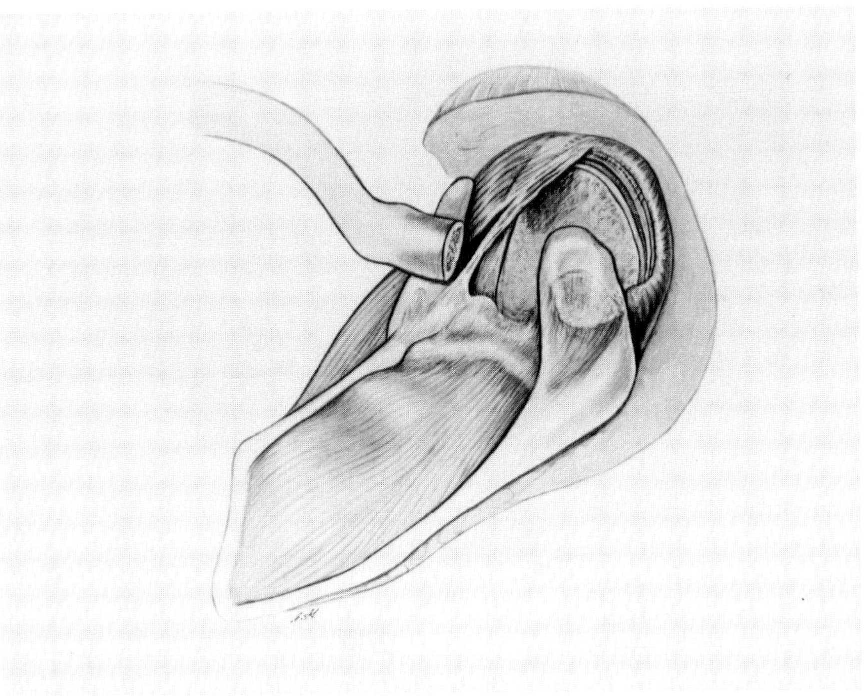

**Fig. 1-43B** With cuff tear arthropathy early distal clavicle excision will improve exposure of the retracted supraspinatus. Supraspinatus adheres to the base of the coracoid and must be freed from the coracoid for tendon mobilization. The supraspinatus is often pulled inferiorly by the intact subscapularis and intact teres minor.

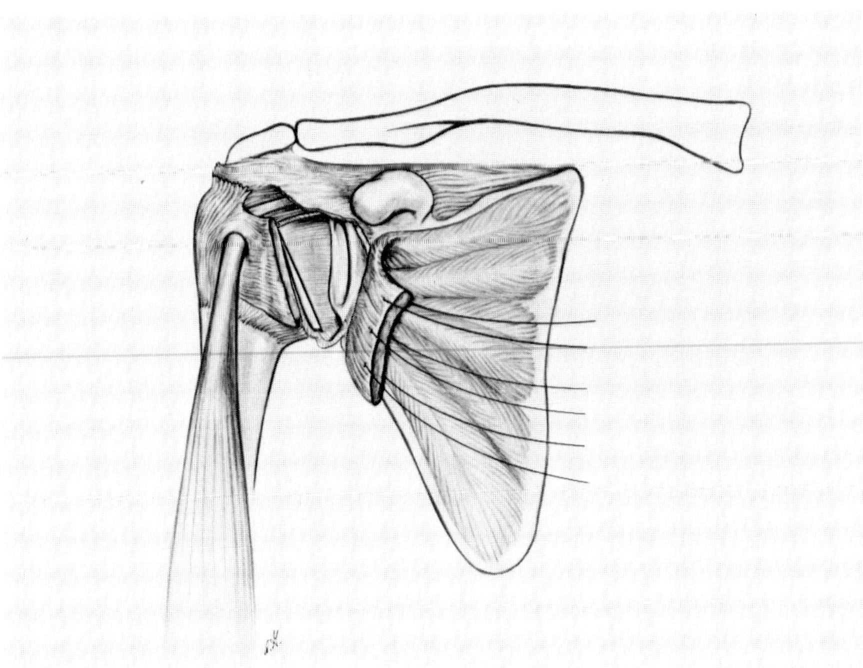

**Fig. 1-43C** In cuff tear arthropathy final mobilization of rotator cuff for repair is done after the head is osteotomized. The supraspinatus often adheres to the undersurface of the acromion and should be freed from the acromion prior to acromioplasty.

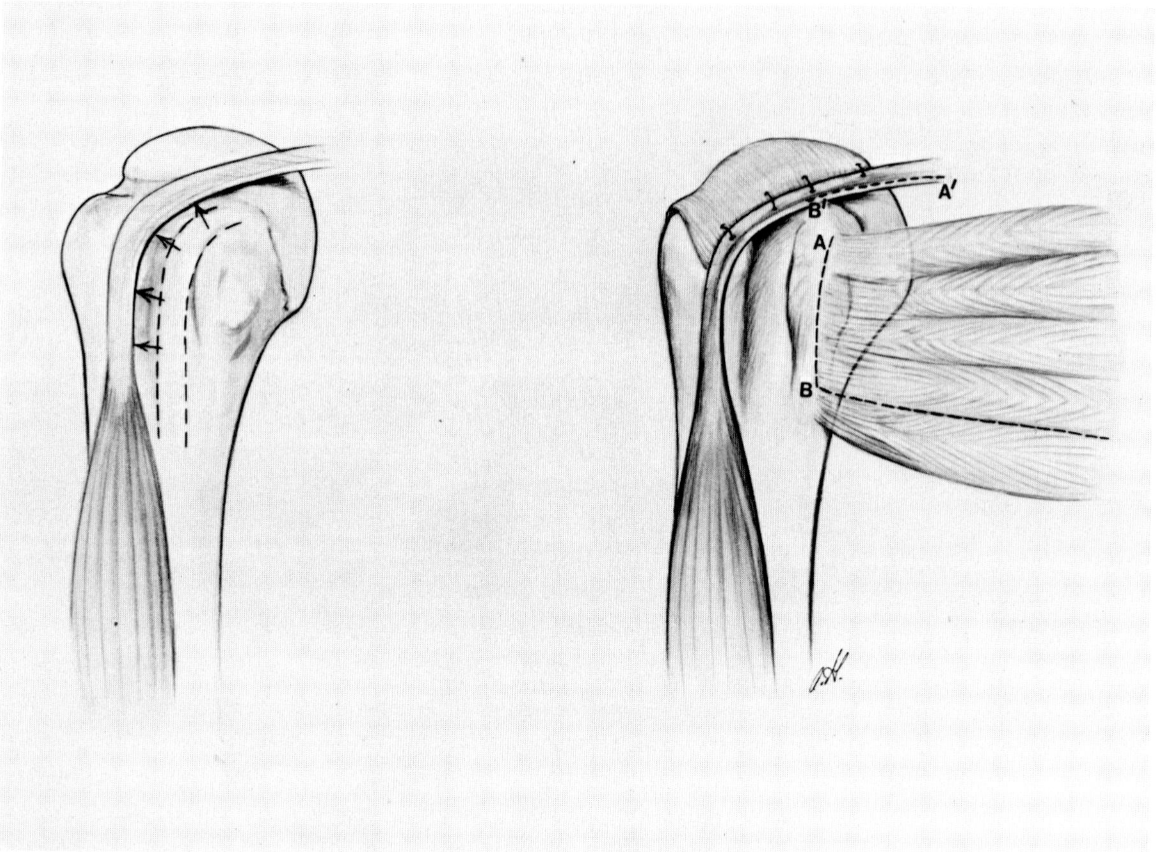


**Fig. 1-43D** With severe cuff deficiency, an intact biceps may be moved posterior to help provide superior or posterior coverage and can be used as a stint into which the mobilized spinati can be sewn. The upper 4/5 of subscapularis can be moved superiorly for additional superior coverage.

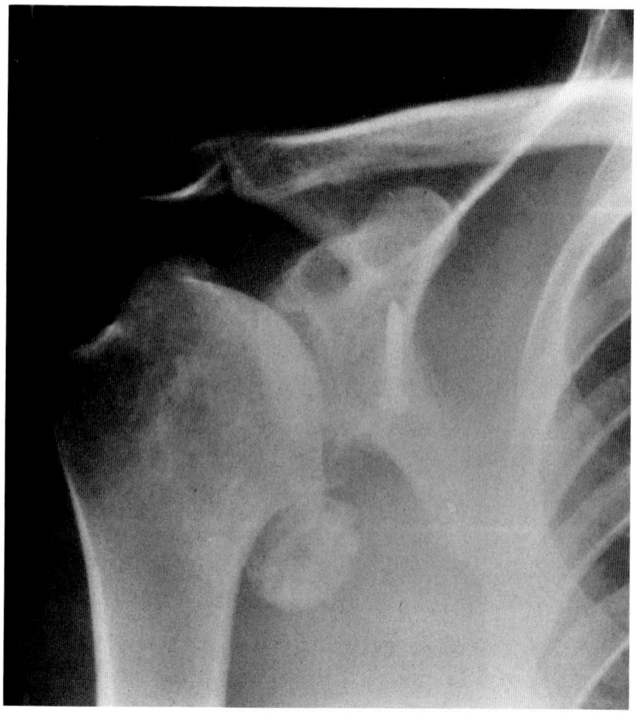

**Fig. 1-44** Degenerative arthritis following multiple dislocations. The patient had a previous Bristow operation.

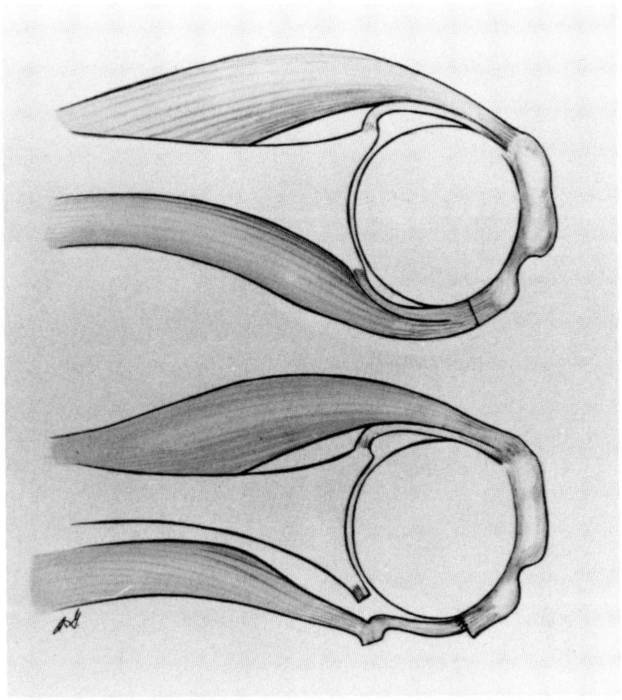

**Fig. 1-45A** The subscapularis-capsular lengthening procedure to provide external rotation. The subscapularis is incised 1½ cm from insertion, the interval between subscapularis and capsule is identified, and the capsule is incised near the glenoid. The subscapularis is then sutured to the lateral capsular flap, effectively adding length to the subscapularis.

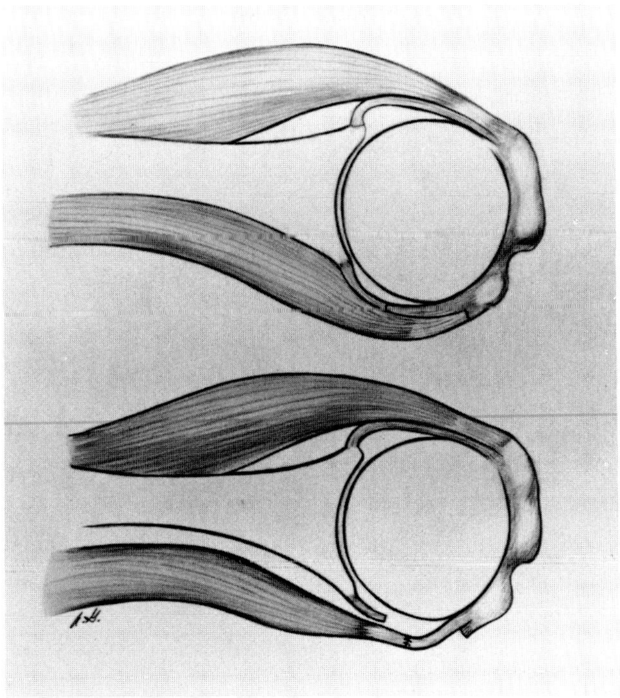

**Fig. 1-45B** The reverse undercutting method of subscapularis lengthening, if the subscapularis and capsule have been incised together at the beginning of the procedure. At the conclusion of arthroplasty, the capsule can be divided near the glenoid insertion, and the capsular-subscapularis interval can be cut in a reverse manner toward the lesser tuberosity insertion. The free end of the capsule is then brought outward and sutured to the original site of subscapularis division, effectively lengthening the subscapularis and enabling more external rotation to be obtained.

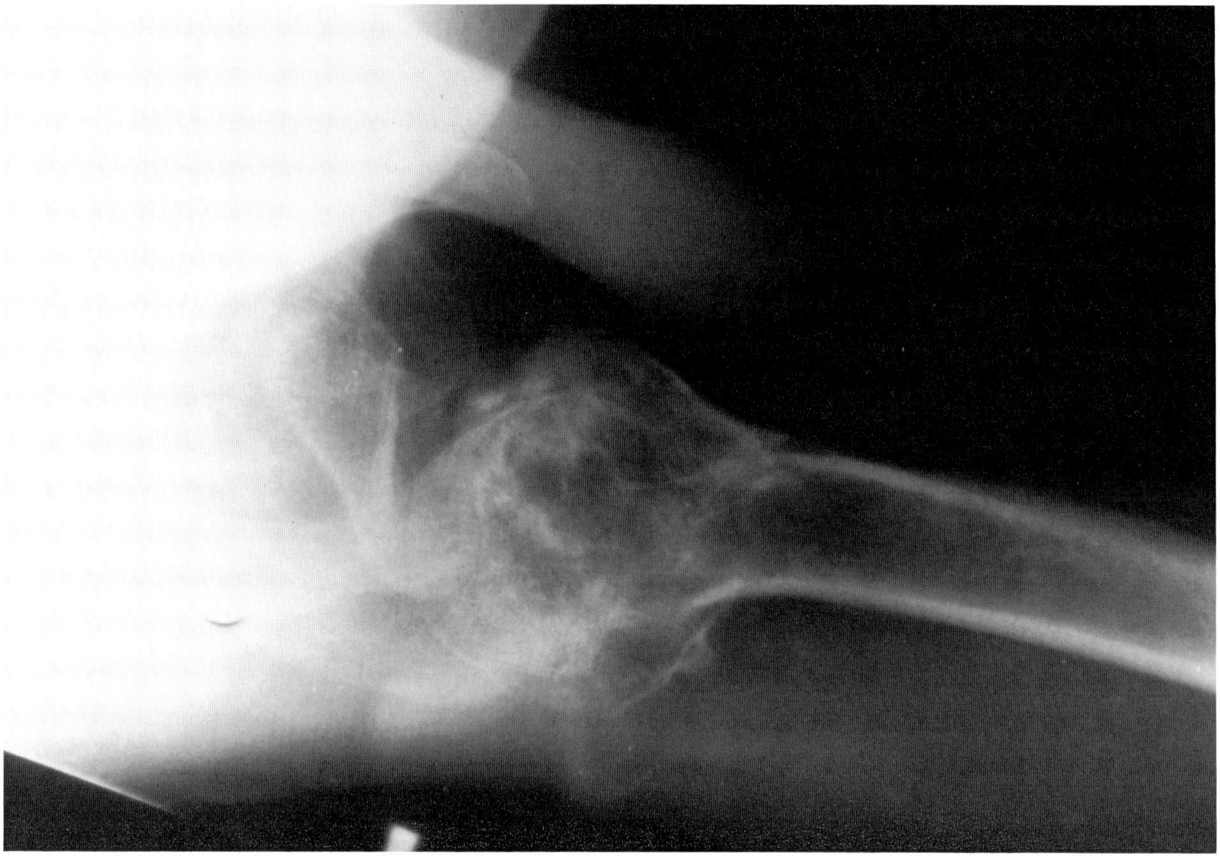

**Fig. 1-46** Posttraumatic arthritis with malunion of the tuberosities and retroversion of the humeral head. Axillary view.

## References

1. Cofield, R.H. Total shoulder arthroplasty with the Neer prosthesis. *J. Bone Joint Surg.* 66A:899, 1984.
2. Neer, C.S. II, and Kirby, R.M. Revision of humeral head and total shoulder arthroplasties. *Clin. Orthop.* 170:189, 1982.
3. Post, M. Constrained total shoulder replacement. In *A.A.O.S. Instructional Course Lectures,* Vol. XXXIV, p. 287, 1985.
4. Neer, C.S. II, Watson, K.C., and Stanton, F.J. Recent experience in total shoulder replacement. *J. Bone Joint Surg.* 64A:319, 1982.
5. Cofield, R.H. Preliminary experience with bone ingrowth total shoulder. Presented at 4th Annual Meeting, American Shoulder and Elbow Surgeons, Los Angeles, California, 1985.
6. Craig, E.V. Continuous passive motion in the rehabilitation of the surgically reconstructed shoulder. Presented at the 2nd Open Meeting, American Shoulder and Elbow Surgeons, New Orleans, Louisiana, 1986.

# Elbow Arthroplasty

# 2

Peter Gearen

## Historical Perspective

An accurate chronicle of the development of total elbow arthroplasty must begin with a review of the surgical techniques that preceded it. Synovectomy for inflammatory arthritis was first discussed in the American literature by Goldtwait in 1900.[1] Radial head excision, in conjunction with synovectomy, was introduced by Smith-Peterson in 1943; this combination has remained popular because significant pain relief and increased function are generally produced.[2] The most comprehensive review of this procedure may be found in Chapter 116 of the *Textbook of Rheumatology*.[3]

Resection arthroplasty, long reported in the literature, has found few proponents over the years because it can result in instability and affords inconsistent pain relief.[4,5] However, there is little doubt that a successful result is more likely following a primary resection arthroplasty than if this operation is performed to salvage a failed total joint replacement.

Interpositional arthroplasty, using numerous types of materials, has been reported over the last six decades.[6] Fascia and skin are the two materials most frequently used. In 1947, MacAusland demonstrated excellent long-term results using fascia in over 100 patients.[7] Other authors have reported good or fair results in over 70% of patients when fascia is used.[8] The results of cutis, or skin interposition arthroplasty, have paralleled those of fascial interposition.

Hemiarthroplasty, in which one of the two articular surfaces is replaced, has not enjoyed significant support and has generally been superceded by total elbow arthroplasty.[9] The introduction of methyl methacrylate in the early 1970s diminished the problem of early prosthetic loosening; this apparently improved the outlook for successful elbow replacement. Implant designers, encouraged by this improvement, intensified their efforts toward elbow prostheses.

The earliest designs had relied upon fully constrained metal hinges.[10,11] A significant number of early and late complications, the most common of which was loosening, caused this type to be abandoned. The development of a constrained metal to plastic hinge did not significantly improve the results.

During the last decade, less constrained implants have been introduced. The current state of the art includes both semiconstrained and completely unconstrained designs. The semiconstrained designs most often couple a metal-to-polyethylene articulating interface with a loose snap-fit hinge, allowing variable amounts of medial/lateral laxity.[12–14] The unconstrained, or "resurfacing" designs also provide a metal/plastic articulation; stability is provided by the retained bone stock requiring the meticulous preservation or reconstruction of the soft tissue envelope.[15,16,17]

## Prosthetic Selection

The rapid evolution of total elbow prosthetic design over the last 10 years was predicated on the high failure rate of the early constrained designs combined with a rigorous biomechanical evaluation of elbow kinematics.[18,19] Presently, two basic types of arthroplasty are available.

### Anatomic/Resurfacing Type

Surgeons in the United States, Japan, Europe, and the British Commonwealth have independently developed various forms of resurfacing design. A common feature in these designs is the lack of an articulating/coupling mechanism. Generally, a minimal amount of bone is removed from the humerus and ulna; stability is achieved by soft tissue and osseous balance. Satisfactory results have been reported in 80–90% of cases using these resurfacing designs.[20,21,22] The principal complications are related to instability (subluxation or dislocation), ulnar nerve injury, and deep infection.

### Semiconstrained Type

The semiconstrained designs are generally used for elbows that lack the ligamentous stability or sufficient bone stock that is necessary to support an unconstrained design. Such deficiencies may occur secondary to rheumatoid disease, posttraumatic degenerative arthritis, or previous failed elbow arthroplasty.

## Indications/Contraindications

There are several pathologic conditions for which total elbow arthroplasty may be recommended. These include rheumatoid arthritis, degenerative arthritis, posttraumatic arthritis, and disease states resulting in bone loss.

In the past, replacement arthroplasty in patients with rheumatoid arthritis was recommended only after the failure of medical management and nearly complete destruction of bone and ligamentous stability. With the advent of resurfacing designs, which are highly dependent upon the original anatomy, earlier surgical intervention has often been recommended. Extrapolating from this, the ideal patient is one with pain unresponsive to medical therapy and with complete loss of articular cartilage, but with adequate remaining bone stock, ligamentous stability, and range of motion.

Idiopathic and posttraumatic degenerative arthritis unresponsive to conservative management are relative indications for total elbow arthroplasty. The reported results in this group have been less satisfactory than in rheumatoid patients, but the procedure may be indicated in selected cases.

Bone loss with unacceptable pain, instability, or diminished range of motion may result from tumor resections or traumatic loss. Therapeutic alternatives must be individualized in these cases. Another indication may be the failure of previous arthroplasties of any type. Generally, the instability and bone loss in these cases mandate a more constrained prosthesis. It has been said that previous interpositional arthroplasty is an absolute contraindication to resurfacing arthroplasty.[15]

The recognized contraindications to joint replacement arthroplasty of the elbow are the presence of infection, a history of neuropathic arthropathy, or a physically demanding life style. Certain anatomic problems may preclude the use of resurfacing designs. Finally, there is little wisdom in the performance of total elbow arthroplasty for the patient with an elbow arthrodesis or a painless, functional ankylosis.

## Research

Recent advances in total elbow arthroplasty have been rapid and dramatic, as with total knee arthroplasty. The most important of these has been the development of prostheses that more clearly adhere to the normal elbow kinematics. Present research involves the refinement of instrument designs that will make uncemented, press-fit arthroplasties more viable surgical alternatives. The ultimate goal is a biologically stabilized, isoelastic material that reproduces the normal elbow kinematics. Some researchers are currently experimenting with the use of allograft supplementation in cases of diminished bone stock.

## Surgical Technique

### Resurfacing Arthroplasty

After induction of general or regional anesthesia, the patient is positioned on the table one of three ways. The common technique is supine positioning with a sandbag placed under the scapula. Some surgeons have placed the patient in a lateral position with the elbow flexed over a bolster, whereas others operate with the patient prone. A tourniquet is essential.

Although numerous incisions have been described, currently most surgeons choose a variation of the Kocher posterolateral approach for resurfacing procedures (Figs. 2-1–2-4). This incision begins 8 cm proximal to the joint just posterior to the supracondylar bony ridge and extends distally over the anconeus for 6 cm along the subcutaneous border of the ulna. The interval between the anconeus and the extensor carpi ulnaris is developed; the anconeus is then reflected from the lateral aspect of the proximal ulna in continuity with the triceps muscle tendon unit. The insertion of the triceps is reflected from the tip of the olecranon exposing the posterolateral aspect of the joint. The lateral collateral ligament is released from its origin on the humeral lateral epicondyle, and the joint capsule is then incised. The radial head is excised at this point.

The elbow may then be hinged on the intact medial collateral ligament, thus affording excellent exposure of the joint and providing a soft tissue envelope that is compatible with the resurfacing-type procedures. The ulnar nerve is generally left undisturbed during this approach.

Preparation of the joint surfaces depends entirely on the specific type of resurfacing implant to be used. Most prosthetic designs do not replace the radial articulating surface. Should the design call for a radial head replacement, a conservative radial head excision should be performed. The distal humerus is prepared to receive the specific type of resurfacing device. The preparation for these more commonly used devices is shown in Figures 2-5–2-11.

Finally, the ulnar fossa is prepared to receive the implant after establishing the position of the ulnar medullary canal (Figs. 2-12–2-15). The bone resection and contouring of the ulnar fossa depends on the shape of the chosen components. The canal may be identified by using the dorsal prominence of the midshaft of the ulna as a guide. Care must be taken not to penetrate the cortex. A thorough synovectomy is performed, and stripping of the anterior capsule proximally in the distal humerus should be done if additional extension is necessary.

A trial reduction begins with the insertion of the ulnar component. This is followed by the implantation of the stemmed radial head component (if desired) and finally by the implantation of the stemmed or resurfacing humeral component.

Great care must be taken during the trial reduction to assure adequate motion and stability. If inadequate bone has been removed, and the device is unconstrained, the triceps may pull the ulna posteriorly in extension. In addition, if inadequate bone has been removed, increased tension may be placed on the medial collateral ligament, and the prothesis will serve as a shim, thus causing medial subluxation of the ulna. The optimal combination of components established by trial reduction will allow reattachment of the radial collateral ligament to its insertion on the lateral epicondyle when the elbow is placed in full extension. Under these circumstances, the medial collateral ligament should be taut. If the radial head is replaced (as in some designs), the extent of resection determines the component thickness. The appropriate size produces stable contact between the capitellum and the radial head throughout the complete arc of motion. Valgus instability may result from too thin a component.

Following the trial reduction, the bone surfaces are prepared in a standard fashion. The ulnar (and radial) component is cemented first. Great care must be taken to remove all excess cement, reintroduce the humeral trial, and allow polymerization with the elbow in maximum obtainable extension.

After fixation of the ulnar (and radial) components, the humeral trial is removed, and the actual implant is cemented in place, once again placing the joint in full extension as the cement cures (Figs. 2-16–2-20).

The tourniquet is deflated prior to closure, and all bleeders are electrocauterized. Gel foam may be used to eliminate dead space and aid in hemostasis.

Soft tissue repair must be meticulous and depends upon the surgical approach (Fig. 2-21). Generally, the collaterals and triceps should be reattached by using drill holes and heavy absorbable sutures. In contracted joints, the elbow is both flexed and extended in order to ensure that there is adequate excursion of the triceps; if not, the sutures are replaced in a way that allows for adequate excursion. Most surgeons have found triceps lengthening unnecessary as 40–60° of increased flexion can be achieved with the triceps intact.

## Rehabilitation

For the resurfacing designs, most surgeons use a long arm splint until the wound has healed, followed by a hinged cast brace for 4–12 weeks to assure extrinsic stabilization. Active motion is begun early in the rehabilitation. Passive motion is never required.

## Revision Procedures

The reported complication rate for revision total elbow arthroplasty is 46%.[20] This statistic makes it apparent that this procedure should be performed by the well-versed surgeon armed with a full complement of instruments and prostheses.

Revision total elbow arthroplasty should be reserved for cases where there is a material failure (e.g., broken axle), instability, or aseptic loosening of the original prosthesis. Conventional wisdom would suggest that the new prosthesis must resolve the problem for which the revision was deemed necessary.

## Technique

Sound preoperative planning is crucial to the successful outcome of revision elbow arthroplasty. Specific instruments may be required to remove a failed articulated prosthesis; the initial operative record or hospital chart will identify the type of prosthesis. The troublesome problem of inadequate bone stock is often present in these cases, and contingency planning (autogenous or allogeneic bone graft) is mandatory. Finally, a full complement of prostheses should be available; a stemmed, semiconstrained design is the most commonly used revision prosthesis.

A number of surgical caveats have been offered in an effort to prevent operative or perioperative difficulties with revision elbow arthroplasty.[24] Skin coverage must be a *preoperative* consideration. Flaps may be required prior to or as part of the revision procedure. The ulnar nerve should be exposed routinely during a revision to prevent injury. A soft tissue envelope including the triceps should be elevated as a unit as in the primary procedure. Finally, preservation of bone stock is of paramount importance. Osseous defects should be grafted.

The postoperative management depends on the adequacy of the soft tissues and design of the implant. If there is any concern about postoperative stability, a long arm cast is acceptable for the first few weeks.

## Acknowledgment

The author is very grateful to Mr. Thomas Wadsworth, Bernard Morrey, M.D., and Rowland Pritchard, M.D. for their significant contributions to this manuscript. This chapter represents a condensation of their efforts.

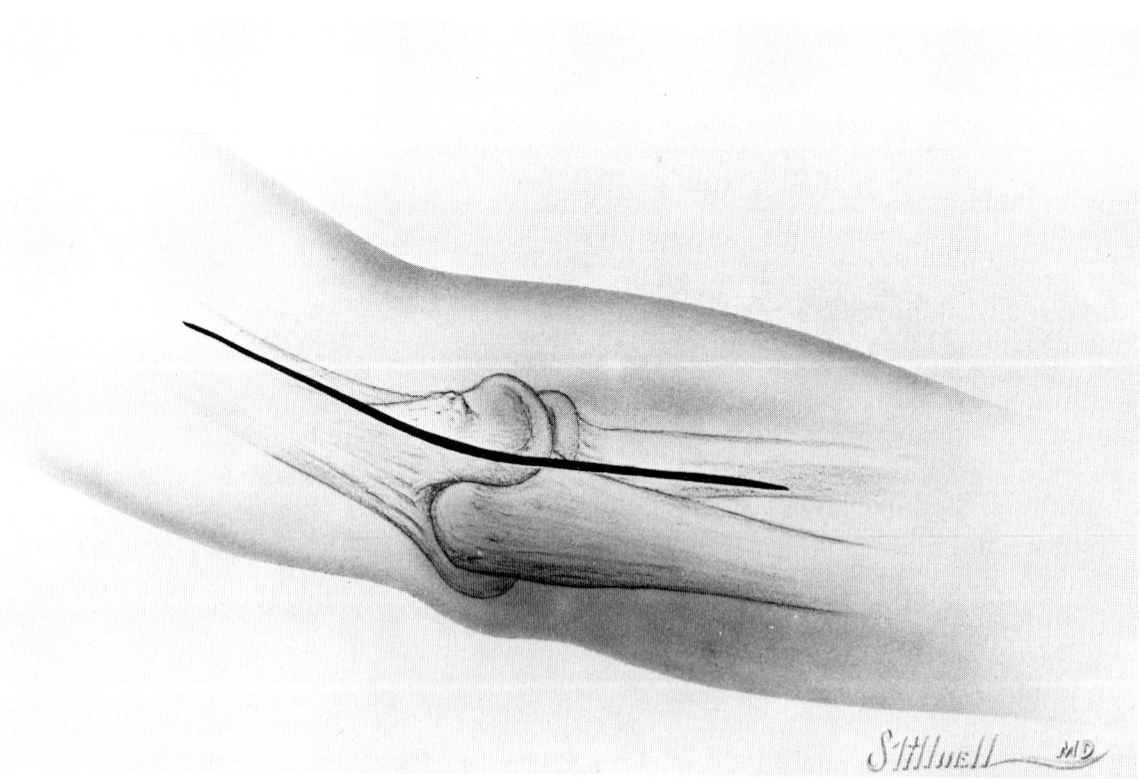

**Fig. 2-1** The Kocher posterolateral approach for resurfacing procedures begins 8 cm proximal to the joint just posterior to the supracondylar bony ridge. It extends distally over the anconeus for 6 cm along the subcutaneous border of the ulna.

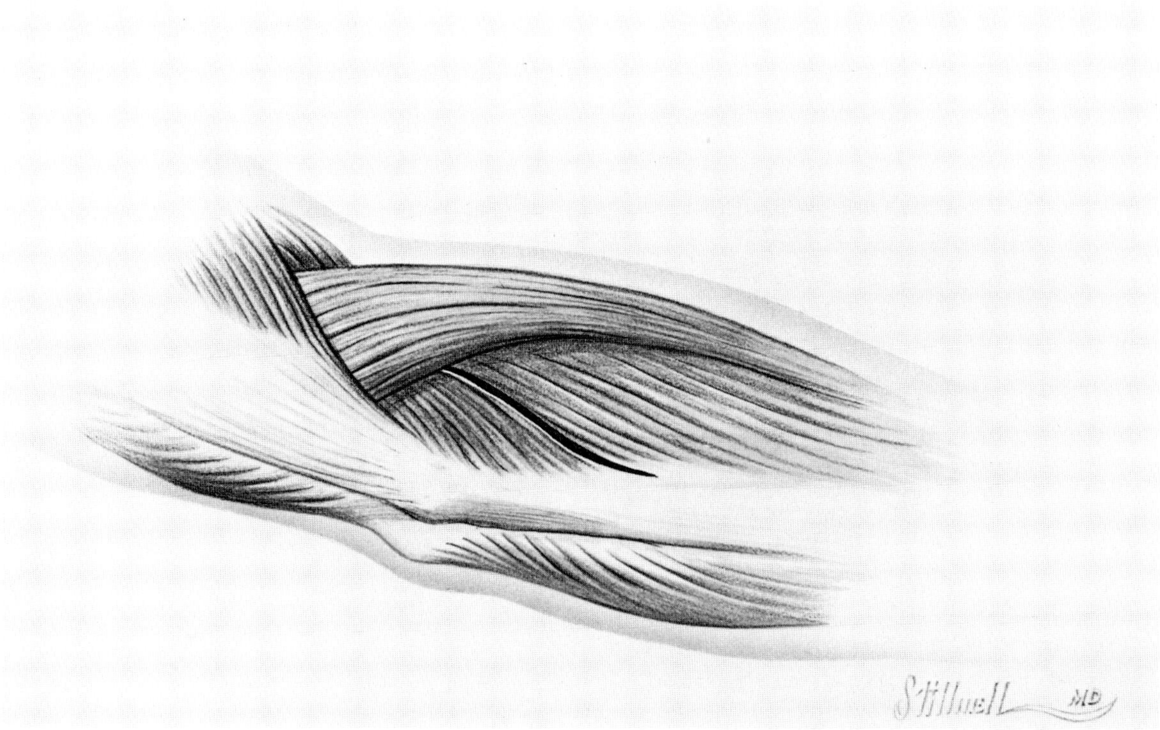

**Fig. 2-2** The interval between the anconeus and the extensor carpi ulnaris is developed.

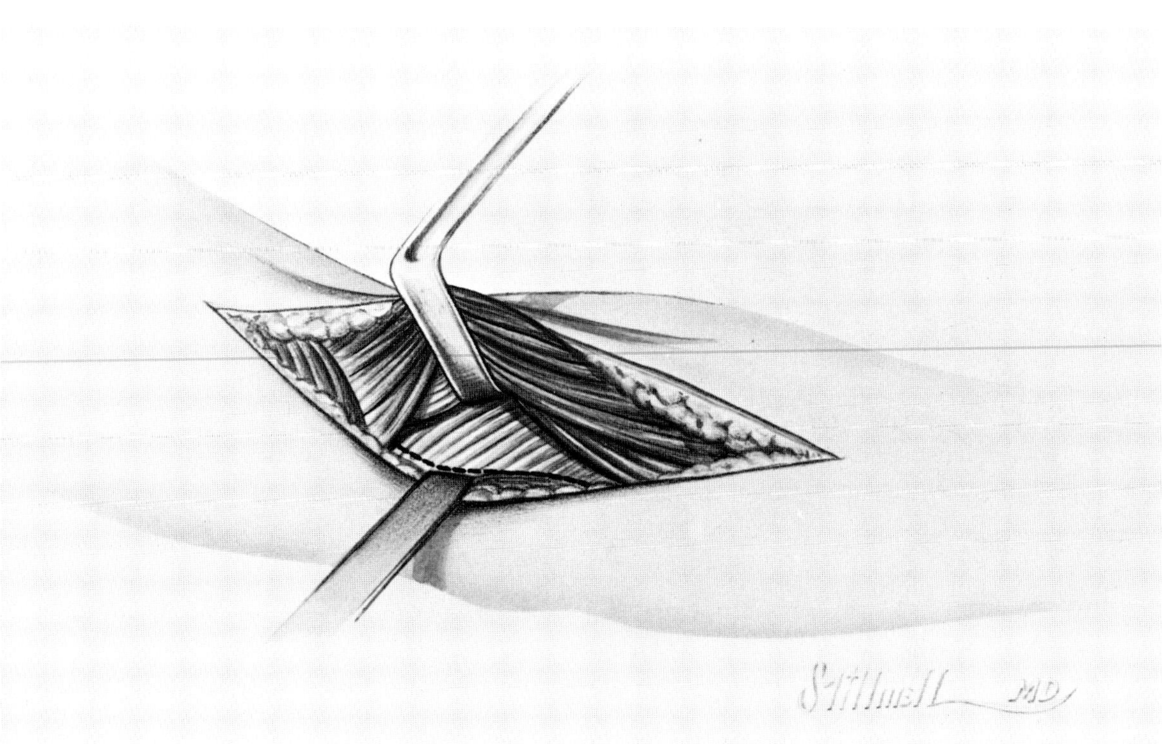

**Fig. 2-3** The anconeus is then reflected from the lateral aspects of the proximal ulna in continuity with the triceps muscle tendon unit.

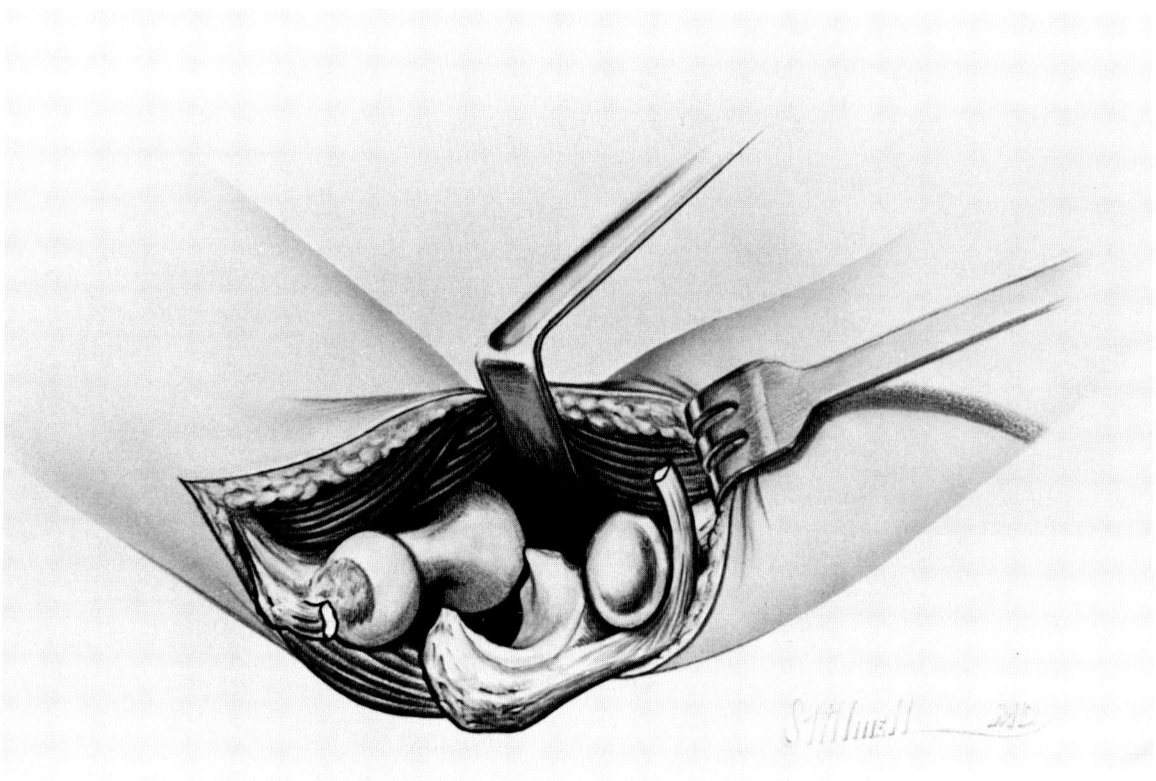

**Fig. 2-4** The lateral collateral ligament is released from its origin on the humeral lateral epicondyle and the joint capsule is incised for complete joint exposure.

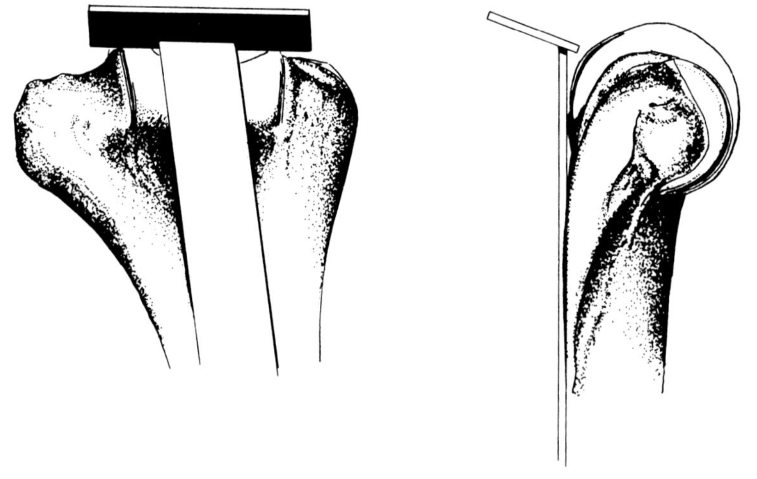

**Figs. 2-5–2-11** Preparation of the joint surfaces depends entirely on the specific type of resurfacing implant to be used. Most prosthetic designs do not replace the radial articulating surface. Should the design call for a radial head replacement, a conservative radial head excision should be performed. The distal humerus is prepared to receive the specific type of resurfacing device. The preparation for these more commonly used devices is as shown.

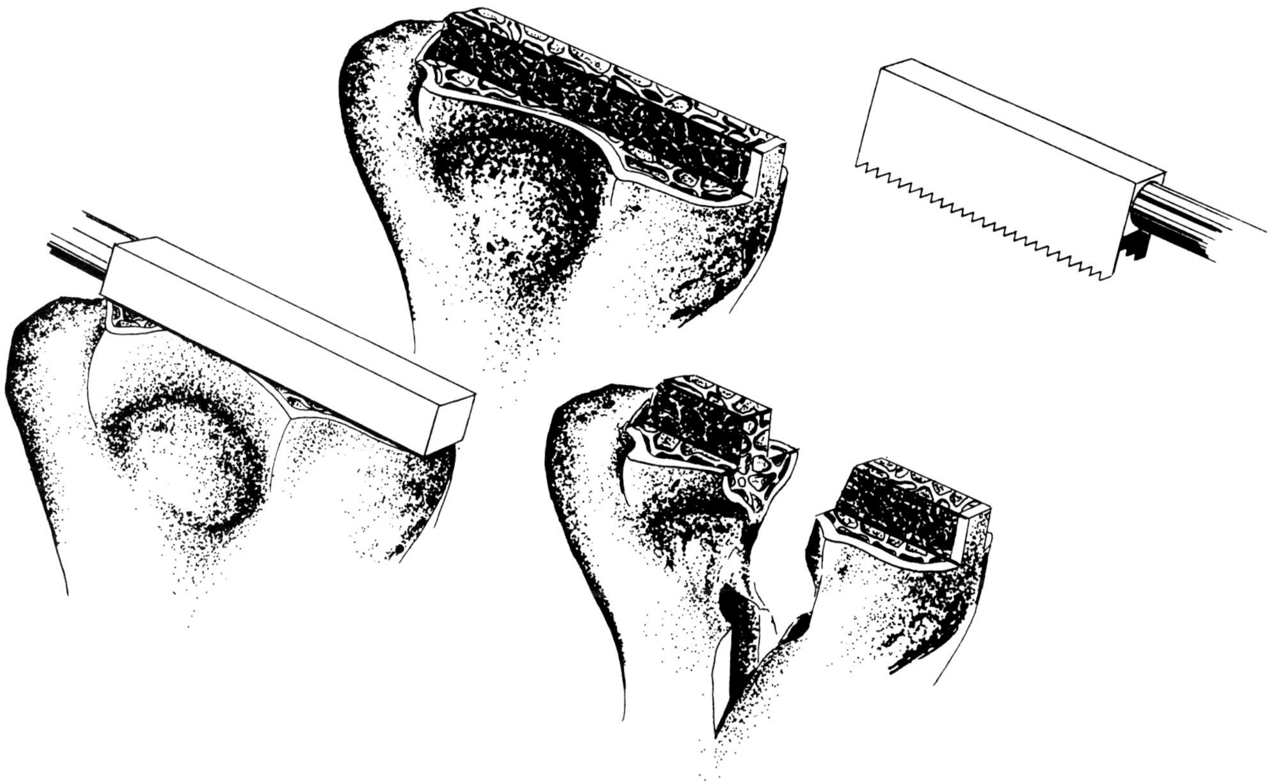

Fig. 2-6

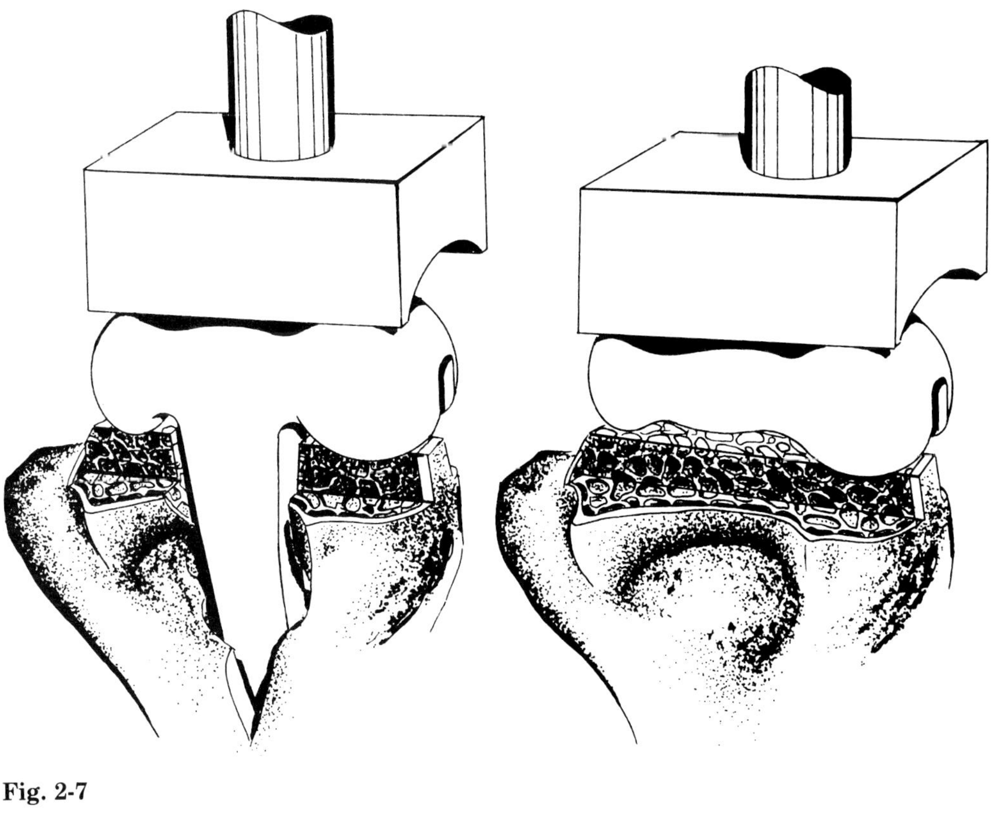

Fig. 2-7

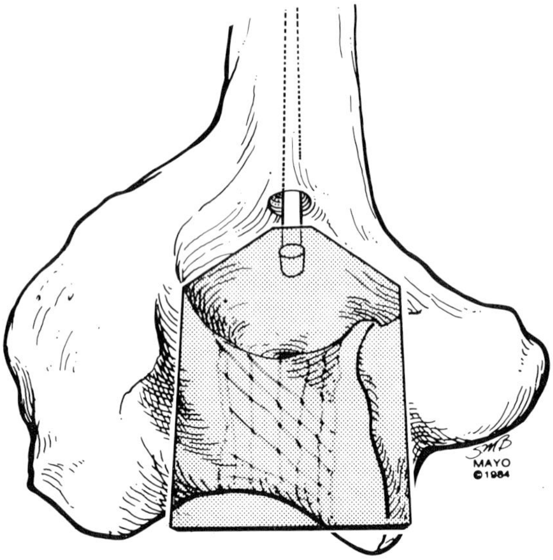


Fig. 2-8

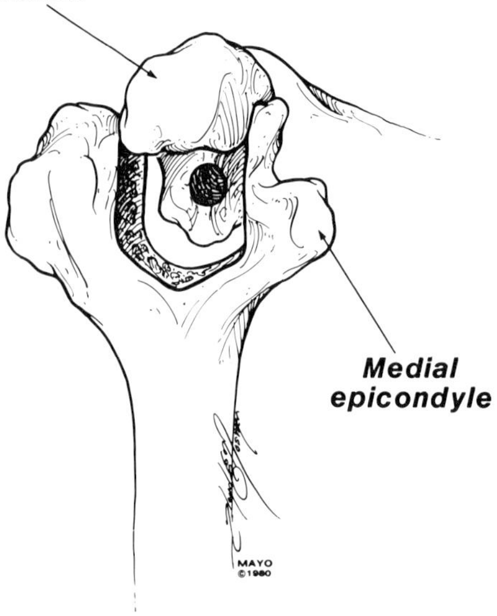


Fig. 2-9

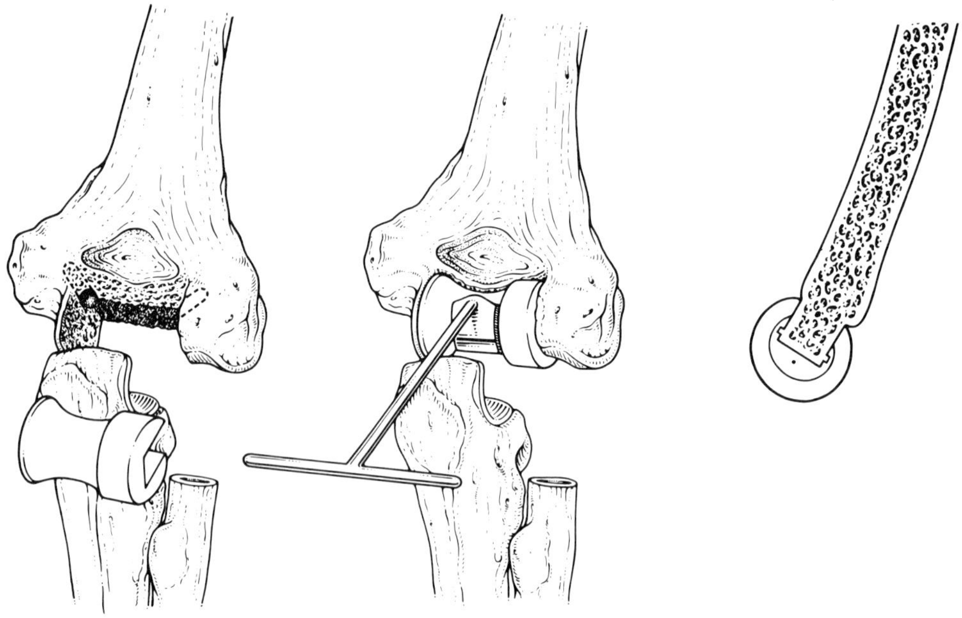

Fig. 2-10

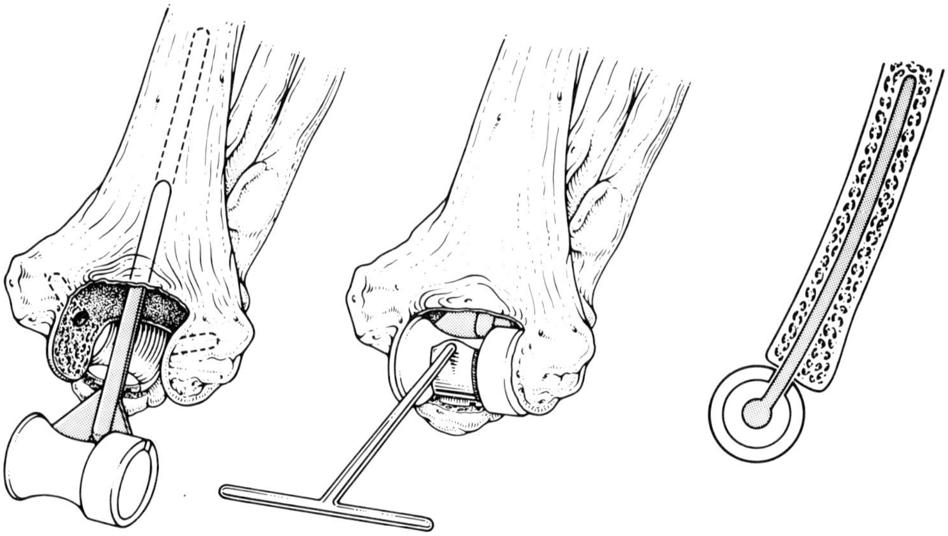

Fig. 2-11

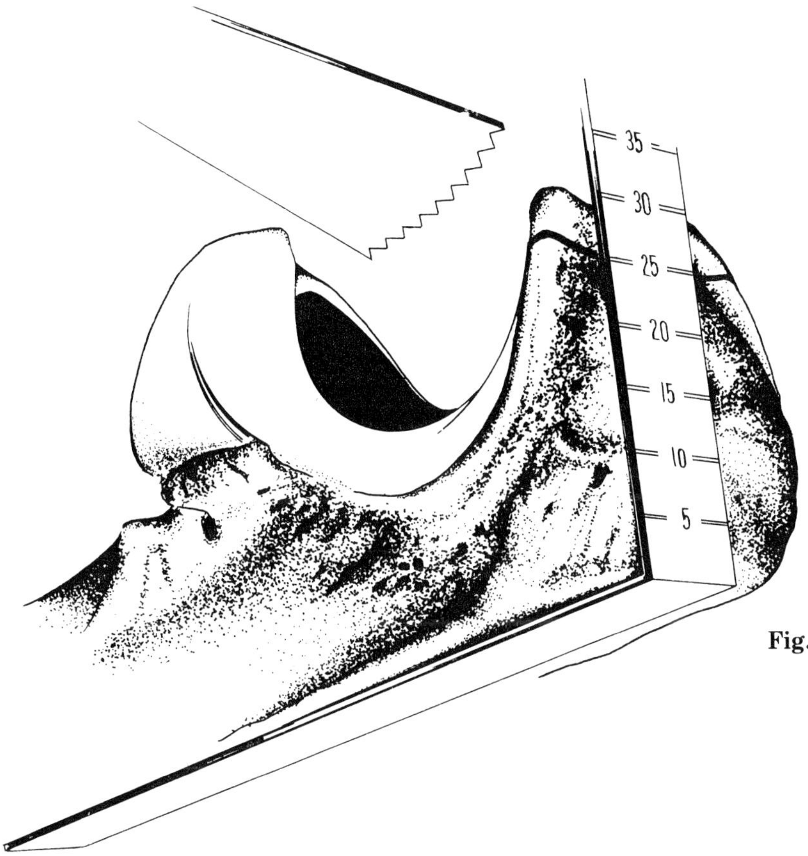


Fig. 2-12

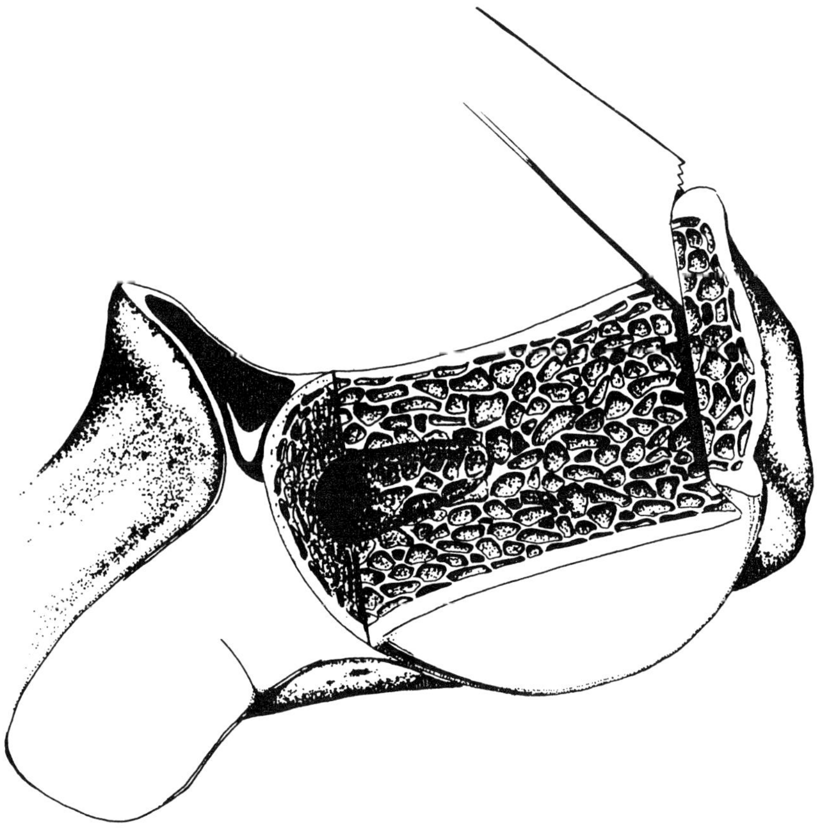

Fig. 2-13

**Figs. 2-12–2-15** The ulnar fossa is prepared to receive the implant after establishing the position of the ulnar medullary canal. The bone resection and contouring of the ulnar fossa depends on the shape of the chosen components. The canal may be identified by using the dorsal prominence of the midshaft of the ulna as a guide. Care must be taken not to penetrate the cortex. A thorough synovectomy is performed, and stripping of the anterior capsule proximally in the distal humerus should be done if additional extension is necessary.

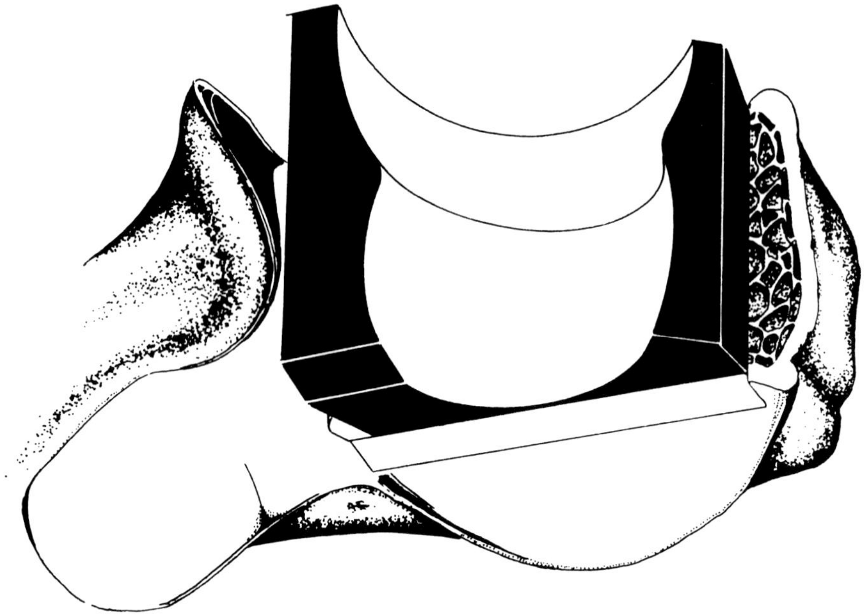

Fig. 2-14

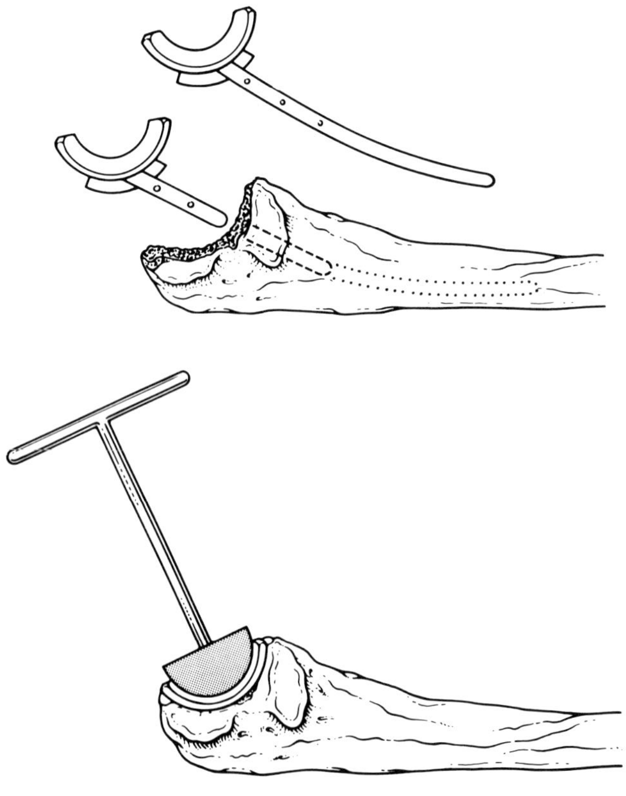

Fig. 2-15

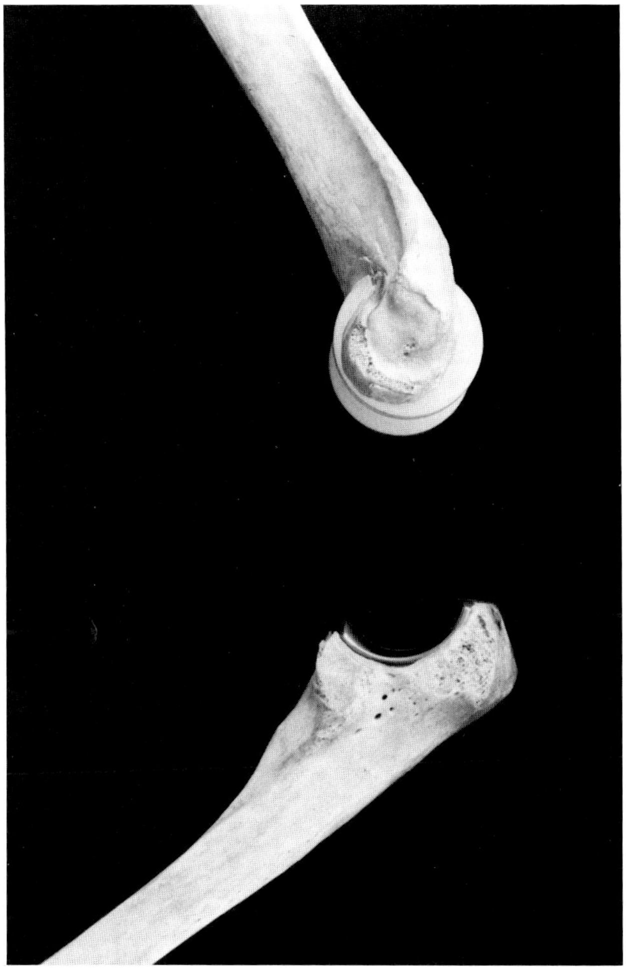

Fig. 2-16

Fig. 2-17

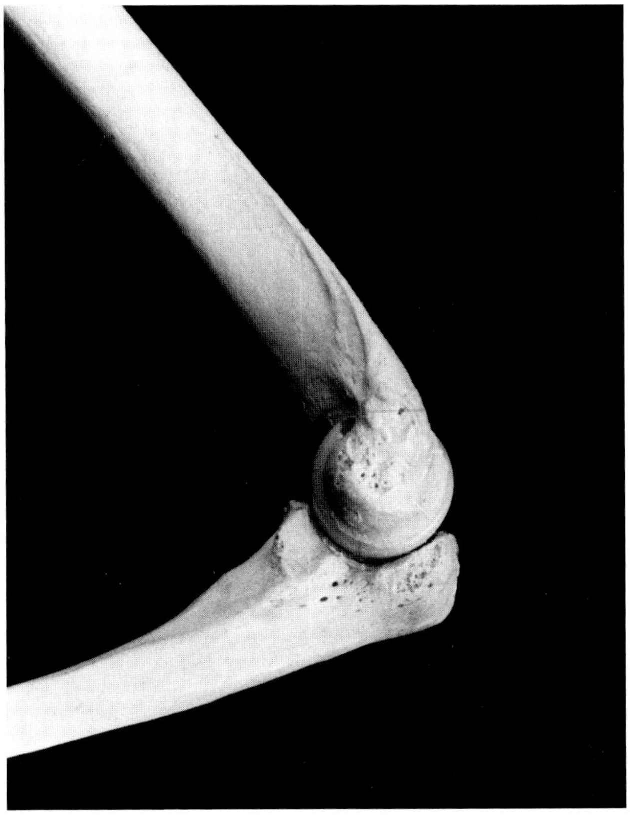

**Figs. 2-16–2-20** Following trial reduction, the bone surface is prepared in standard fashion. The ulnar (and radial) component is cemented first. After fixation of the ulnar and radial components, the humeral trial is removed, and the actual implant is cemented in place, once again placing the joint in full extension as the cement cures.

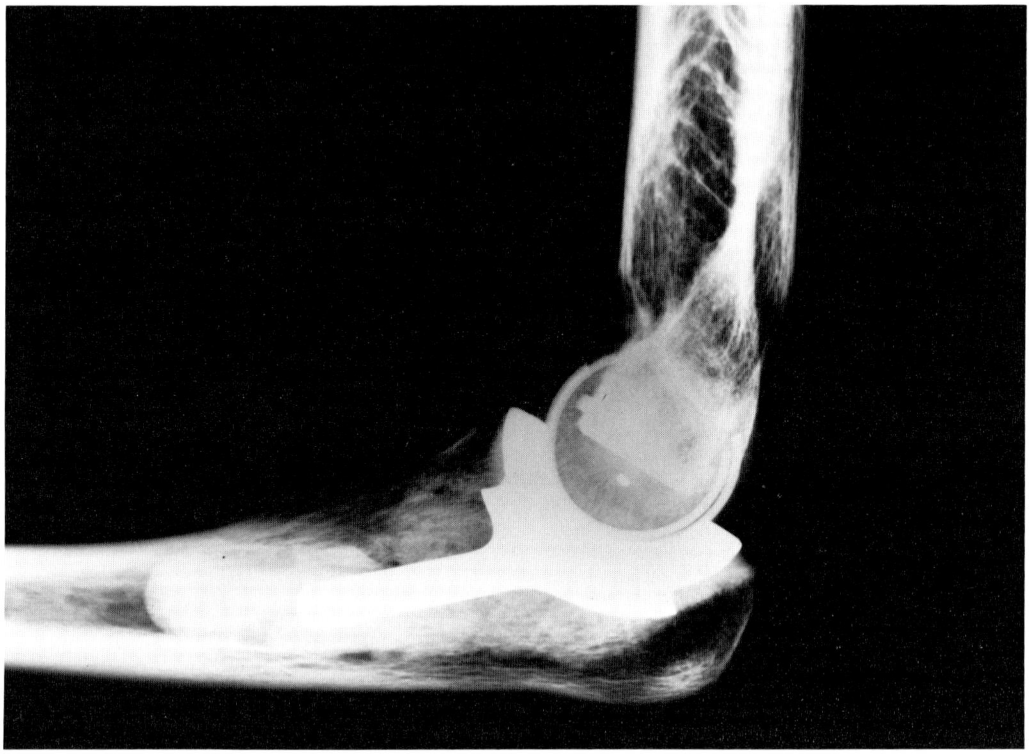

Fig. 2-18

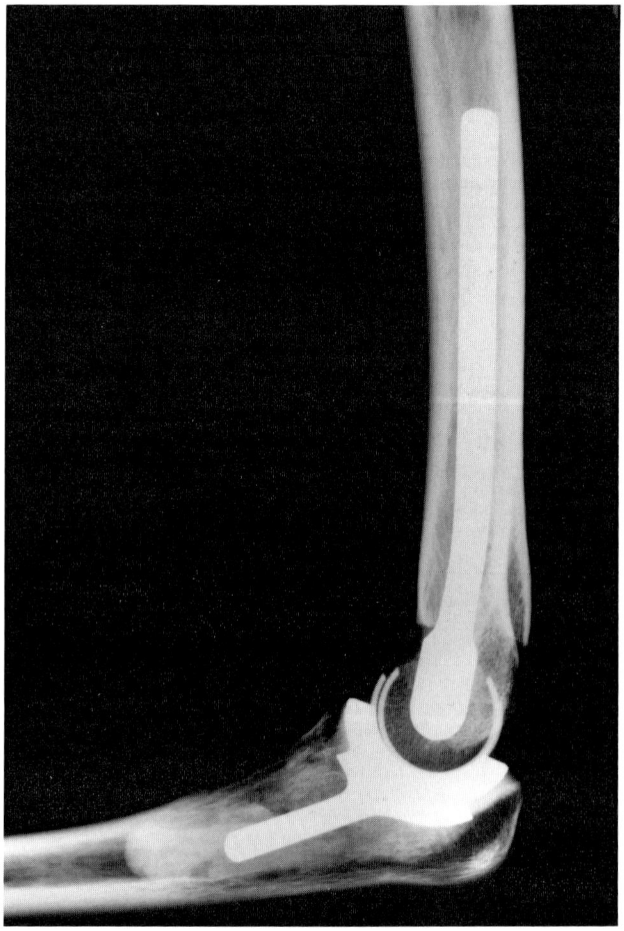

Fig. 2-19

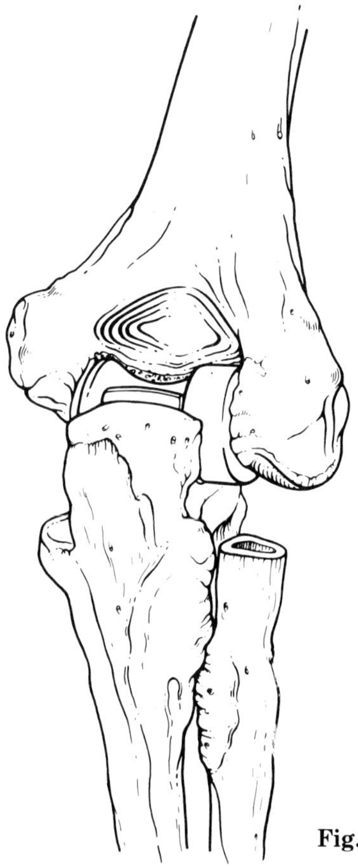

Fig. 2-20

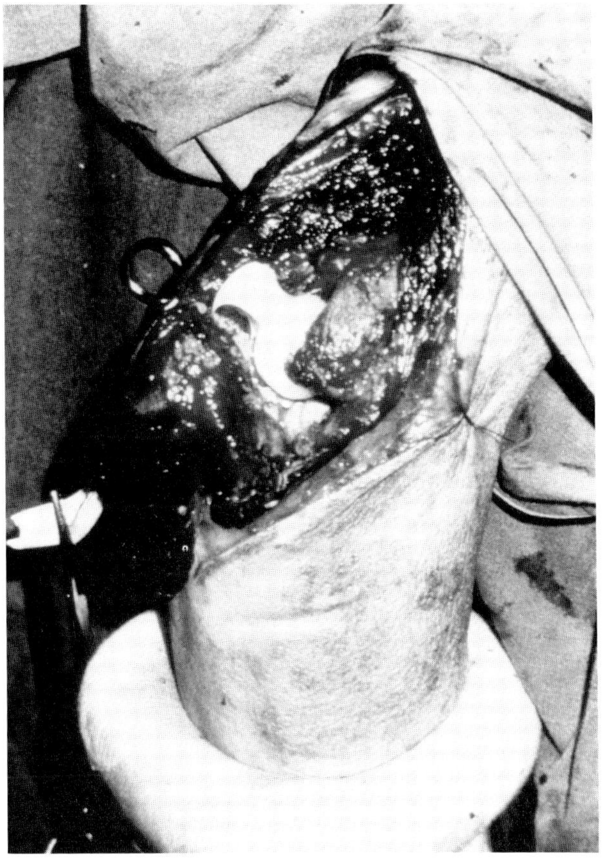

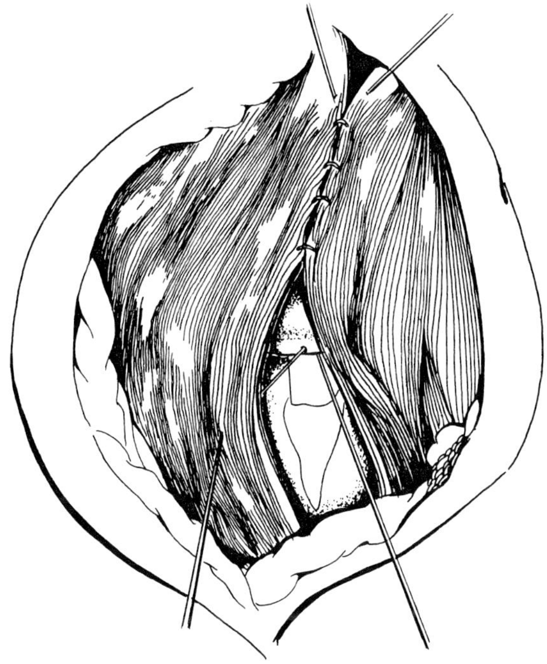

**Fig. 2-21** Soft tissue repair must be meticulous and depends upon the surgical approach. Generally, the collaterals and triceps should be reattached by using drill holes and heavy absorbable sutures.

## References


1. Goldtwait, J.E. Knee joint surgery for non-tubercular conditions. A report of 38 operations for synovial fringes, injured semi-lunar cartilage, loose cartilage, coagula, exploratory incision, etc. *Boston Med. Surg. J.* 143:286, 1900.
2. Smith-Peterson, M.N., Aufranc, O.E., Larson, C.B: Useful surgical procedures for rheumatoid arthritis involving joints of the upper extremity. *Arch. Surg.* 46:764, 1943.
3. Ewald, F.C. Reconstructive surgery and rehabilitation of the elbow. In Kelly, W.N., Harris, E.D., Ruddy, S., Sledge, C.B. (Eds.), *Textbook of Rheumatology.* Philadelphia: W.B. Saunders, 1981, 1921–1943.
4. Dickson, R.A., Stein, H., and Bentley, G. Excision arthroplasty of the elbow in rheumatoid disease. *J. Bone Joint Surg.* 58B:227, 1976.
5. Haas, J. Functional arthroplasty. *J. Bone Joint Surg.* 26:297, 1944.
6. MacAusland, W.R. Mobilization of the elbow by free fascia transplantation with report of 31 cases. *Surg. Gynecol. Obstet.* 23:223, 1921.
7. MacAusland, W.R. Arthroplasty of the elbow. *New Engl. J. Med.* 236:97, 1947.
8. Knight, R.A., and Van Zandt, I.L. Arthroplasty of the elbow. An end result study. *J. Bone Joint Surg.* 34A:610, 1952.
9. Barr, J.S., and Eaton, R.G. Elbow reconstruction with a new prosthesis to replace the distal under the humerus. A case report. *J. Bone Joint Surg.* 47A:1408, 1965.
10. Dee, R. Total replacement arthroplasty of the elbow for rheumatoid arthritis. *J. Bone Joint Surg.* 54B:88, 1972.

11. Gschwend, N. Arthroplasty of the elbow using the GSB prosthesis. In *Proceedings of the Twelfth Congress of the International Society of Orthopaedic Surgery and Traumatology, Tel Aviv, October 9–12, 1972*. Amsterdam: Excerpta Medica.
12. Inglis, A.E., and Pellicci, P.M. Total elbow replacement. *J. Bone Joint Surg.* 8:1252, 1980.
13. Pritchard, R.W. Flexible elbow joint replacement. *Orthop. Trans.* 1:109, 1977.
14. Schlein, A.P. Semi-constrained total elbow arthroplasty. *Clin. Orthop. Rel. Res.* 121:222, 1976.
15. Ewald, F.C. Non-constrained metal to plastic total elbow replacement. In Inglis, A.E. (Ed.: Upper extremity joint replacement), *Symposium on Total Joint Replacement of the Upper Extremity,* 1979. St. Louis; C. Mosby Co., 1982.
16. Kudo, H., Iwano, K., and Watanabe, S. Total replacement of the rheumatoid elbow with a hingeless prosthesis. *J. Bone Joint Surg.* 62A:277, 1980.
17. Pritchard, R.W. Anatomic surface elbow arthroplasty. A preliminary report. *Clin. Orthop.* 179:223, 1983.
18. London, J.T. Kinematics of the elbow. *J. Bone Joint Surg.* 63A(4):529, 1981.
19. Morrey, B.F., Askew, L.J., An, K.N., and Chao, E.Y. A biochemical study of normal functional elbow motion. *J. Bone Joint Surg.* 63A:83, 1981.
20. Davis, R.F., Weiland, A.J., Hungerford, D.S., Moore, J.R., and Volenec-Dowling, S. Non-constrained total elbow arthroplasty. *Clin. Orthop.* 187:154, 1984.
21. Ewald, F.C., Scheinberg, R.D., Poss, R., Thomas, W.H., Scott, R.D., and Sledge, C.B. Capitellocondylar total elbow arthroplasty. Two to five year follow-up in rheumatoid arthritis. *J. Bone Joint Surg.* 62A:1259, 1980.
22. Rosenberg, G.M., and Turner, R.H. Non-constrained total elbow arthroplasty. *Clin. Orthop.* 187:154, 1984.
23. Morrey, B.F., and Bryan, R.S. Reimplantation revision for failed total elbow arthroplasty. American Academy of Orthopaedic Surgeons Annual Meeting, Atlanta, Georgia, February, 1984.
24. Morrey, B.F. Revision joint replacement. In Morrey, B.F. (Ed.), *The Elbow and Its Disorders*. Philadelphia: WB Saunders, 1985, pp. 570–581.

# Wrist Arthroplasty

# 3

Robert G. Volz

## Historical Perspective

Wrist arthroplasty is a relatively new procedure in the surgeon's armamentarium. The factors that account for this are the lack of suitable materials to serve as a replacement or substitute for a damaged or diseased carpus and the relatively infrequent need for the preservation of painfree motion at the carpus. In the late 1960s, however, with early successes being documented in the use of silastic in the reconstruction of arthritic joints, attention was turned to the carpus, where a silastic spacer was designed and implemented by Swanson. Early breakage of this material when used at the carpus due to the appreciable stresses that can be observed at this articulation had a limiting effect upon the wide acceptance of this form of arthroplasty. During the early 1970s, an improved grade of silastic material became available that had greater resistance to tear propagation, the method by which silastic material generally breaks.

The first cementable nonconstrained articulating total wrist prothesis was designed by Meuli in Bern, Switzerland in 1971. The principle of the application of this type of prosthesis paralleled that of the cemented hip implant. The successes that had been observed with the latter prosthesis prompted the application of a cementable implant composed of a metallic, high-density polyethylene interface. In 1973, a total wrist prosthesis was designed at the University of Arizona Health Sciences Center by Volz. The prosthesis was also fabricated of a cobalt chrome alloy that articulated against a high-density, polyethylene interface, with both components being secured by methyl methacrylate cement to the supporting bony bed.

During the early and mid-1970s, these three prostheses represented the most popularly employed implants for treatment of damaged or diseased wrist joints. Because of the restraint placed upon artificial joint developers and manufacturers by the enactment of the Device Legislation Act in 1976, progress has been slow in the refinement and creation of more sophisticated implants. However, during the past several years there have been several other implants that have been made available for investigational use only. These include implants designed by Beckenbaugh, Taleisnik, and Hamas.

## Prosthetic Selection

Presently, the issue of prosthetic selection is a very subjective one, for both silastic and cemented total joint prostheses appear to give comparable results provided patient selection has been carefully arrived at. Because many hand surgeons have not been trained or are not familiar with the use of methyl methacrylate cement, preference is given to the use of the silastic wrist spacer. Certainly, the indications for use of a silastic wrist spacer include the patient with far-advanced inflammatory arthritic changes to the carpus, particularly the patient with rheumatoid arthritis. Care should be taken to identify, however, the degree of stress that will be placed upon the upper extremity, particularly in the use of crutches or other walking aids or in the act of arising from a sitting position. Patients who are apt to subject their wrist to extremes of motion do run a greater risk of failure of the silastic material, although the incidence of this complication is, perhaps, no greater than 2–4%. Individuals who present with the diagnosis of osteoarthritis and who exhibit sturdy bone stock are more appropriate candidates for some type of cementable total wrist arthroplasty. Because aseptic loosening of the implantable components has been reported to be quite low, in the neighborhood of 2–3% with a mean follow-up of 6 years, these devices appear to be reasonably durable. Obviously, patients who exhibit poor quality bone stock are not suitable candidates for cementable total wrist arthroplasty due to the fact that there is not sufficient strength to support the implant against the stresses that might be encountered with activities of daily living.

## Indication

The indication for any type of wrist arthroplasty is, first of all, a sufficient degree of disability confined to the carpus where hand and finger function are appreciably compromised. It should further be stated that the most appropriate form of treatment for far-advanced destructive changes to the carpus is an arthrodesis. However, it has been pointed out that bilateral arthrodeses of the wrist offer a significant degree of compromise to hand and upper extremity function, particularly in areas of personal hygiene and in vocations and avocations that require some degree of wrist motion. Thus, only in individuals who, because of vocational or avocational needs, require the preservation of some degree of wrist motion should wrist arthroplasty be considered as the primary form of treatment. Additionally, patients who exhibit diffuse arthritic change, not only at the carpus but at the hand, are also considered appropriate candidates since it is well-documented that a small degree of painfree motion at the wrist tends to augment fine motor control in activities of daily living.

## Contraindications

Numerous contraindications exist with reference to the performance of wrist arthroplasty. Patients who are engaged in heavy manual labor are not considered appropriate candidates because of the problem of breakage of the implant, dislocation, or aseptic loosening of any cemented device. Patients who are engaged in vocational or avocational activities that also place an extraordinarily great demand upon a considerable arc of motion at the wrist are also inappropriate candidates for the previous reasons. Prior infection in the site of prosthetic implantation, inadequate bone stock, and the absence of intact wrist extensors should also be considered absolute contraindications for such surgery. It cannot be overemphasized that the preservation of intact wrist extensors is essential if the implant's stability and performance are to be maintained. As a general rule, patients presenting with a painful wrist have lost a significant arc of extension. This extension augments grip strength and fine motor control of the hand and fingers and, therefore, is one of the prime goals of any type of wrist arthroplasty. Intact wrist extensor function is, therefore, essential to an acceptable result.

## Present and Future Research

Because aseptic loosening of cemented prosthetic devices represents the single most commonly observed mode of failure, much interest has been generated recently in the use of "biologically fixed" implants. Such implants derive their stability, in part, from a textured or porous surface that provides for an ingrowth of living tissue that subsequently may undergo a metaplastic change into supporting bone. Although experiences with such devices are quite limited at the present, initial impressions remain quite favorable as to their long-term durability. Because of the marked loss of bone that is frequently observed in patients with inflammatory arthritis, such as observed in rheumatoid arthritis, use of cemented devices in such a setting is generally not recommended. Additionally, the technical difficulties associated with extraction of a failed cemented device make the option of using a noncementable wrist prosthesis an extremely attractive one. Presently, no large series of devices designed for press-fit or biological fixation are available for review. But, with the rapid advances that are being observed in the use of various ingrowth surfaces, such studies will soon be making their appearance, thereby enabling the surgeon to make a comparative analysis between cemented and noncemented devices.

## Surgical Technique

As with any type of technically demanding procedure, it is absolutely imperative that the operating surgeon thoroughly prepare himself as to the anatomical and technical aspects of the case. A wide knowledge of the complexities of wrist anatomy and the dynamics of the motor forces that act upon the wrist is essential. Briefly stated, the most difficult aspect of any prosthetic wrist arthroplasty is the ultimate degree of balance that is achieved. Particularly in cases of tendon rupture such as those observed with rheumatoid arthritics, the problem of postoperative wrist balance is critical. Frequently, the surgeon is unable to identify preoperatively deficient or absent motor units and is left with the difficulty of transfers or repairs at the time of prosthetic implantation. Furthermore, it cannot be overemphasized that the preservation of active wrist extensor activity is absolutely mandatory for a satisfactory postoperative result.

The surgical approach to the carpus when a prosthesis is to be inserted is from the dorsum. Curvilinear incisions are to be avoided since they tend to disrupt more of the critical dorsal venous structures than does a straight midline vertical incision. Because healing of such wounds is critical, delicate retraction of skin edges without extensive undermining of skin is a must. Many patients, especially those with rheumatoid arthritis, will present with a significant loss of subcutaneous fat. In such cases, dissection should be developed to provide clear-cut layers for the subsequent wound closure, thereby minimizing any direct communication from the skin to the underlying prosthesis.

In cases where significant distal radial ulnar disease exists, incision of the dorsal retinaculum overlying the extensor carpi ulnaris is carried out to permit adequate exposure of the distal end of the ulna. Following resection of no more than 5 mm of the distal ulna, the dorsal retinaculum is resutured in a vest-over-pants arrangement, thereby tending to stabilize the distal end of the ulna to prevent dorsal displacement with pronation.

In the surgical approach to the carpus, the third compartment is entered through the dorsal retinaculum. Care is taken to retract the extensor digitorum communis tendons to the ulnar border while the extensor carpi radialis, brevis, and longus and the extensor pollicis longus are retracted radialward. The dorsal capsule is carefully identified and is reflected radialward through the creation of a U-shaped incision that begins proximally over the distal radial plate and extends distally to nearly the base of the fourth metacarpal. The distal radius and underlying carpus are now visualized. Because volar subluxation of the carpus is a frequent finding in patients with rheumatoid arthritis, enhancement of exposure of the carpus is gained by first removing the distal radial plate by use of a reciprocating saw. This initial cut is made at right angles to the long axis of the radius. Once this plate is removed, the subluxated carpus is better visualized. Next, the necessary segments of the carpus are excised either separately or in toto. This includes the scaphoid, the lunate, the head of the capitate, the radial portion of the hamate, and the lesser multangular.

The exposure now permits preparation of the remaining carpal and distal radial beds for the particular prosthesis to be inserted. Once prosthetic insertion has been accomplished, careful closure is mandatory for few layers of tissue exist between skin and the implant. If capsular closure is impossible owing to insufficient soft tissue, reinforcement of the defect by use in part or all of the retinaculum is possible. It is desirable, however, to retain some dorsal retinaculum to anchor extensor tendons, thereby lessening the problem of postoperative bow stringing.

The soft tissues over the dorsum of the hand are loosely fixed to the deeper tissues, thereby giving rise to the development of a sizeable hematoma should adequate drainage of the wound not be carried out. It is, therefore, desirable to use some type of suction drainage placed within the subcutaneous or intercapsular regions. The application of a carefully applied moistened pressure dressing is also critical in the prevention of postoperative swelling.

## Revision Surgery

The most frequently observed indication for prosthetic removal is either breakage or sinkage of a silastic implant or the mechanical loosening of a cemented device. Occasionally, however, cases of postoperative imbalance of the wrist, especially a posture of fixed ulnar deviation and wrist flexion, may serve as the sole indication for a revision surgery. Although the surgical approach is essentially unchanged, several additional points are worthy of mention. First, if a cemented device is to be removed and the components cannot freely be extracted without jeopardizing the intact cortical bone, the potential for the creation of a fracture of the cortex can be lessened by the creation of a longitudinal saw cut over the respective prosthetic stem. This will allow the cortical shell to expand slightly as the device is tapped from its bed. Cerclage suture fixation may be used as is deemed necessary. As in any case of deep periprosthetic infection, it is mandatory that all foreign material be removed if resolution of the infection is to be anticipated.

In cases where prosthetic removal is to be followed by arthrodesis, freshening of the devascularized bony surfaces is critical. We have found that some degree of initial stability of an interpositional bone graft can be achieved by reconstituting the carpal/metacarpal height ratio (this is approximately 0.54:1). The insertion of such a proportioned interpositional bone graft derives its stability by reestablishing sufficient soft tissue capsular tension. The option to further stabilize the arthrodesis graft site by use of a pin or plate remains an issue of personal surgical judgment.

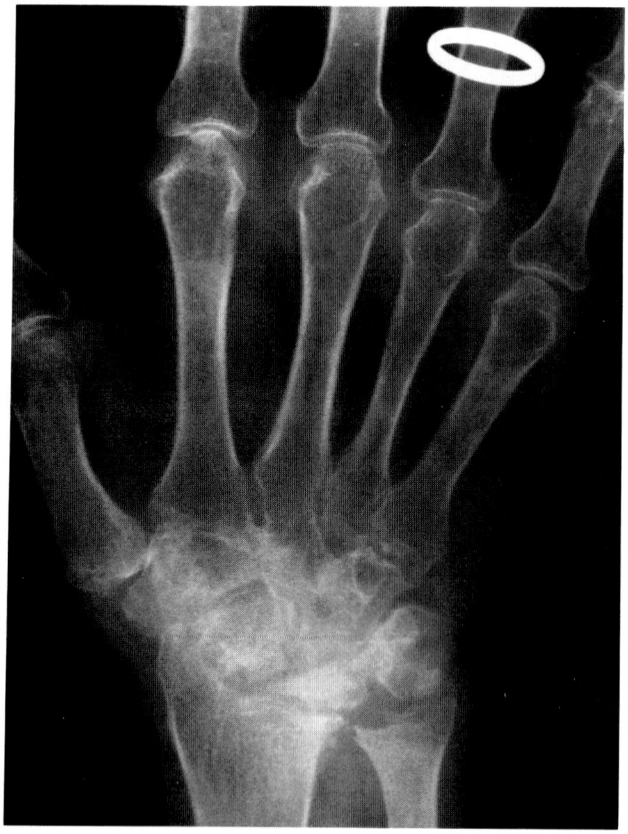

**Fig. 3-1** When diffuse arthritic changes exist at the carpus, the treatment options include arthrodesis or wrist arthroplasty. Elimination of pain at the wrist enhances power-gripping activities and fine motor control of the fingers.

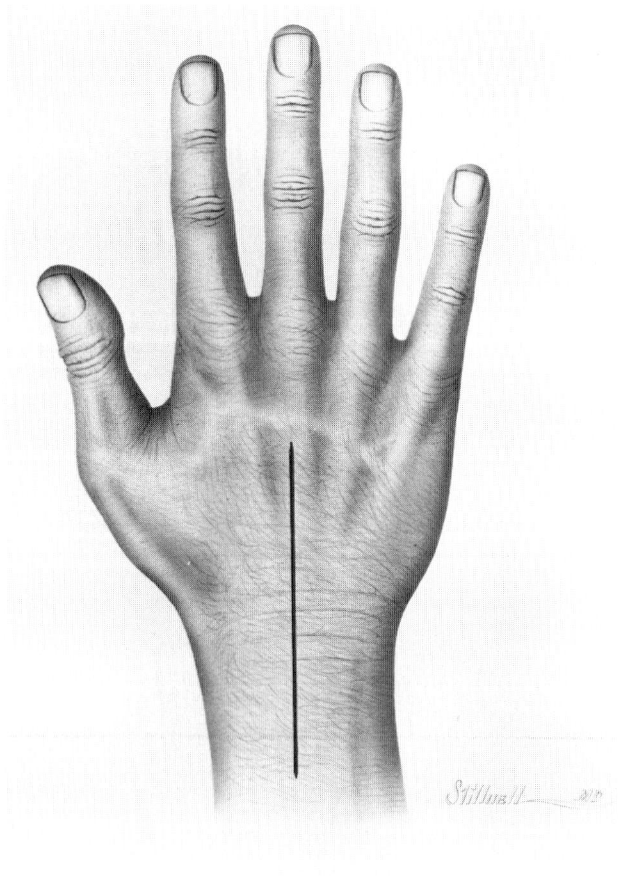

**Fig. 3-2** A dorsal midline surgical incision is made beginning distally over the third metacarpal and progressing proximally, approximately 2 in. from the distal radial plate of the radius. Care should be taken to preserve all subcutaneous venous structures. Dissection is carried down to expose the dorsal retinaculum, which is divided through the third compartment.

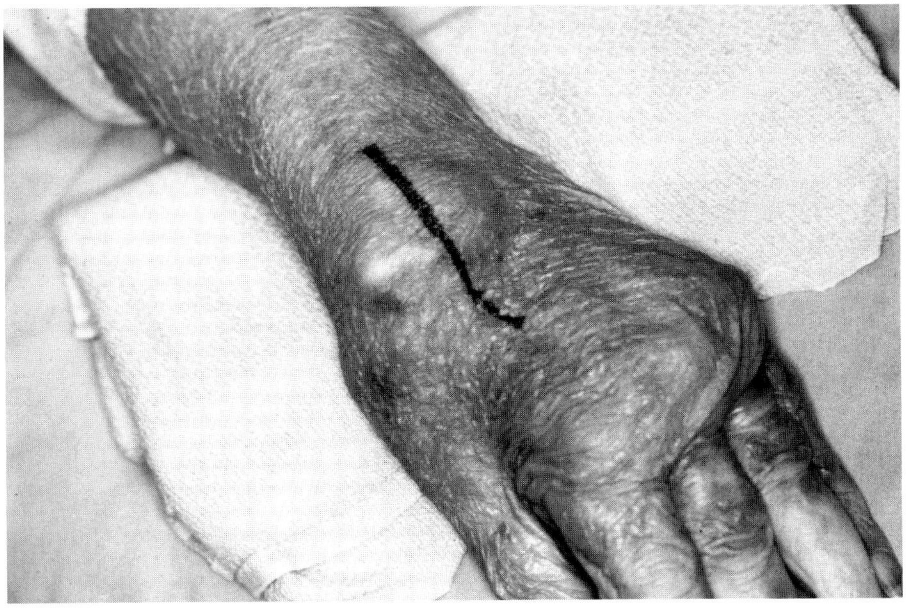

Fig. 3-3

Fig. 3-4A

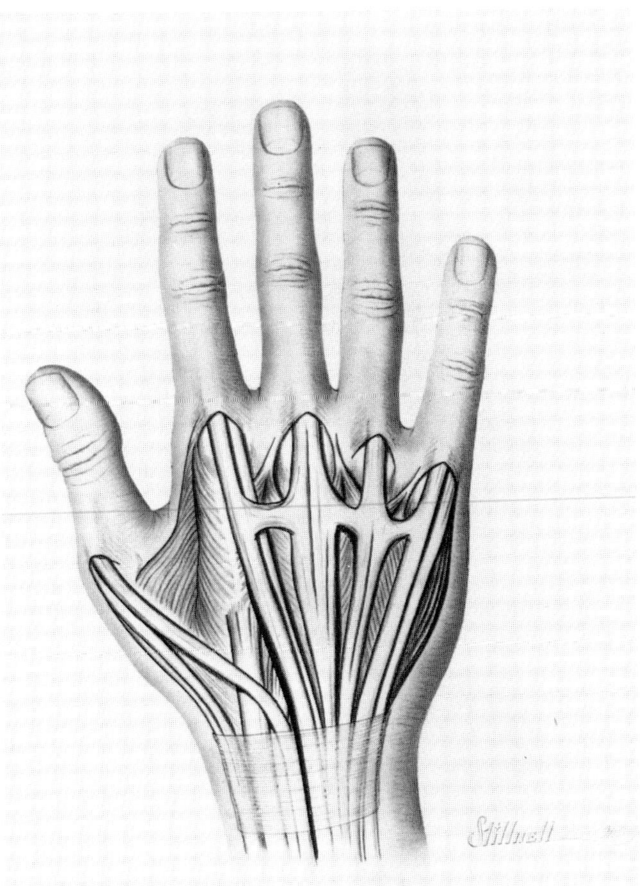

Fig. 3-4B

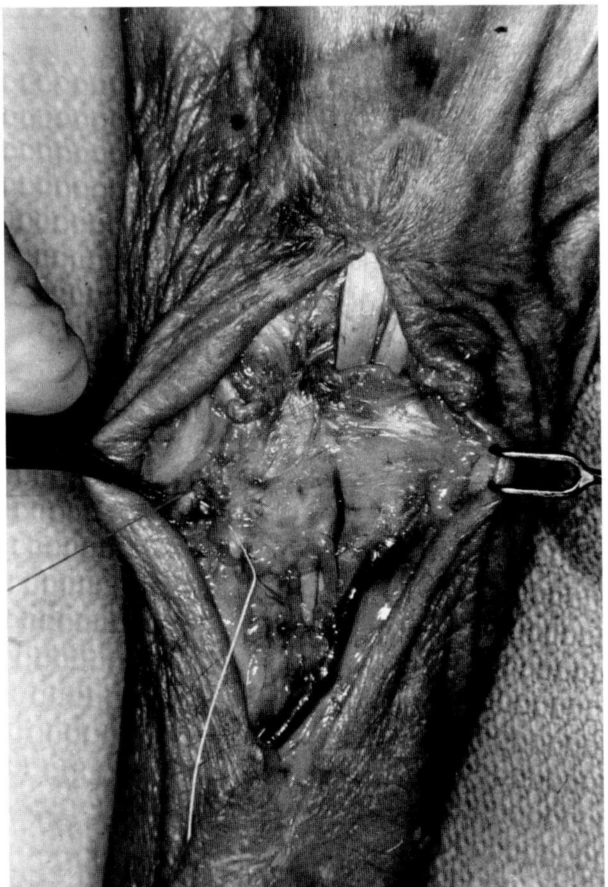

**Figs. 3-3–3-5** A straight dorsal incision in line with the third metacarpal should be utilized in the exposure of the carpus in wrist arthroplasty. All venous structures should be preserved.

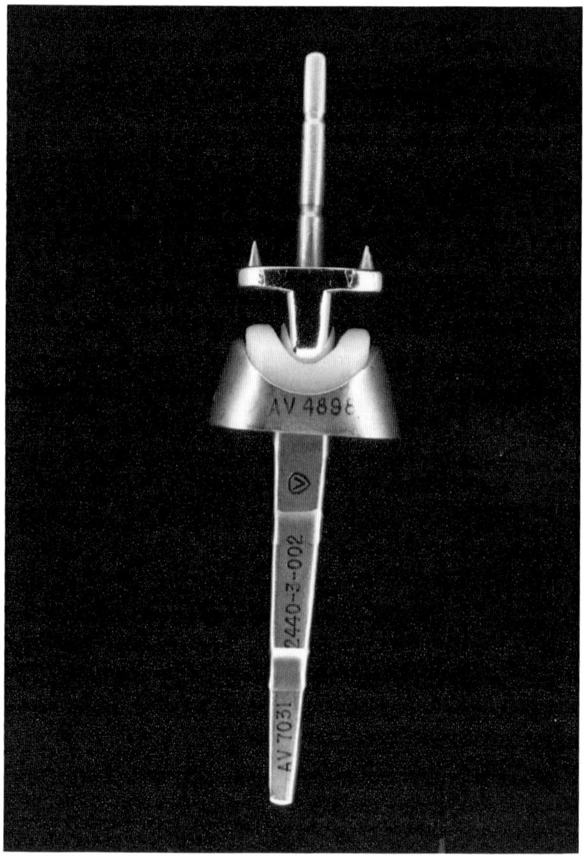


**Fig. 3-6** The articulated, semiconstrained total wrist prosthesis designed at the Arizona Health Science Center. The interface provides for 90° of flexion-extension and 50° of radial-ulnar deviation. The metacarpal component is "press fitted" into the third metacarpal-carpal bed; the radial component is cemented into the distal radius.

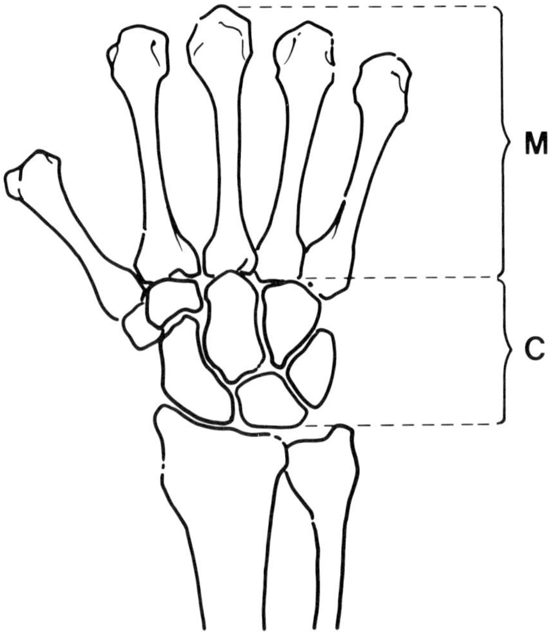


**Fig. 3-7** The normal height of the carpus can be expressed as a ratio of the length of the third metacarpal. This ratio is normally 1:0.54 ± 0.03. Restoration of this ratio when altered by disease is critical if sufficient tension is to be regained in the flexor and extensor tendons.

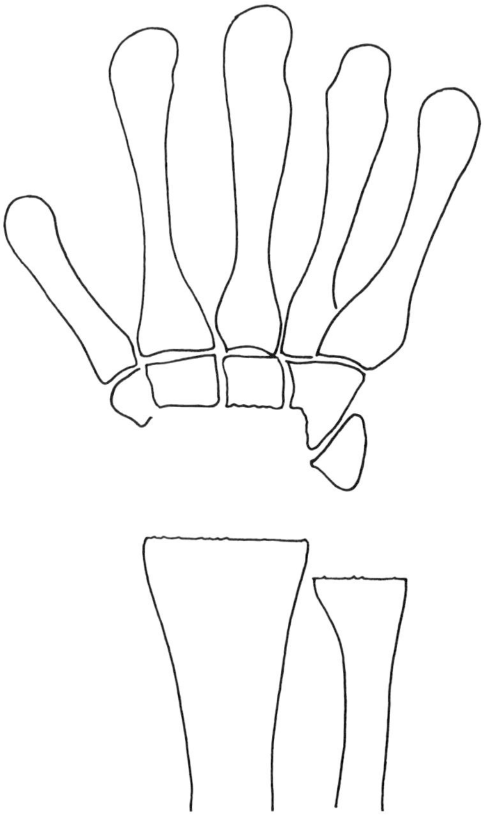

**Fig. 3-8** Resection of the distal radial plate, the scaphoid, lunate triquetrum, proximal half of the capitate, and a small portion of the hamate will provide sufficient space for the implantation of a prosthesis. If disease involves the distal radial-ulnar joint, the distal 1 cm of the ulna should be resected.

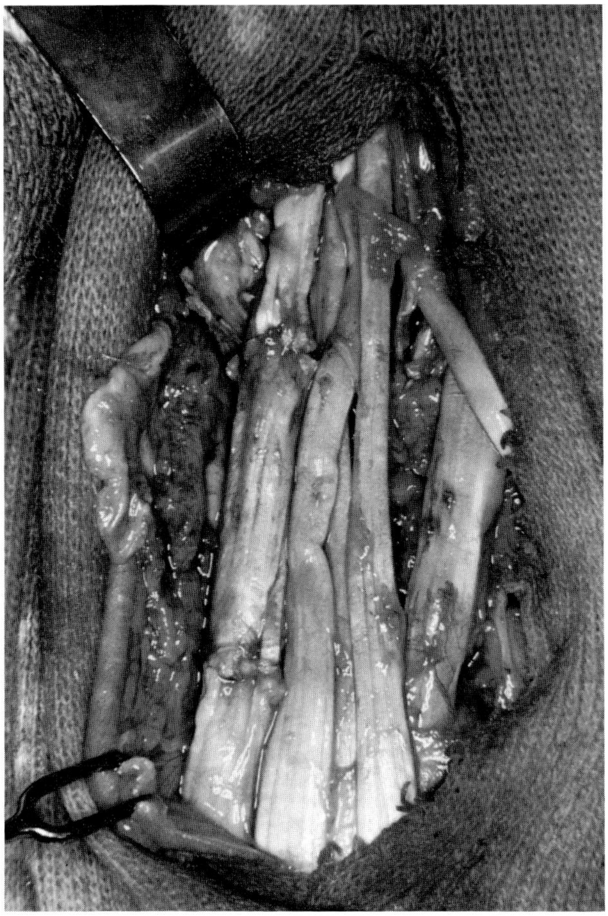

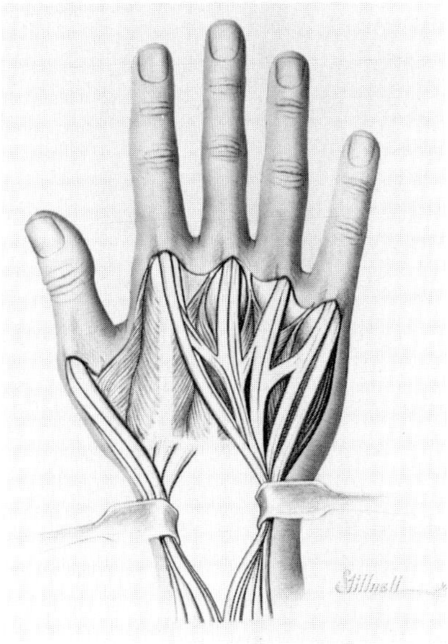

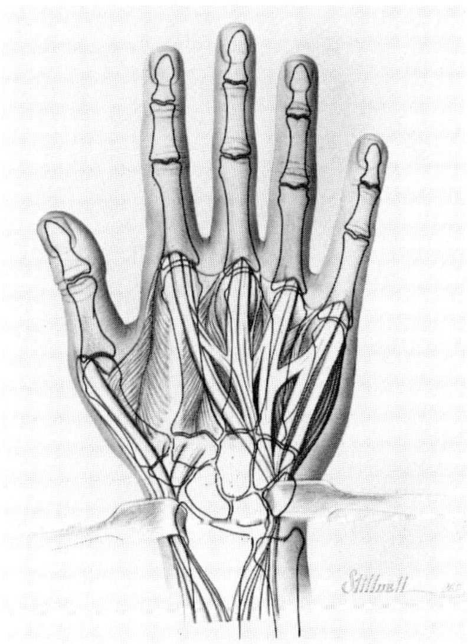

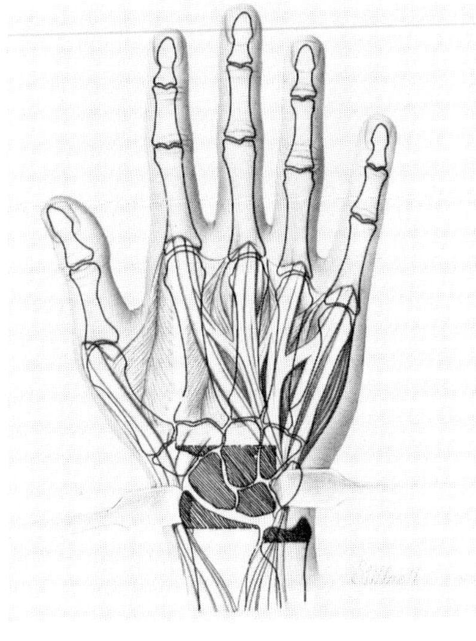

**Fig. 3-9** The distal end of the ulna is further identified by soft tissue dissection. The extensor carpi ulnaris is retracted ulnarward; the extensor digitorum comminus is retracted radialward. By careful dissection, the capsule and all soft tissue attachments to the distal end of the ulna are dissected free, and approximately 1 cm of the distal end of the ulna is resected by use of a reciprocating saw. The extensor pollicis longus is now freed from Lister's tubercle and is retracted radialward with the extensor carpi radialis, brevis, and longus. The common extensors to the fingers are retracted ulnarward. The dorsal capsule is now adequately exposed, and a U-shaped incision is made overlying the base of the lesser multangulum, the capitellum, the lunate, and the scaphoid. This segment of dorsal capsule is reflected radialward. Exposure of the underlying carpus and the distal radial plate has now been facilitated. By use of a reciprocating saw, the distal radial plate is now amputated. By use of a reciprocating saw, or rongeur, the proximal pole of the capitate is removed along with the lunate and scaphoid. A small portion of the hamate may also require removal.

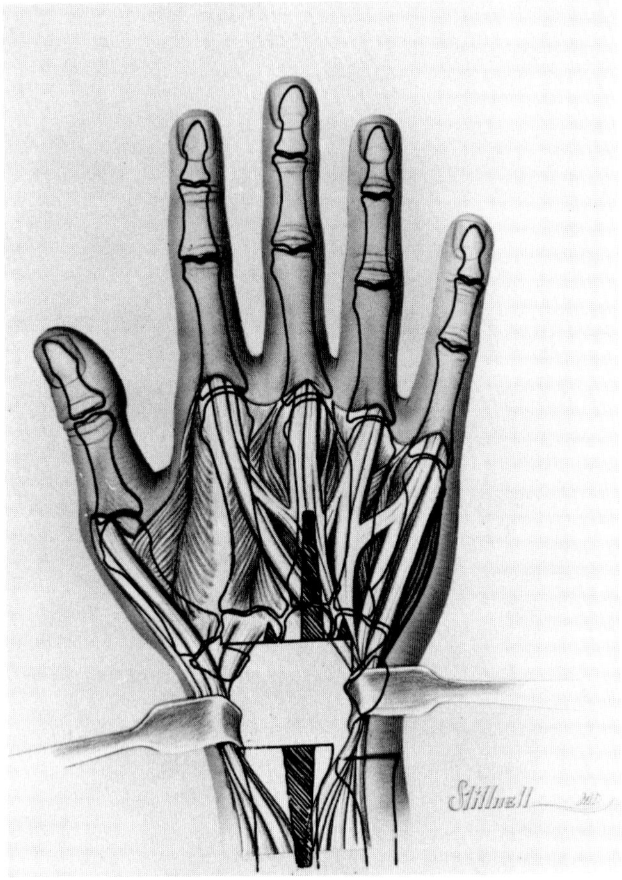

**Fig. 3-10** A trial fit of the prosthetic device is next performed after insertion of the metacarpal component, followed by insertion of the radial component. The wrist should be placed through an adequate arc of motion, and any soft tissue tethering should be identified.

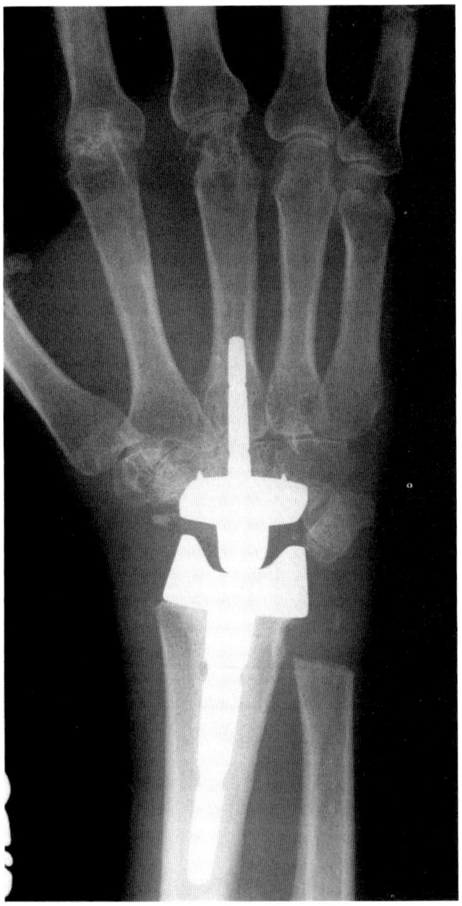

**Fig. 3-11** Shown implanted is a total wrist arthroplasty. The matacarpal component has been "press fitted"; the radial is secure by methyl methacrylate cement.

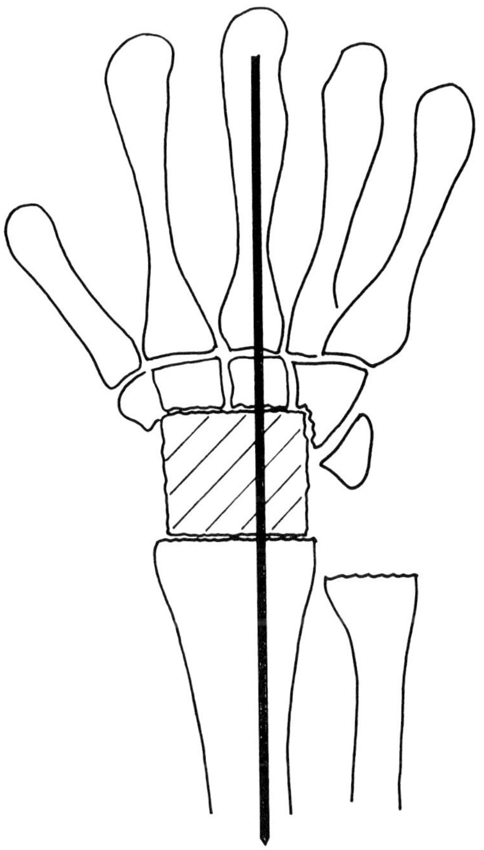

**Fig. 3-12** Diagram of a reconstructed wrist following removal of a failed implant. The interpositional bone graft is sufficiently proportioned to reconstitute the metacarpal/carpal ratio.

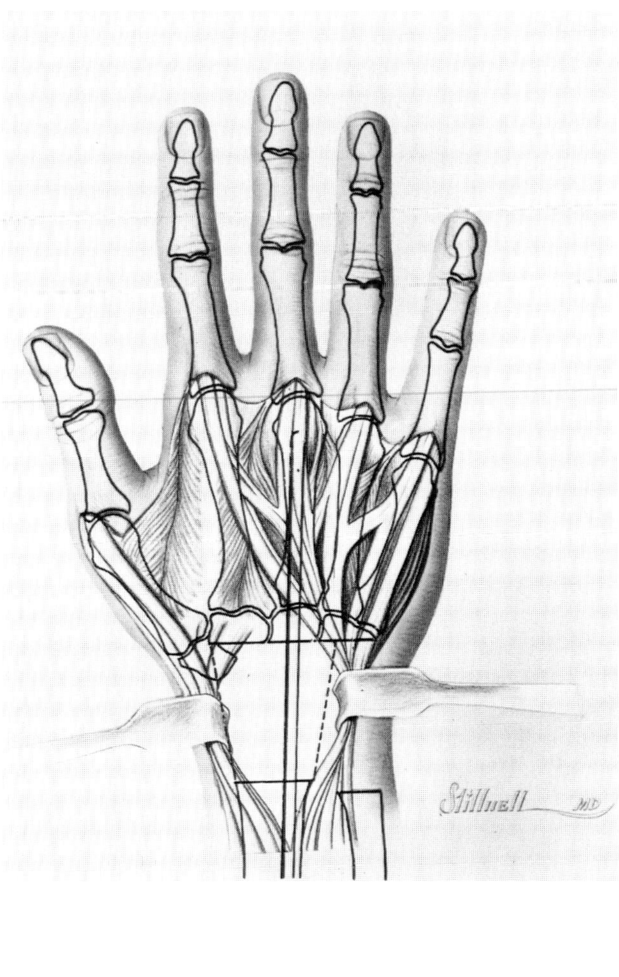

**Fig. 3-13** When revision surgery is necessary and prosthetic removal is indicated to be followed by arthrodesis, a longitudinal incision may be placed through the dorsal cortex of the third metacarpal and the distal radius. Cemented prosthetic devices may now be tapped free without fear of comminution of the outer cortical shell. Exposed prosthetic bed surfaces are freshened by use of a reciprocating saw until healthy-appearing bone has been identified. An appropriately sized bicortical graft taken from the anterior portion of the iliac crest is now harvested. This is inserted within the prior prosthetic bed and fashioned to reconstitute the normal metacarpal/carpal ratio. The degree of dorsiflexion of the wrist can be controlled by further precise shaping of the interpositional graft material. Once sufficient stability has been achieved, a Steinmann pin may be driven into the medullary canal of the third metacarpal and advanced until it secures the bone graft to the distal portion of the radial shaft. The wound is then carefully closed in layers, with the placement of a subcutaneous drain.

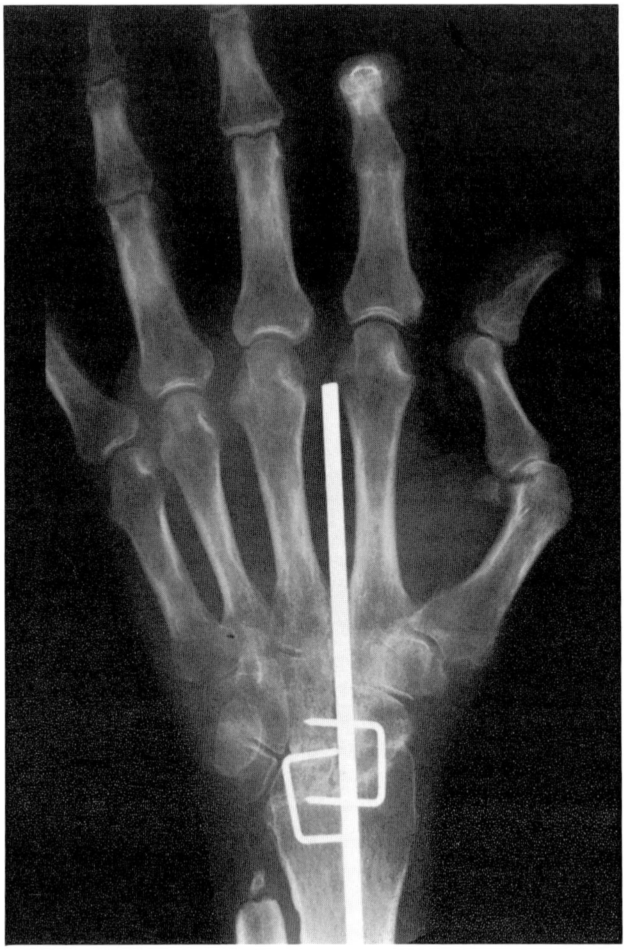

**Fig. 3-14** Radiograph of an arthrodesed wrist following removal of a failed implant arthroplasty.

# Arthroplasty of the Hand

# 4

Susan M. Craig

The concept of joint replacement in the hand has a long history. Factors peculiar to the small joints of the hand and to the demands placed on them, however, have made practical application of hand joint replacement a development of the last two decades. This chapter is a review of current techiques for replacement of these small joints, indications for and constraints on hand joint replacement, as well as potential pitfalls and complications. In addition, two of the multiple operations for hand joint replacement are explained and illustrated.

## Joint Replacement

Joint replacement in the hand takes several forms. *Resection arthroplasty* refers to direct excision of degenerated joint surfaces with protected healing followed by guarded motion. Resection arthroplasty is appropriate in situations where there is excellent soft tissue support, minimal surrounding deformity, and where the amount of joint surface to be resected is not excessive. In these selected circumstances, resection arthroplasty results in a painless, functioning joint and excellent long term prognosis.

Currently the most popular form of joint arthroplasty is the insertion of a *silastic spacer* after excision of arthritic articular surfaces (see Figs. 4-1 through 4-16). This approach carries resection arthroplasty one step further and controls from within the scar formation, allowing early motion. Successful use of the silicone spacer also relies on surrounding soft tissue support, although its inherent stability, when the prosthesis is correctly inserted, permits simultaneous soft tissue reconstruction such as correction of boutonniere or hyperextension deformities. Because digit length is maintained, postoperative motion can begin as early as patient comfort permits, even before suture removal. Closely supervised early motion encourages encapsulation of the silastic spacer with a pseudosheath similar to that which forms around silastic rods.

The greatest experience with the *cemented hinged arthroplasty* has been at the proximal interphalangeal (PIP) joint. This prosthesis attempts to mimic the hinged uniplanar PIP joint. Consistent problems with loosening, subsidence, and bone erosion have caused a high early and late failure rate, eroding the popularity of this particular joint replacement.

Recent advances in microsurgical techniques have introduced the *vascularized joint transfer* as an alternative in arthroplastic surgery. Rapid bone healing and maintenance of growth potential both represent tremendous advantages of this approach, especially to the young patient with isolated traumatic joint destruction and good soft tissue preservation. This technique also can provide excellent soft tissue cover when both joint and surrounding structures are destroyed.

*Perichondral grafting* is one alternative in joint replacement in the hand whose full potential has yet to be explored. The transfer of cells with cartilagenous potential, usually from the costochondral junction, although limited in its application to patients with degenerative disease, is promising in those with traumatic or congenital problems where soft tissues are functional and preservation of near normal motion is desirable.

## Indications

*Pain* is the most frequently seen indication for joint replacement in the hand; it is commonly associated with radiologic evidence of joint destruction. The loss of normal smooth articular cartilage surfaces may be due to osteo or rheumatoid arthritis; other forms of arthritis, including those associated with psoriasis or gout, as well as those associated with trauma, result in the characteristic narrowing or obliteration of the joint space and in subluxation or actual dislocation of bone as surrounding soft tissue changes occur.

*Joint deformity* is therefore the second most common indication for joint replacement in the hand. This may or may not be associated with joint instability. It is crucial to recognize both instability and deformity preoperatively. Soft tissue reconstruction must be done in conjunction with joint replacement if the joint replacement is to be successful. Patients with rheumatoid arthritis are particularly prone to the early and disabling soft tissue problems of swan neck and boutonniere deformities, subluxing and ruptured extensor tendons, capsular weakness, and ulnar drift; tight intrinsic muculature in the rheumatoid must be released for improved postoperative motion following arthroplasty. The successful function of the replaced joint depends on the support and adequacy of the surrounding soft tissue.

*Failure of a previous procedure* is a third indication for total joint replacement. This includes both failed soft tissue interposition and failed attempts at primary correction of intraarticular fractures. Such a course leads to the final common denominator of pain, requiring joint replacement. However, soft tissue changes surrounding the involved joint and adjacent joints sometimes point to the necessity for total joint replacement even before pain is a factor.

*Stiffness and lack of mobility* do not preclude joint replacements and are often ameliorated by such procedures. The shortening or soft tissue release that accompanies joint arthroplasty is sufficient to allow great improvement in motion not totally attributable to the joint replacement itself.

## Surgical Procedures

In addition to the above-cited indications, selection of appropriate joint arthroplasty depends upon (1) the joint or joints involved, (2) the extent of disease, and (3) the surgeon's experience and personal preference. Two operations among the multiple procedures available have been chosen as illustrative in hand joint arthroplasty.

### Silastic Implant Arthroplasty in the Proximal Interphalangeal Joint

The flexible silastic implant is used in both proximal interphalangeal and metacarpal phalangeal joints; it is made of a medical grade silastic with improved tear resistance that greatly lowers the risk of implant fracture, once a mishap seen with some frequency.

The implant is inserted through a dorsal skin approach usually planned to allow for closure of the joint capsule under an intact skin flap. If possible, the central slip and its attachment to the base of the middle phalanx should be preserved.

The medullary canal reaming should be sufficient to allow the implant to seat without buckling; there should be no impingement when the joint is brought into passive flexion. This relatively loose fit allows for slight motion at the bone-implant interface that reduces implant wear by disseminating shear and compressive forces over a wide surface.

Complications associated with insertion of the silastic spacer are several. As mentioned, implant fracture occurs, although with less frequency than originally seen. Even when fracture occurs, however, the implant acts as an internal stent, and the joint usually remains asymptomatic; removal and implant replacement are not required. Moreover, soft tissue deformities associated with degenerative joint disease such as contracture or boutonniere at the proximal interphalangeal joint can persist or recur postoperatively. Inadequate soft tissue release allows persistent contracture; the extensor tendon must be sufficiently tightened prior to reinsertion to correct a chronic boutonniere deformity. Recurrence or persistence of these problems may be due to operative technique; in addition, appropriate postoperative splinting together with careful supervision as motion is regained help to ensure that the deformity will remain corrected.

Implant dislocation occurs postoperatively; early dislocation is usually a result of a technical misadventure such as overenthusiastic bone shortening, inappropriate spacer size, or poor soft tissue support.

Silastic implant arthroplasty is the most common proximal interphalangeal and metacarpal interphalangeal arthroplasty in use today. The implant has shown itself to be durable and flexible, and the operation provides good pain relief.

## Interposition Arthroplasty in the Thumb Basal Joint

The interposition of soft tissue as a cushion between debrided arthritic joint surfaces provides a biologic spacer eliminating the use of synthetic material. This operation is used in joints whose motion is multiplanar, such as the thumb carpal metacarpal joint. The material used for interposition, whether tendon, freeze-dried fascia, or joint capsule, has no inherent stability and is interposed in conjunction with a stabilizing reconstruction. In the case of the thumb basal joint, volar ligament reconstruction is performed (see Figs. 4-17 through 4-26). The reconstruction of the volar ligament makes use of the radial half of the flexor carpi radialis tendon. The radial and volar aspects of the joint are exposed through a curved incision at the base of the thenar musculature. It is important to release the musculature for full exposure, although the muscle cone must be reattached during closure. When the joint capsule is opened, the joint must be widely exposed by elevating the capsule. This allows for excision of the multiple osteophytes or loose bodies that accumulate at the medial side of the carpal metacarpal joint. Their removal is important to allow the base of the thumb metacarpal to be completely repositioned on the distal trapezium.

The length of available flexor carpi radialis tendon may not provide sufficient bulk for an interposed cushion. When this happens, the palmaris longus tendon may be harvested through the same tendon-exposing incision and used to augment the cushion.

In reconstructing the volar ligament of the carpal metacarpal joint, it is crucial that the cut end of tendon be brought through the dorsum of the thumb metacarpal in a plane perpendicular to the plane of the fingernail. From its volar distal attachment to the index metacarpal, the tendon course mimics the normal anatomy of the volar ligament and, when tightened, holds the thumb securely against the trapezium. If this is not done with care, the thumb metacarpal will sublux radially, and metacarpal adduction will occur, or recur.

Complications of this procedure are usually limited to technical problems. If the joint capsule is not carefully closed over the tendon cushion, the cushion can prolapse dorsally or radially. When the joint capsule proves inadequate for closure, a 4-0 plain suture can be tied to the folded tendon and brought out the dorsal wrist at the base of the index metacarpal. This will anchor the folded tendon in position. Exposure of the carpal metacarpal joint must be extensive, or threading the flexor tendon will be technically impossible.

Postoperative mobility proceeds in an orderly fashion. When the cast is removed 5 weeks postoperatively, gentle flexion-extension exercises are begun. Palmar abductor-adduction follows; the patient is protected in a thumb spica splint until motion is normal, usually 2–3 weeks after cast removal, at which time strengthening is begun.

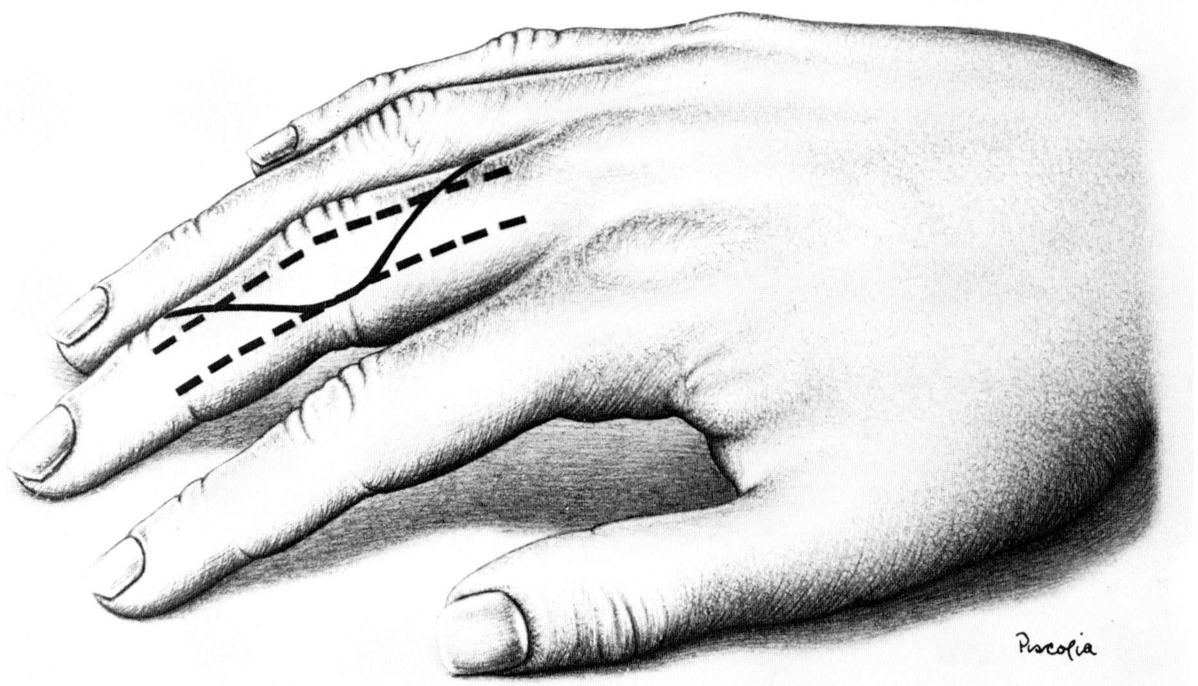
Piscolia

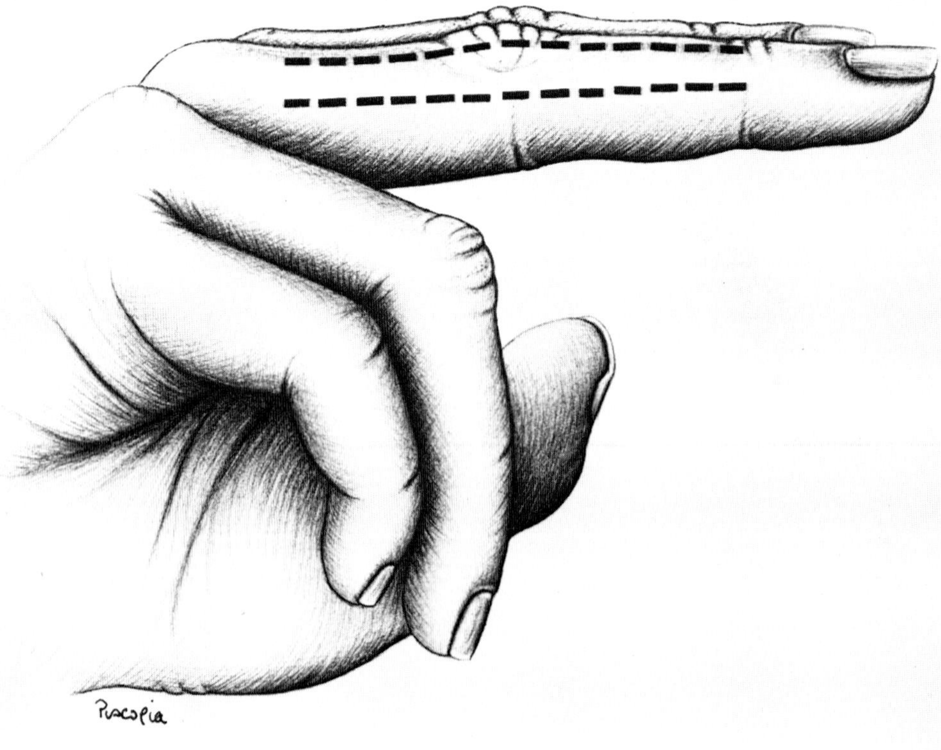
Piscolia

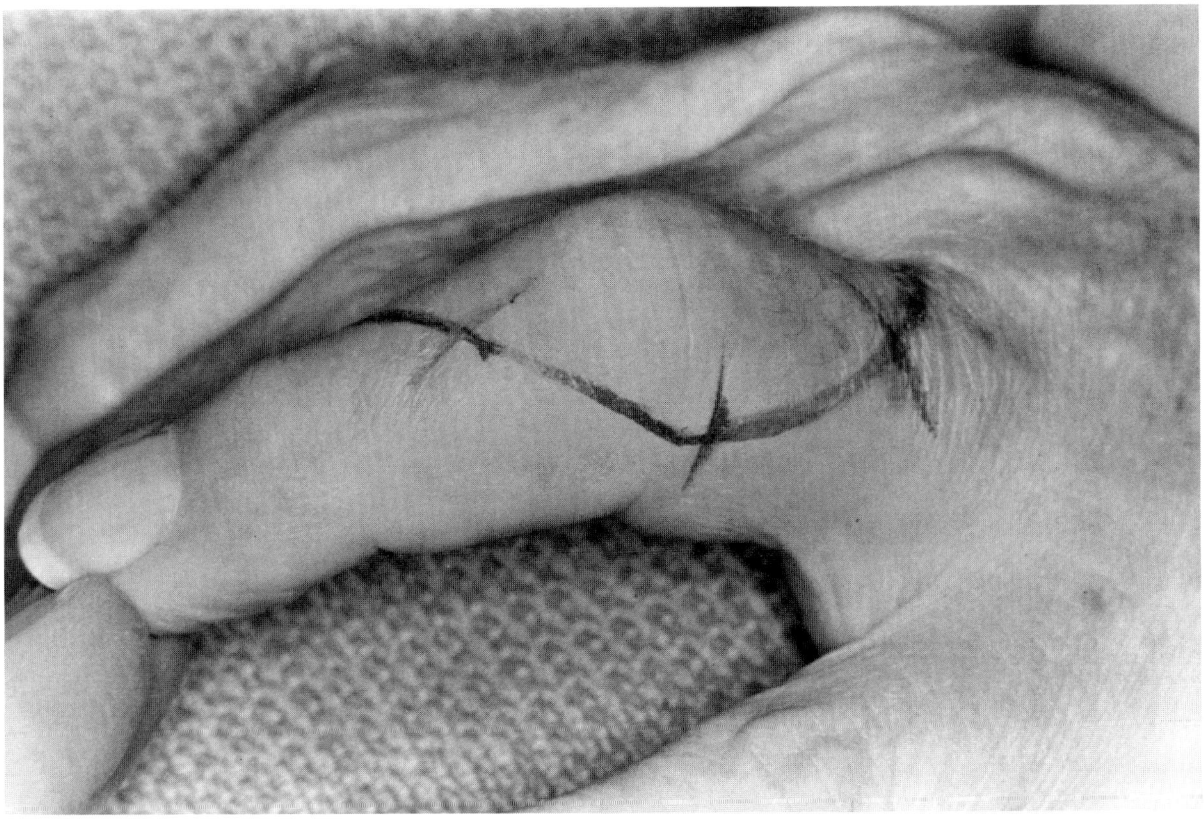

**Figs. 4-1 and 4-2** Proximal interphalangeal joint replacement. The incision is planned to maximize exposure and soft tissue cover. Two midaxial incisions provide excellent exposure but do not allow correction of the attenuated central slip. The incision chosen here is an ulnarly based curvilinear one, with its apex at the midaxial line.

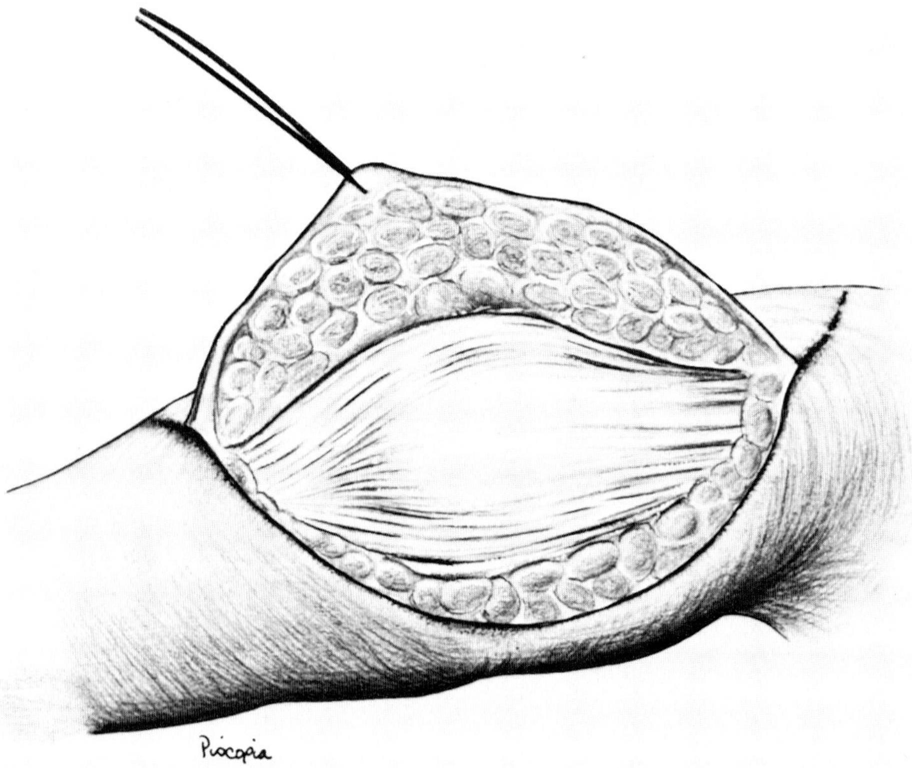
Piscopia

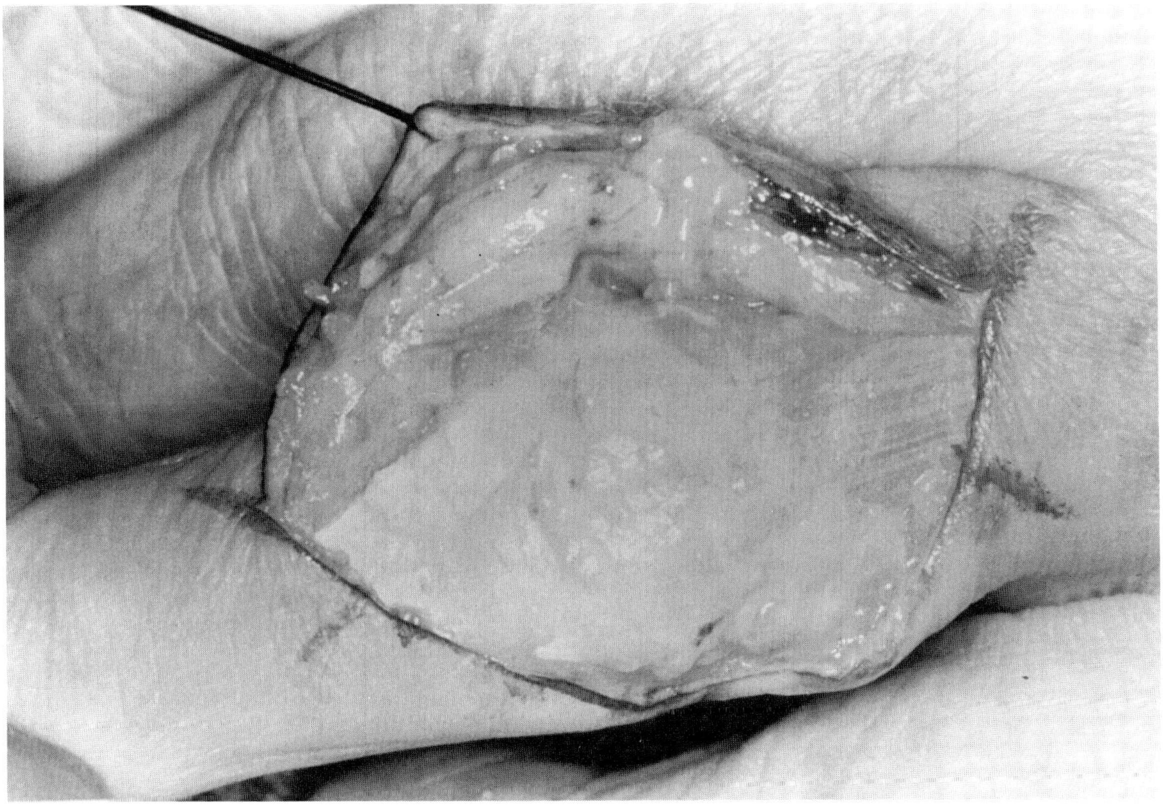

**Fig. 4-3** Proximal interphalangeal joint replacement. Skin and soft tissue are reflected in the areolar tissue plain, leaving intact venous structures. In this patient, a very attenuated central slip was encountered whose distal attachment to the tubercle at the base of the middle phalanx could not be preserved.

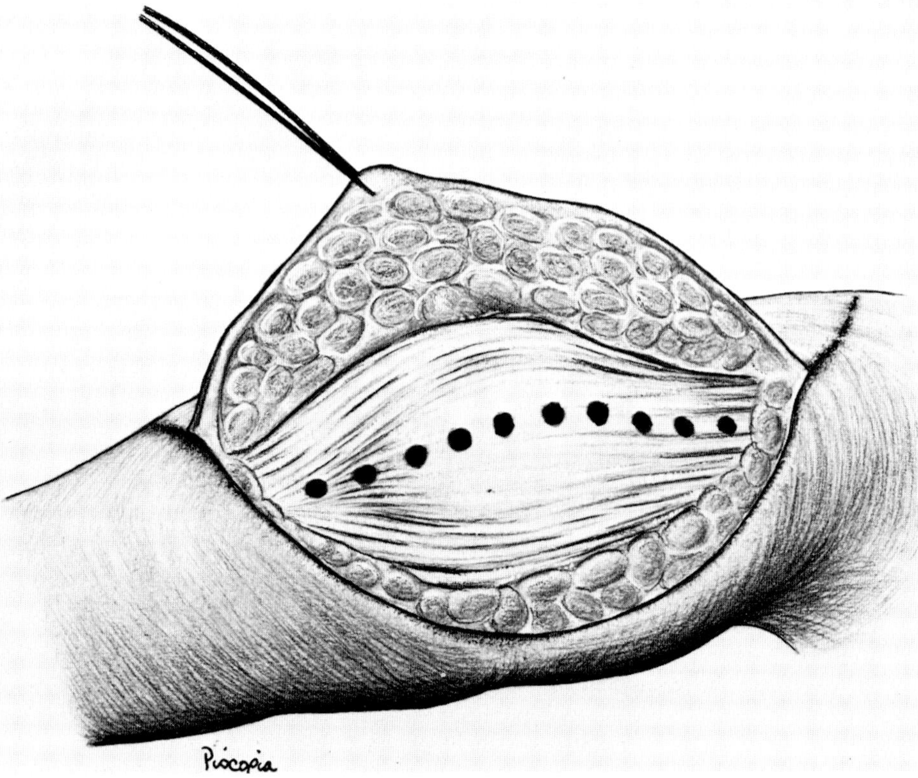

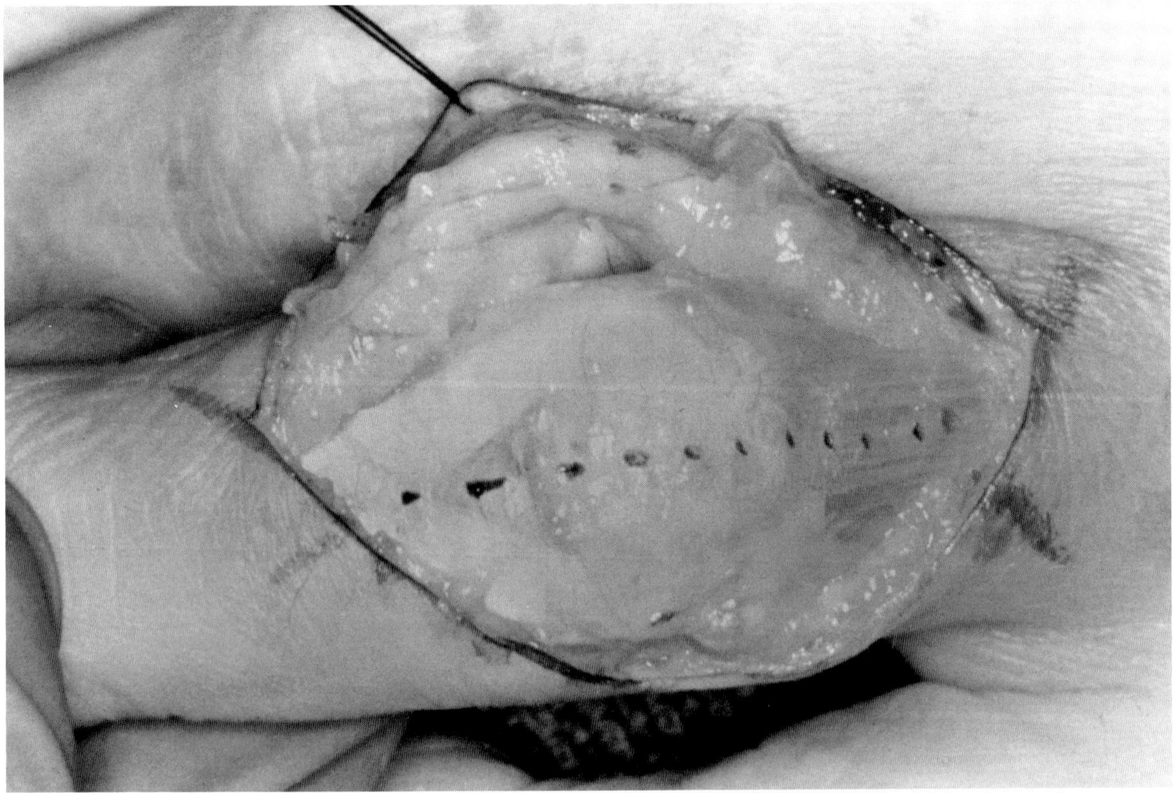

Fig. 4-4

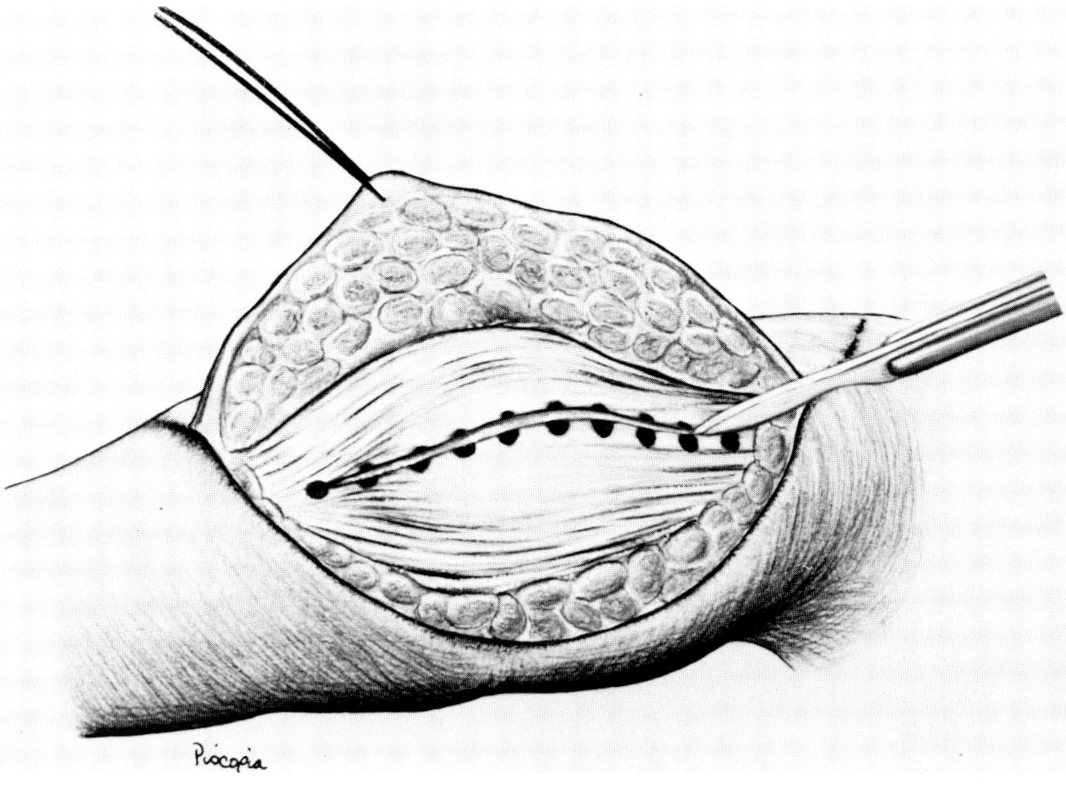

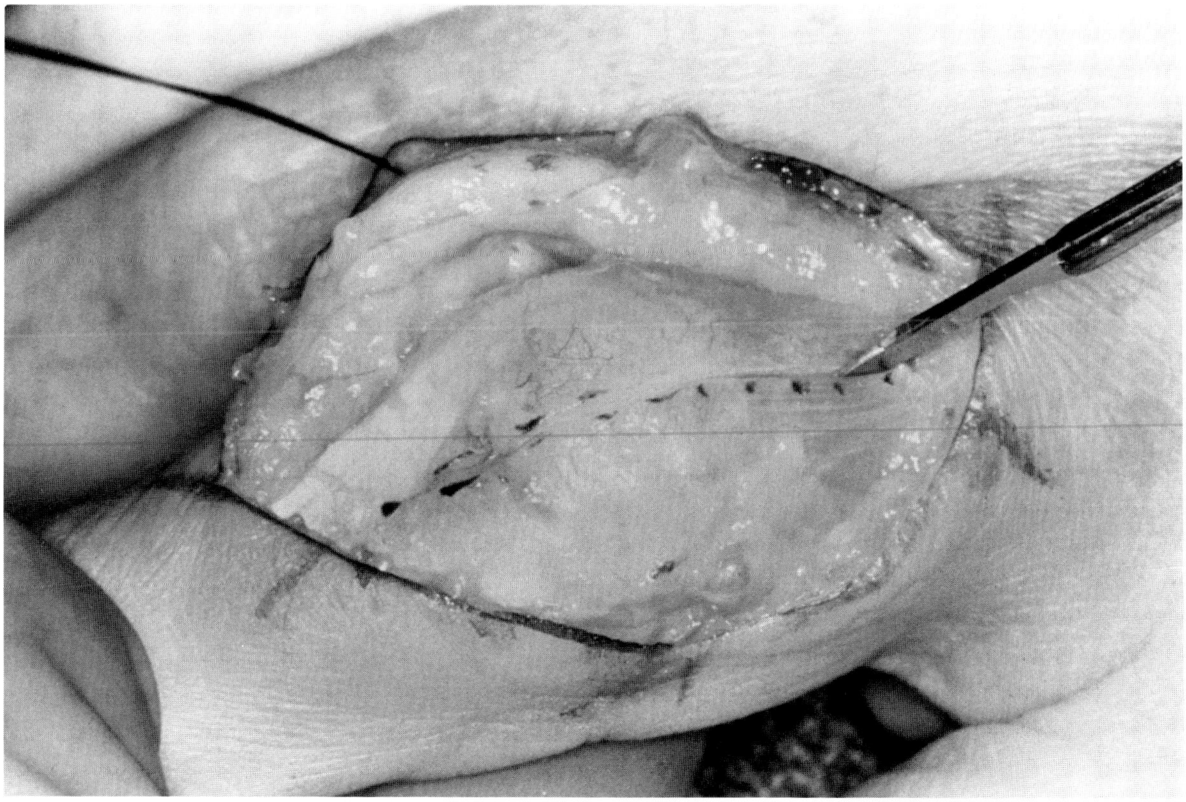

**Figs. 4-4 and 4-5** Proximal interphalangeal joint replacement. The middorsal longitudinal incision is made, exposing the underlying boggy synovium.

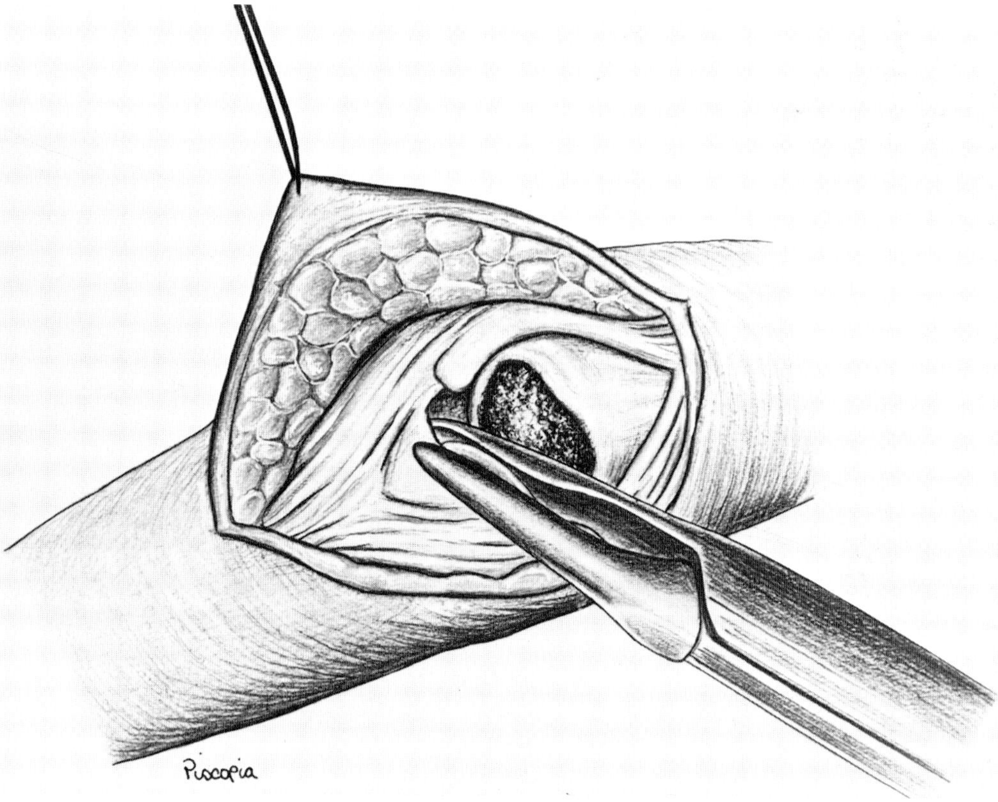


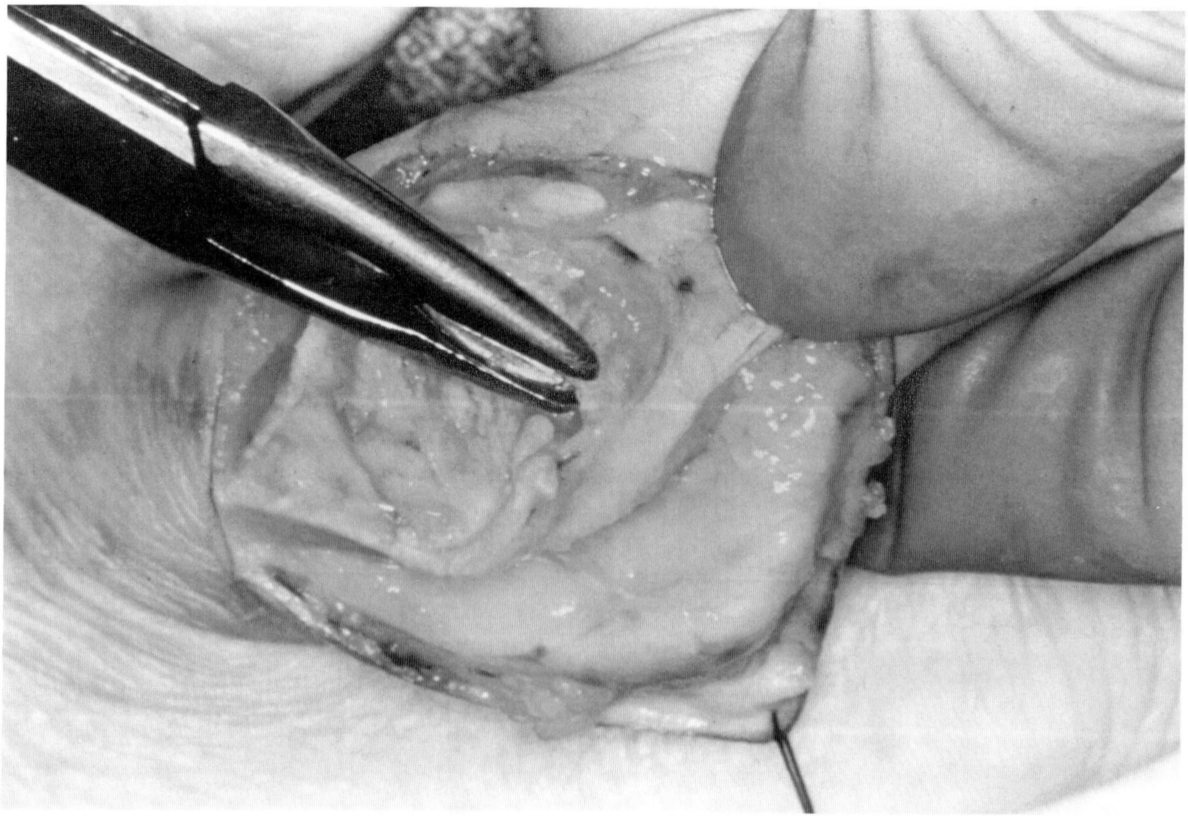

**Fig. 4-6** Proximal interphalangeal joint replacement. A rongeur is used to trim the synovium and expose the worn cartilaginous joint surfaces. Collateral ligaments should, if possible, be preserved.

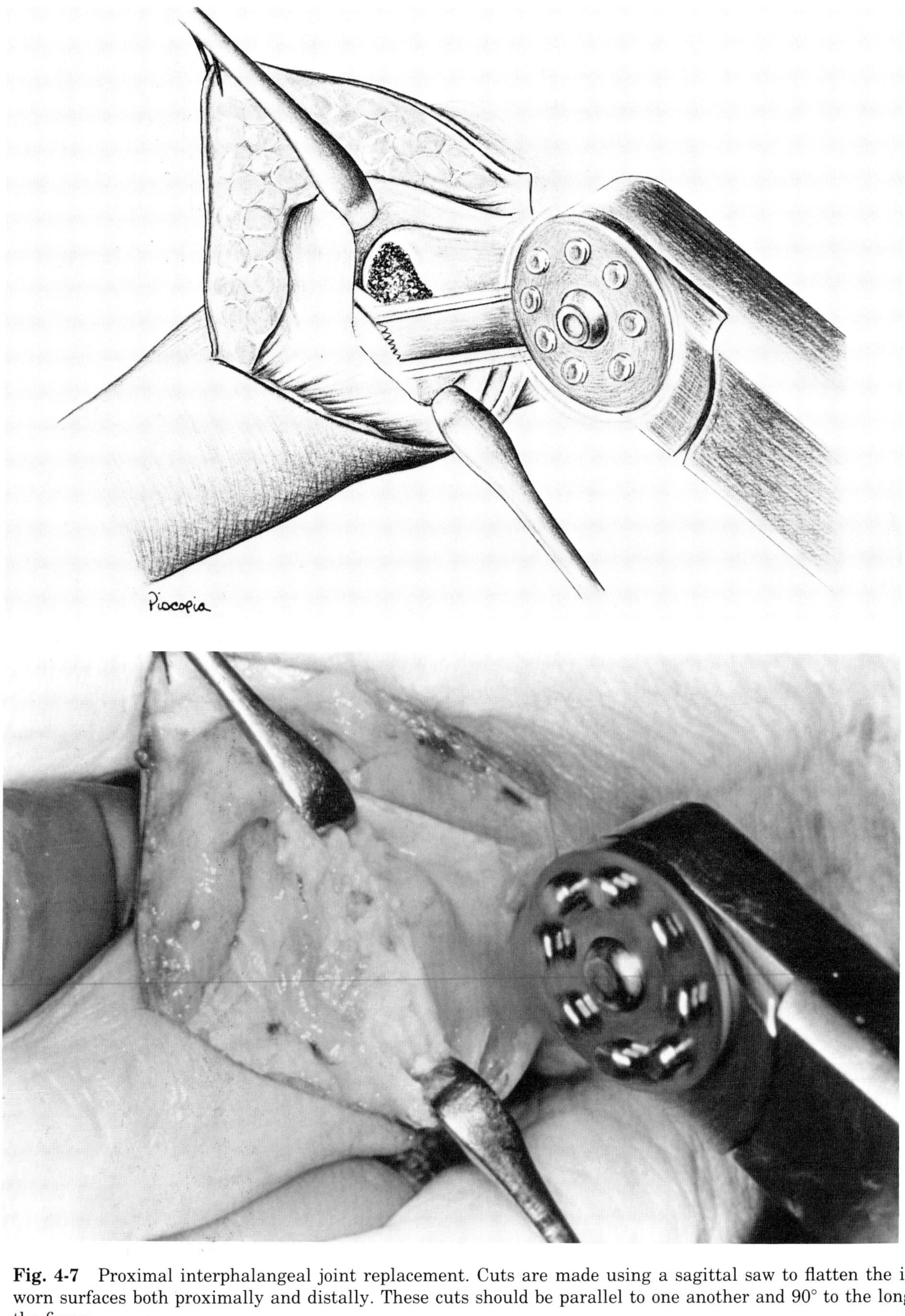


**Fig. 4-7** Proximal interphalangeal joint replacement. Cuts are made using a sagittal saw to flatten the irregular worn surfaces both proximally and distally. These cuts should be parallel to one another and 90° to the long axis of the finger.

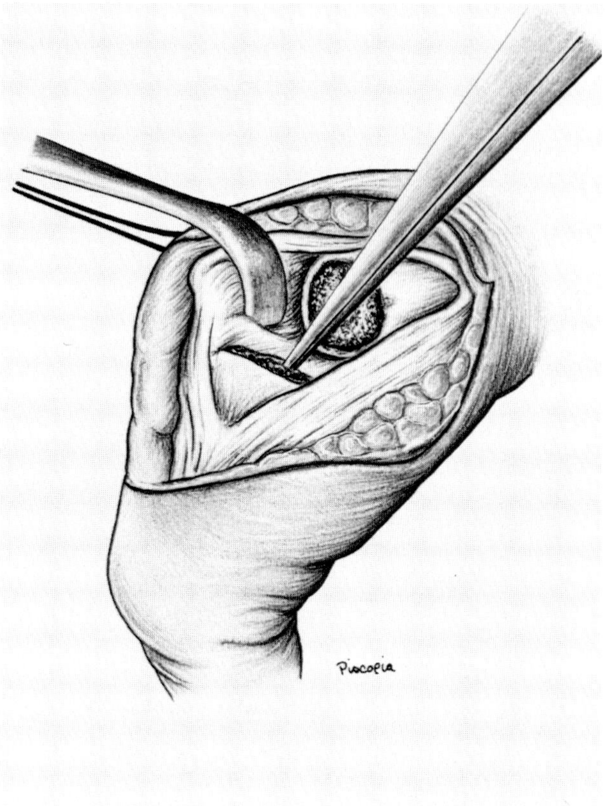

Fig. 4-8

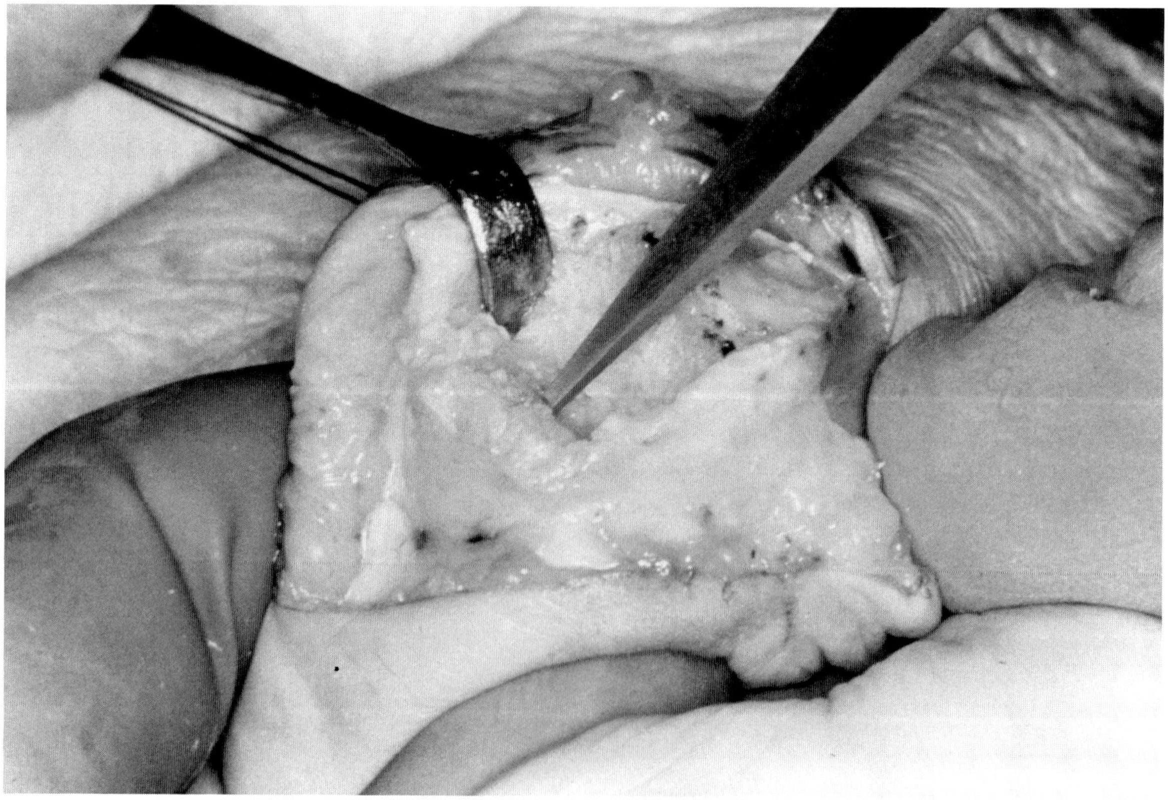

**Figs. 4-8 through 4-11** Proximal interphalangeal joint replacement. The canals of the middle and proximal phalanges are gently reamed using instruments designed with a rectangular base to provide proper seating of the joint spacer.

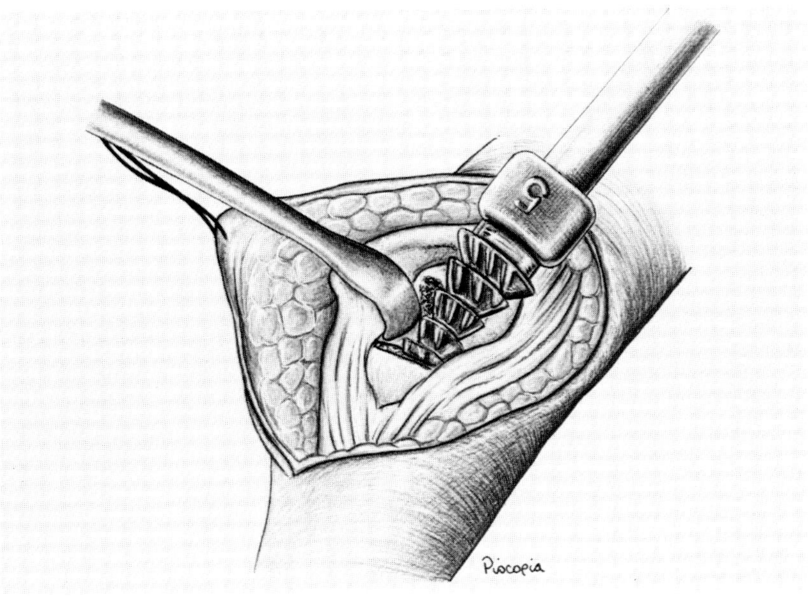


Fig. 4-9

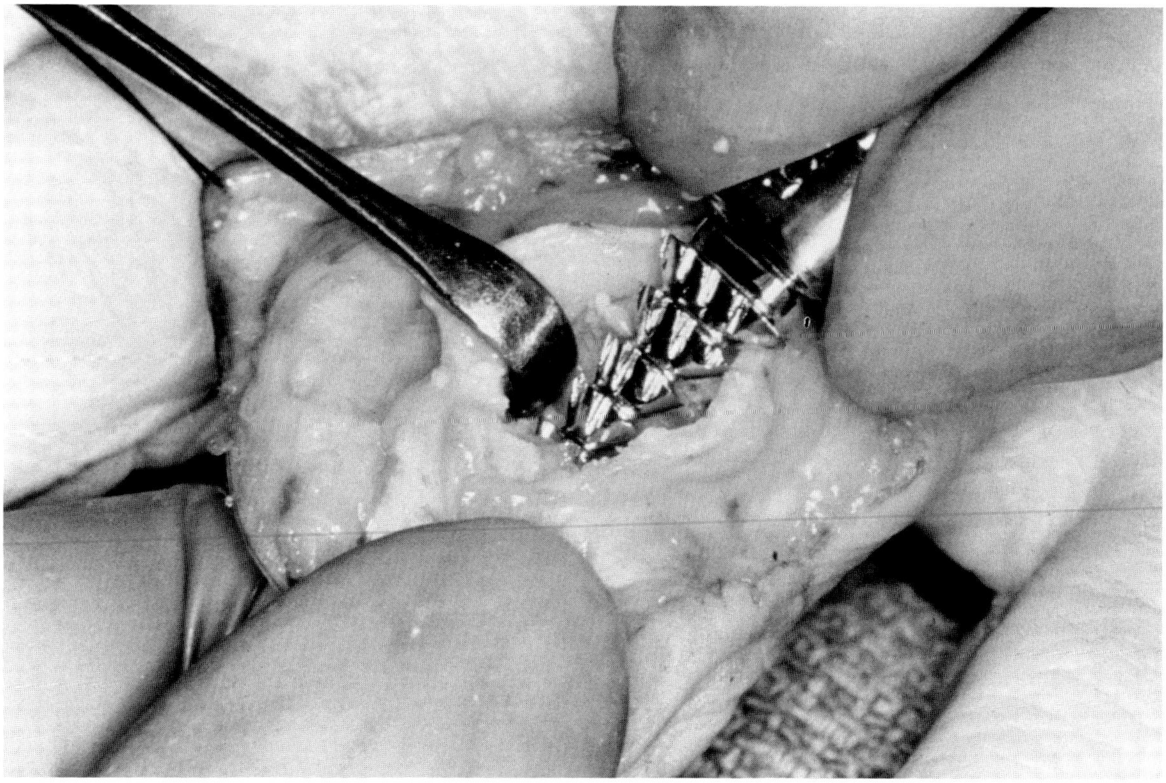

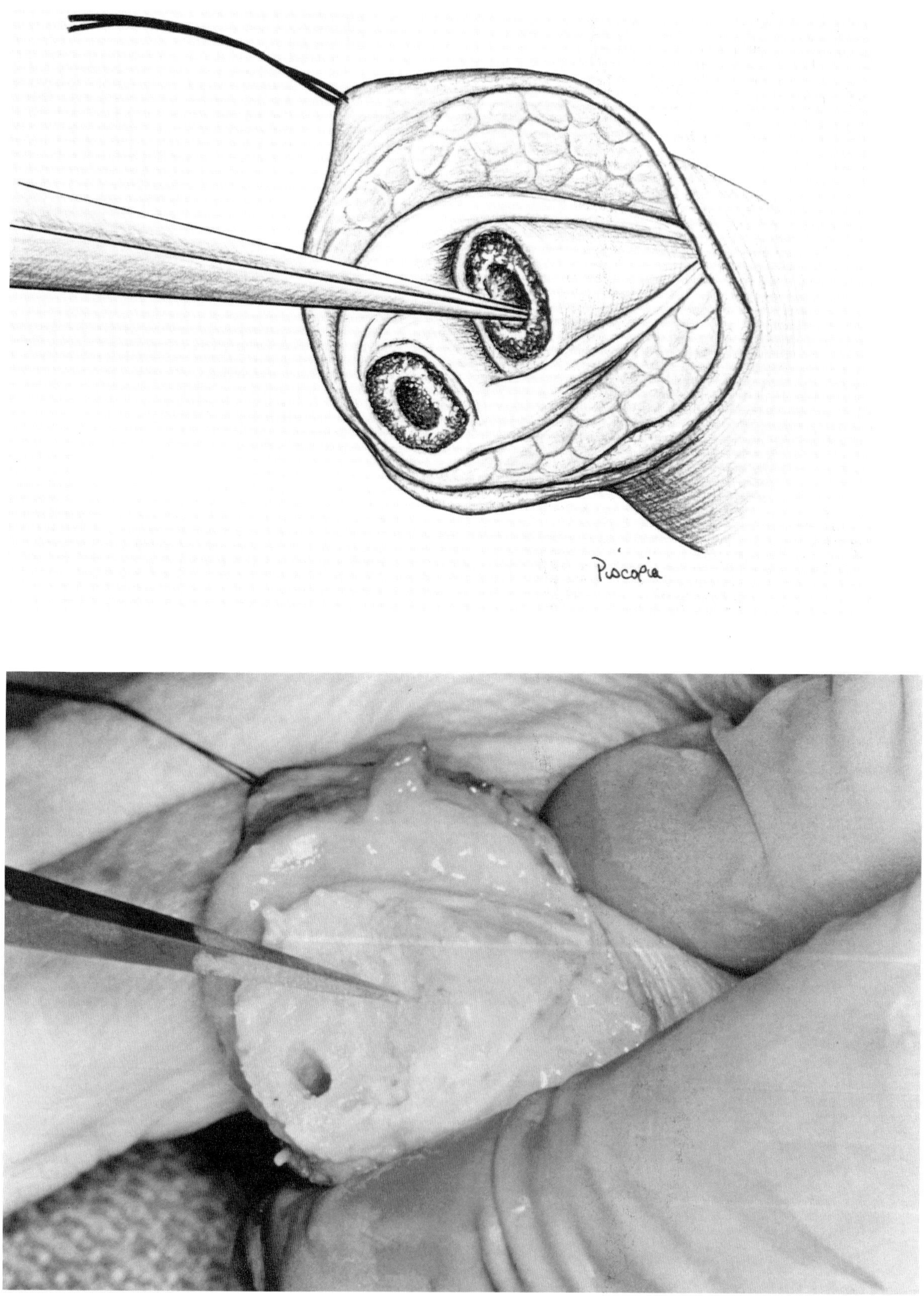

Fig. 4-10

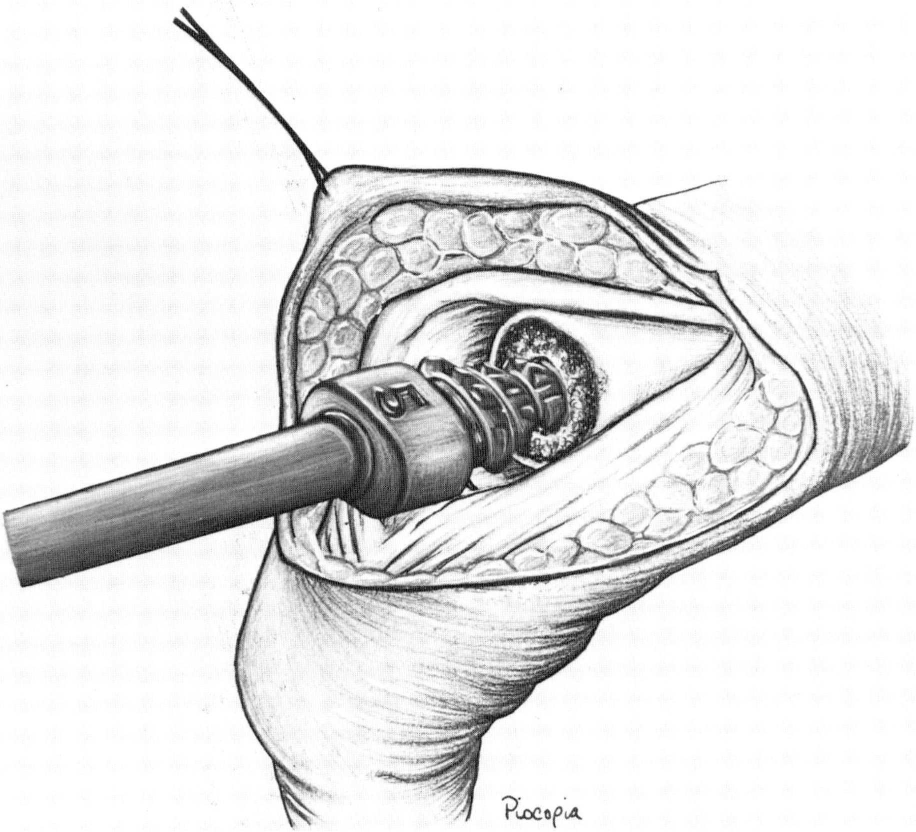

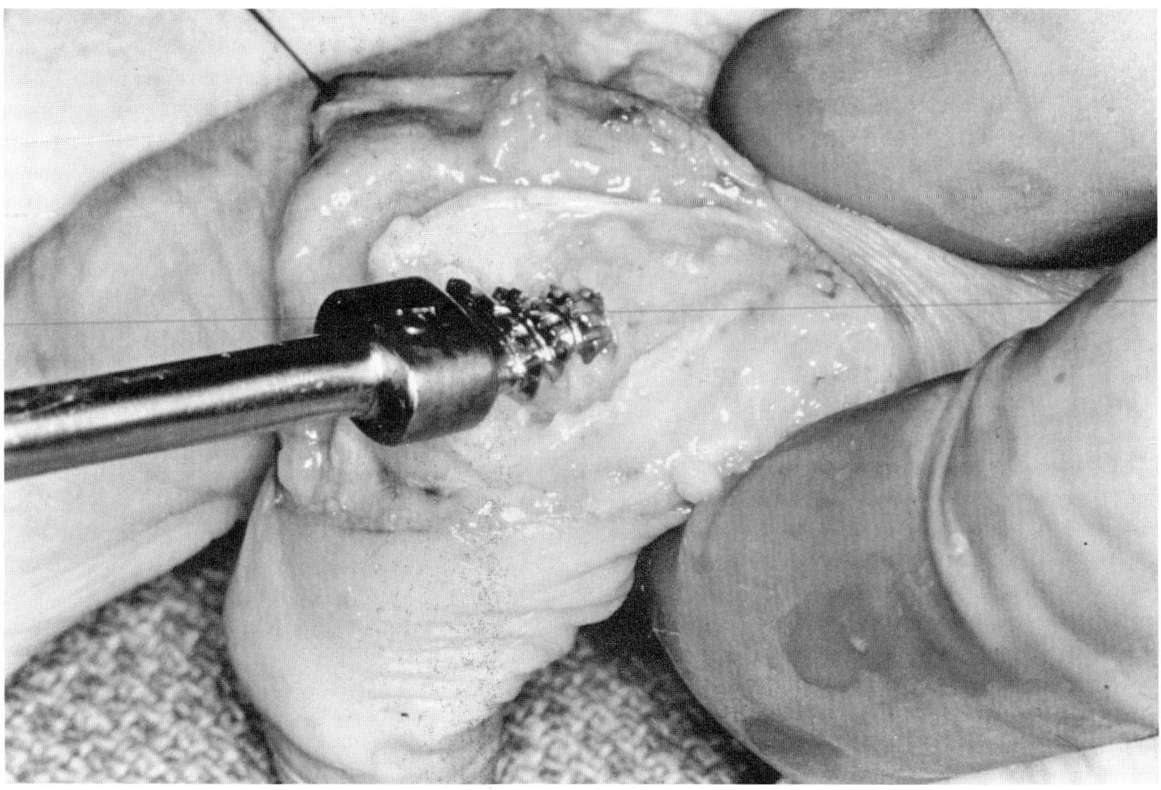

Fig. 4-11

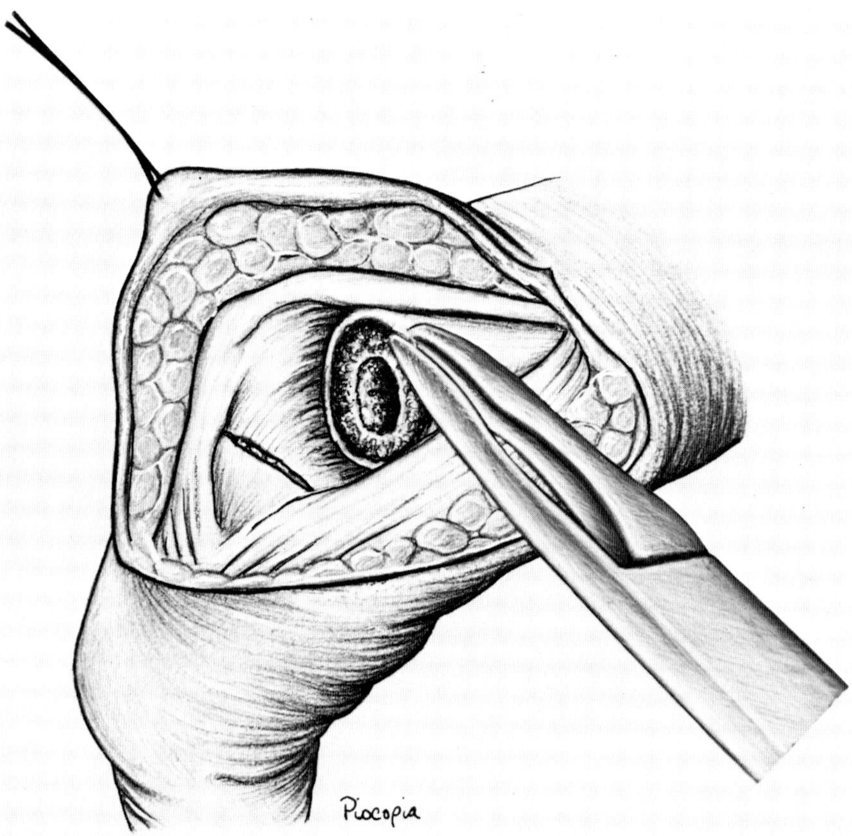

**Fig. 4-12** Proximal interphalangeal joint replacement. Additional soft tissue is then trimmed to allow a neat fit and to prevent interposition of soft tissue between the spacer and medullary canal.

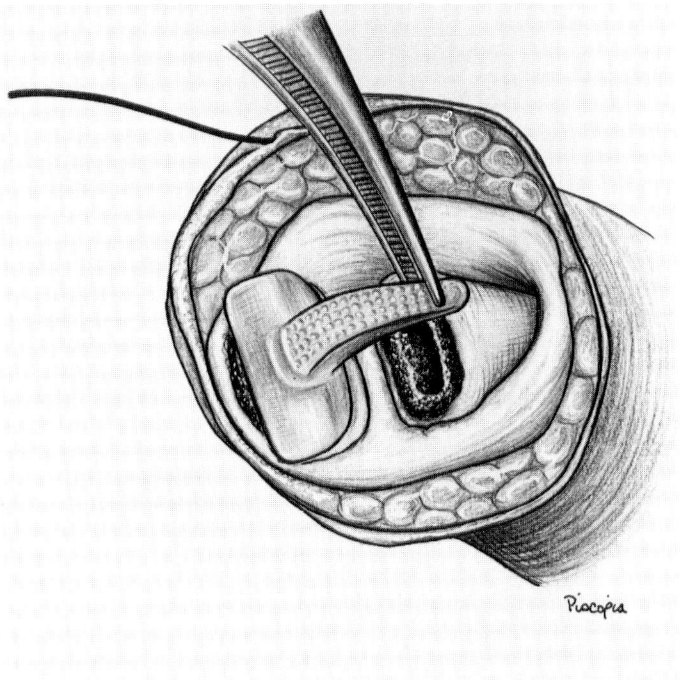

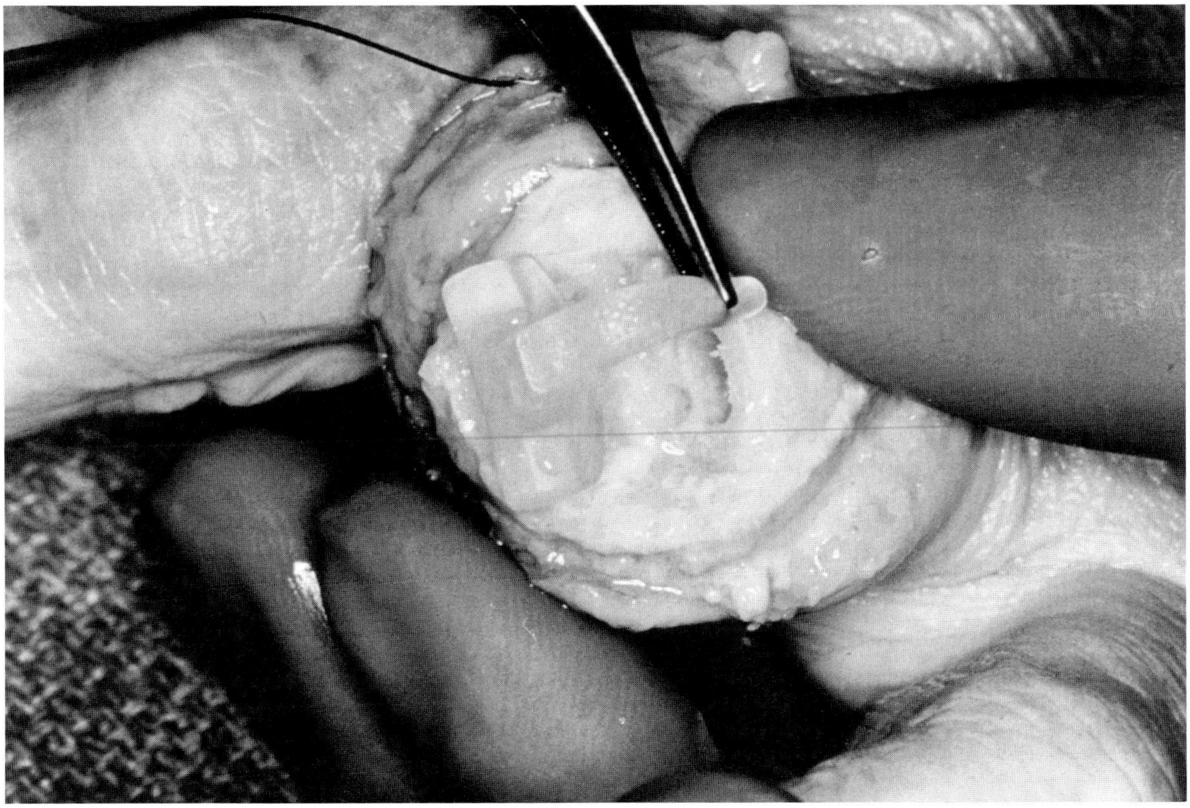

**Figs. 4-13 and 4-14** Proximal interphalangeal joint replacement. A silicone spacer of appropriate size is chosen and gently inserted after irrigation of the canal. The fit should allow the central barrel-shaped post of the spacer to appose the phalanx proximally and distally. Finger motion in flexion and extension is checked passively to assure that there is no buckling or compression of the silicone spacer.

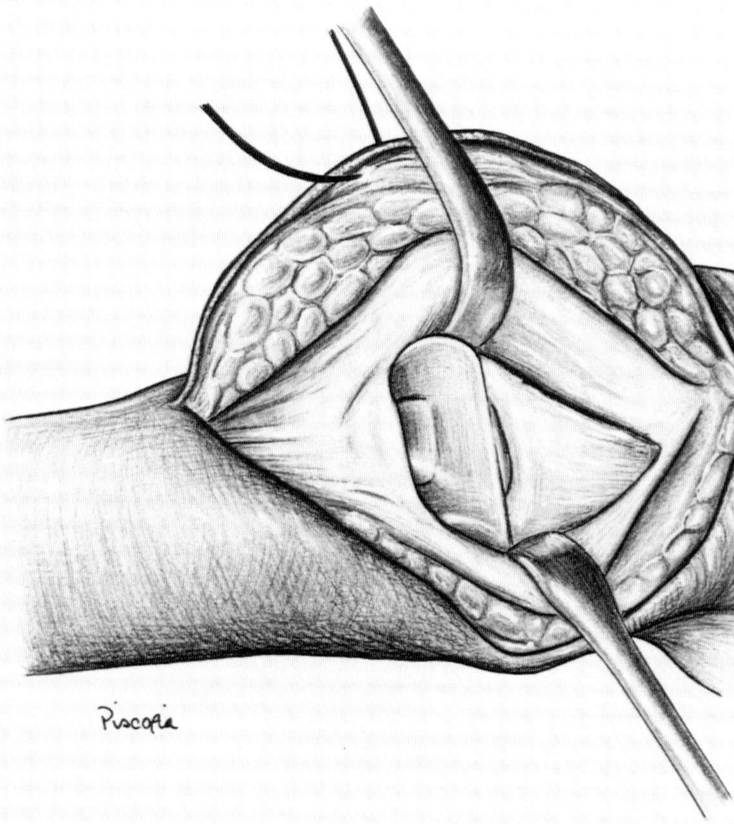


**Fig. 4-14**

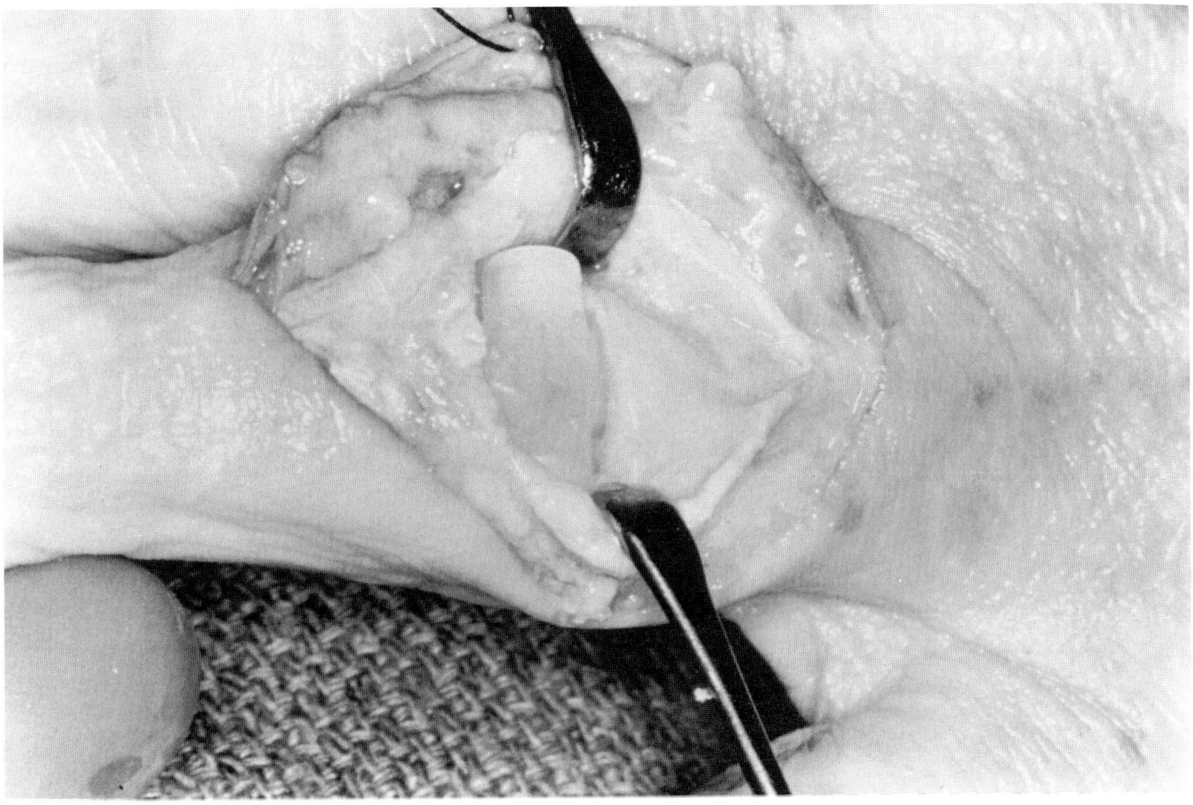

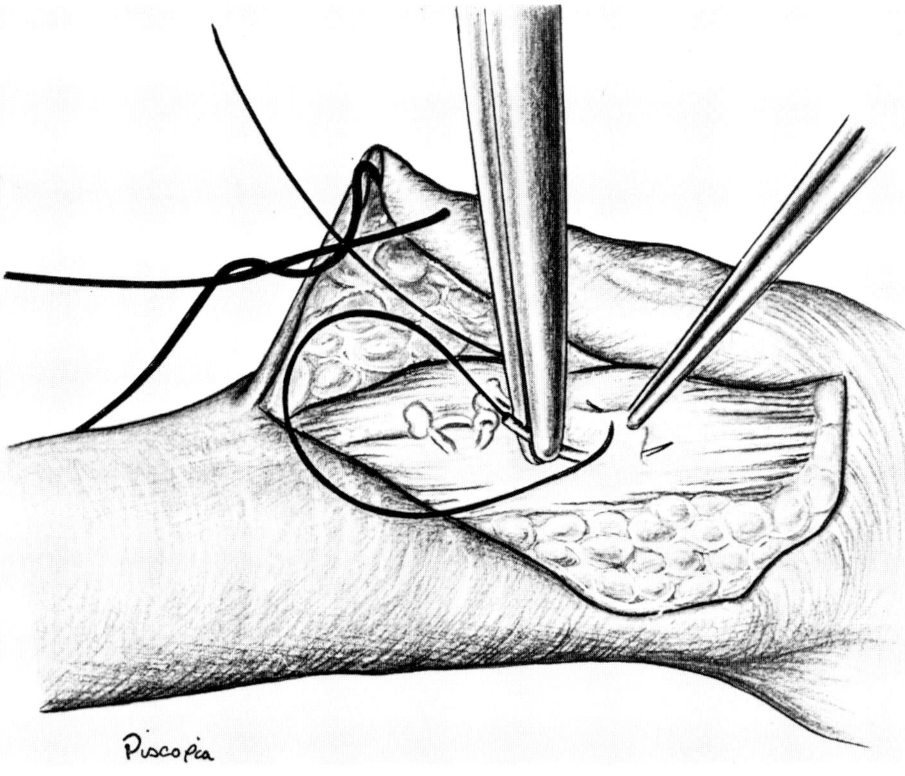


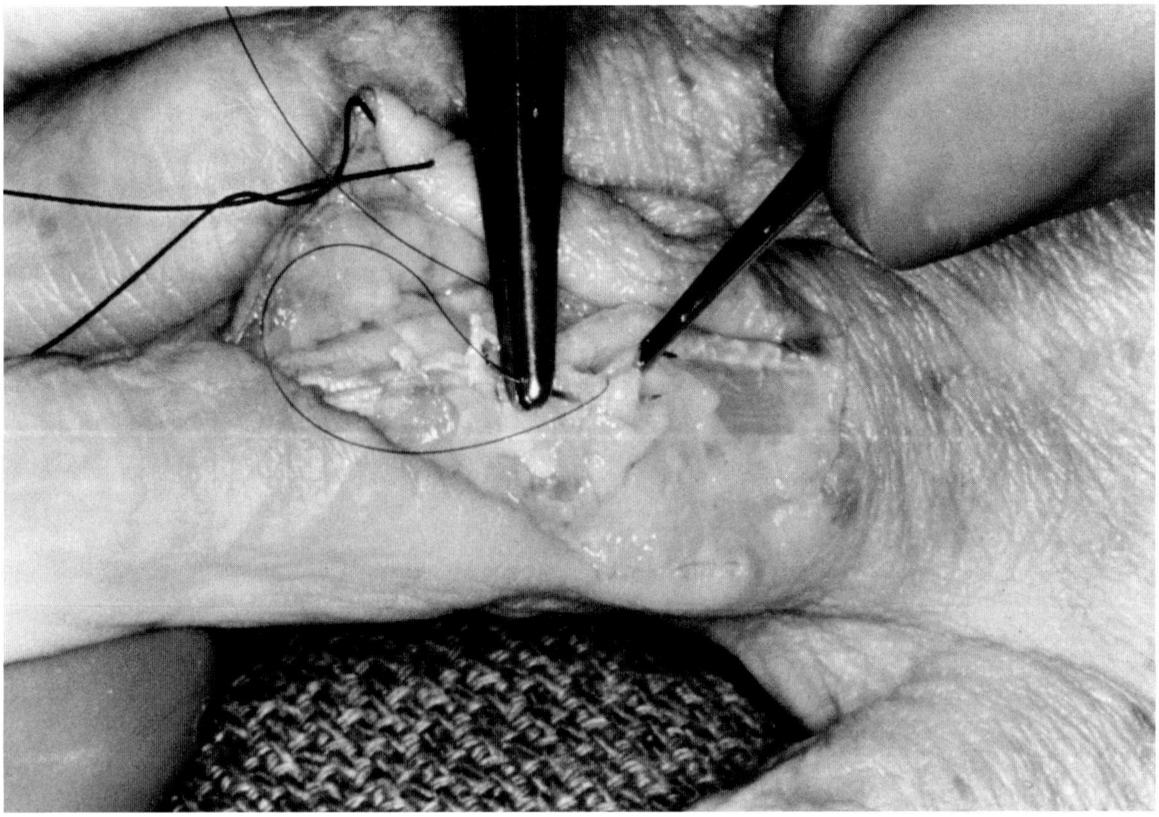

Fig. 4-15

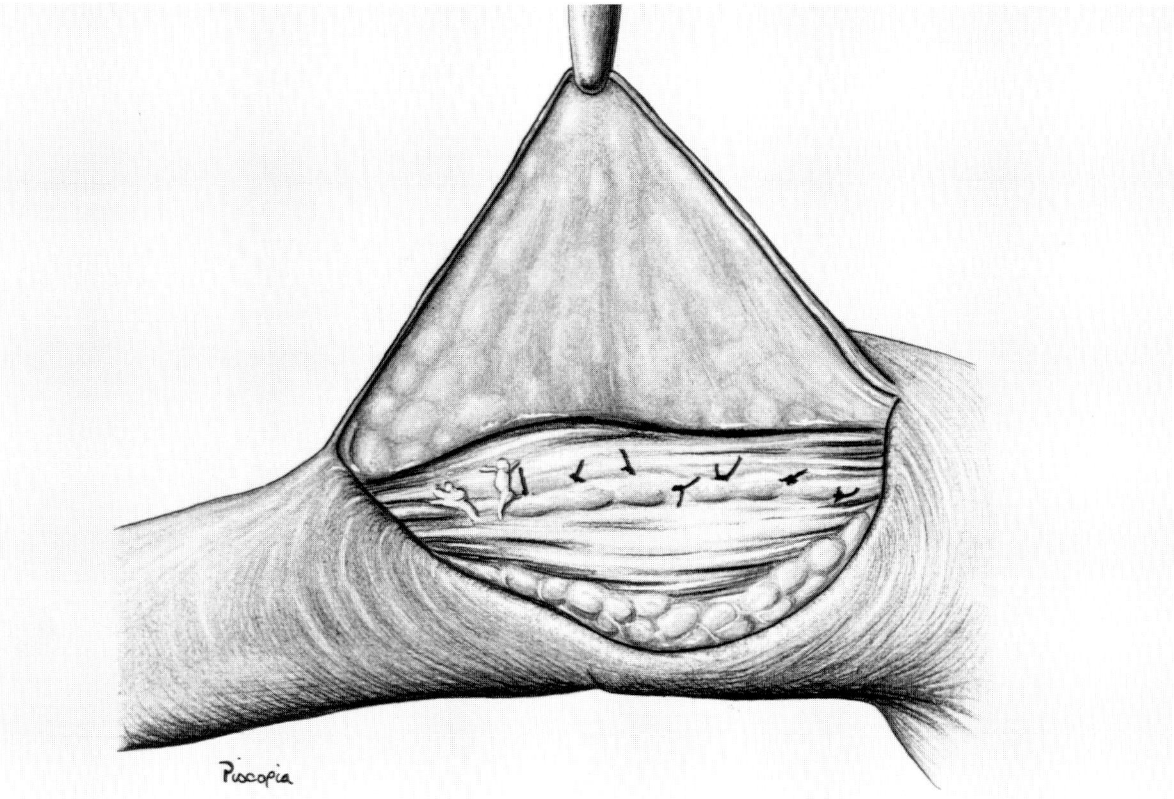

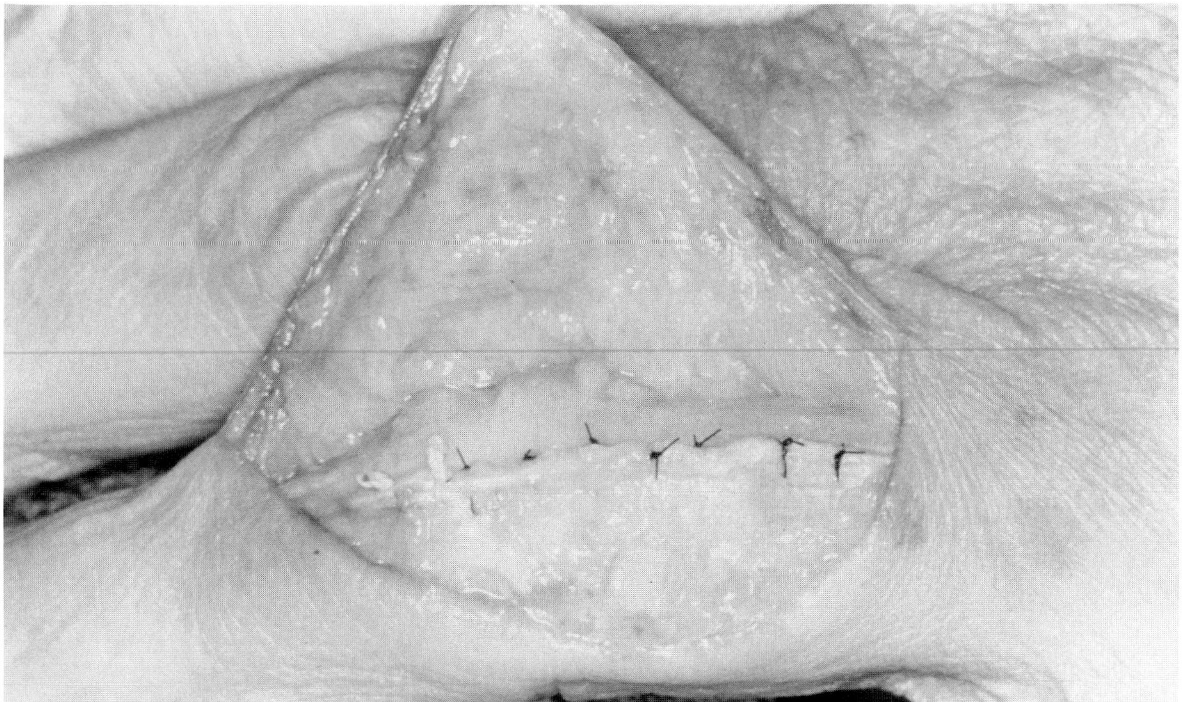

**Figs. 4-15 and 4-16** Proximal interphalangeal joint replacement. The attenuated central slip at this point should be reinserted into the dorsal base of the middle phalanx, and the remainder of the central tendon is coapted. Fine permanent suture, such as clear nylon, is used and will allow the desired early motion.

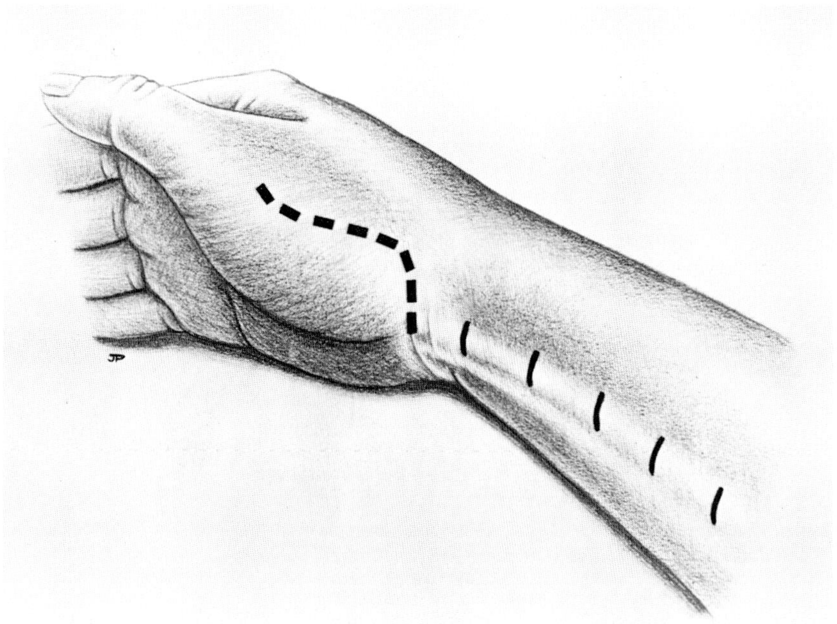

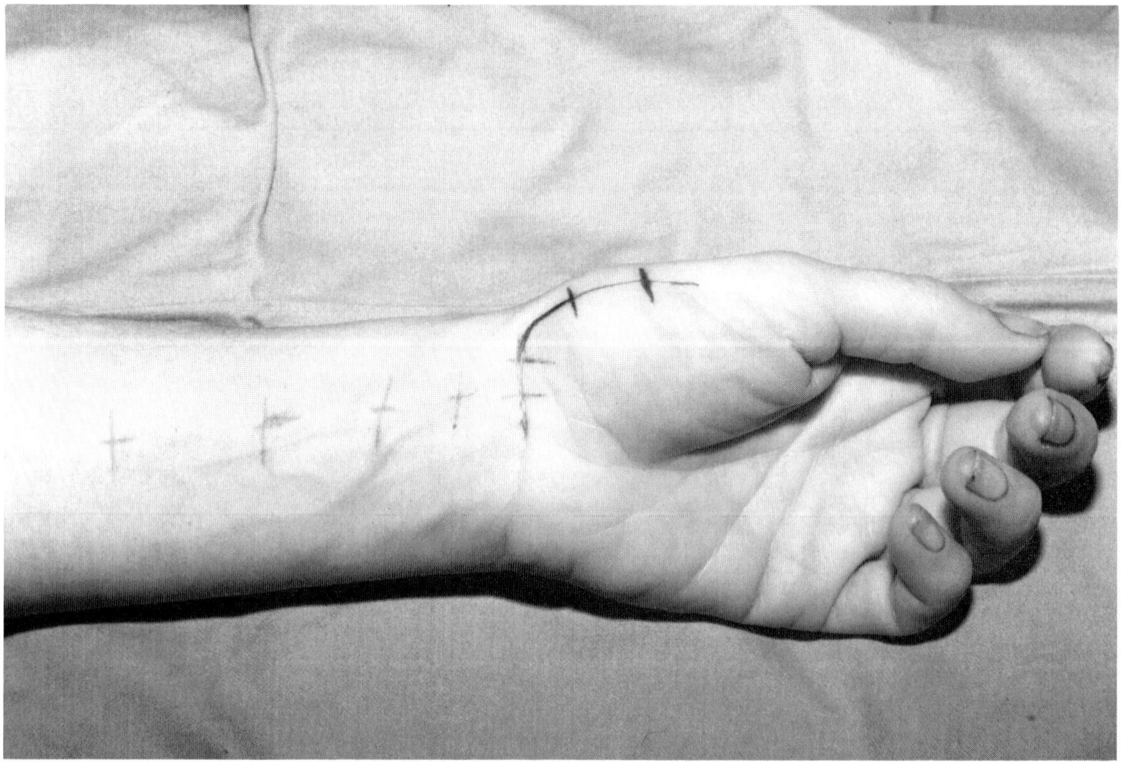

**Fig. 4-17** The incision is planned at the junction of the palmar and dorsal skin, beginning just proximal to the thumb metacarpal phalangeal joint. It turns ulnarward in the distalmost wrist crease. Small transverse incisions are marked at 2 cm intervals along the course of the flexor carpi radialis tendon.

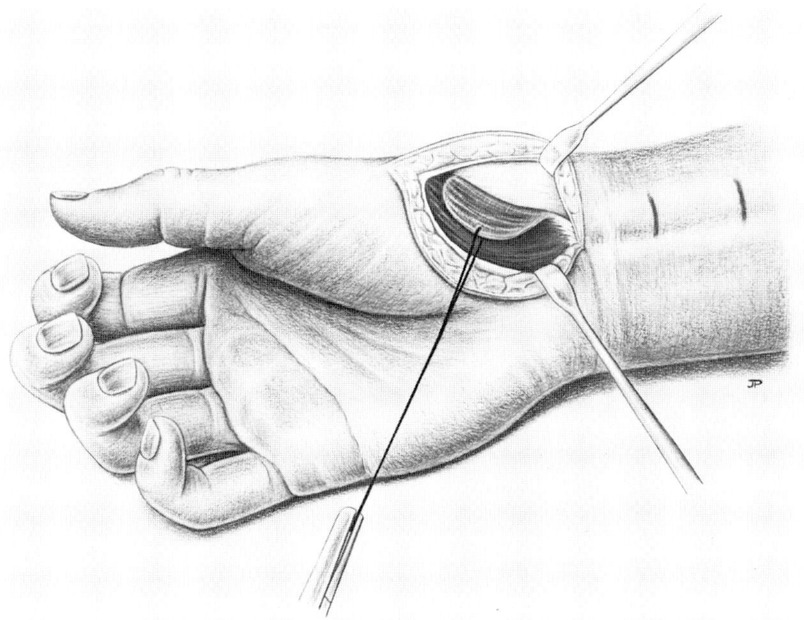

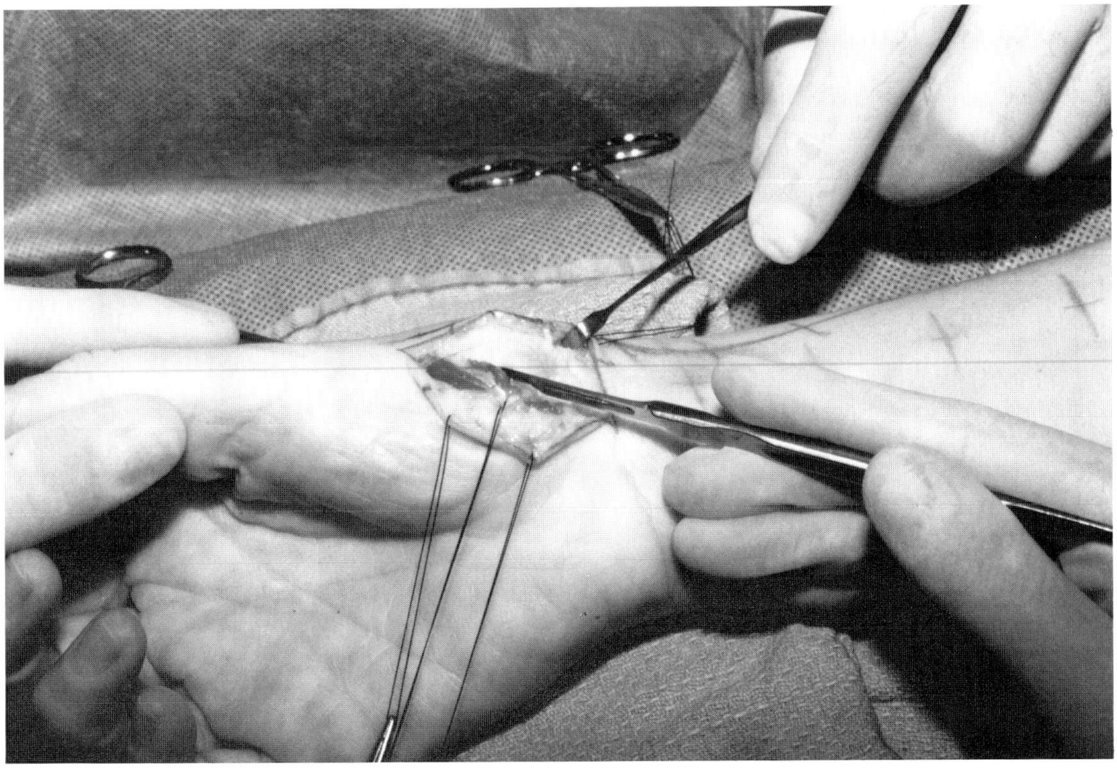

**Fig. 4-18** The thenar muscle core is taken down from its dorsoradial attachment. For complete exposure, its proximal aponeurosis must also be incised at the point where it inserts into the anterobrachial fascia. This segment of the incision must expose the distal end of the radial wrist flexor tendon.

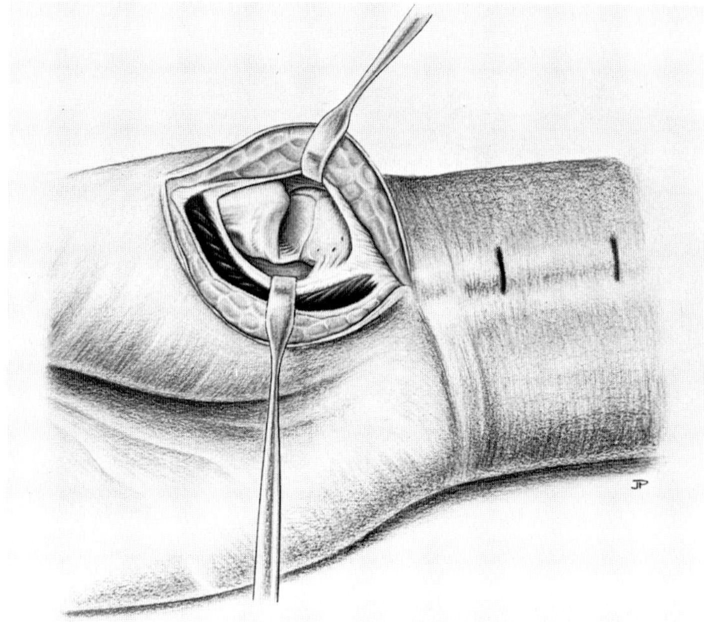

**Fig. 4-19** The joint capsule is opened longitudinally, and a periosteal elevator is used to free it dorsally and volarly. A longitudinal incision allows for capsule closure at the termination of the procedure.

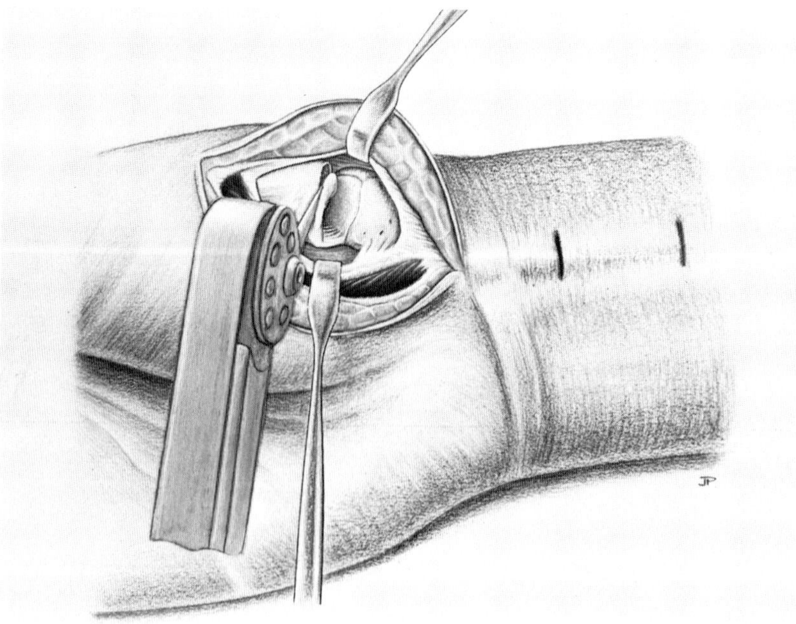

**Fig. 4-20** The base of the thumb metacarpal is trimmed with a saggital saw in a plane perpendicular to the long axis of the bone. The deepest recess of the joint must be visualized, and any osteophytes or loose bodies removed.

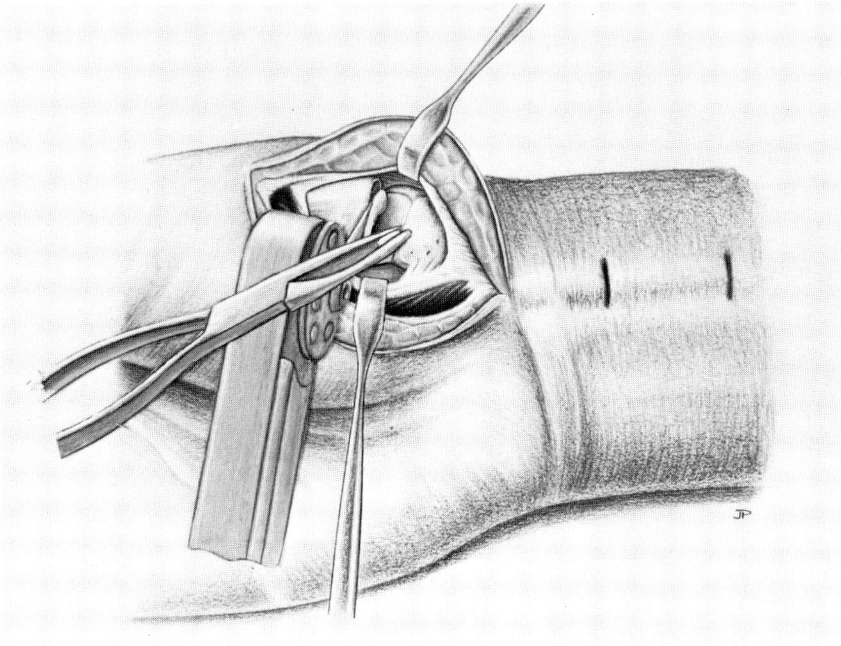

**Fig. 4-21** The distal articular surface of the trapezium may be trimmed with a rongeur or a saw to flatten the surface and remove the worn cartilage.

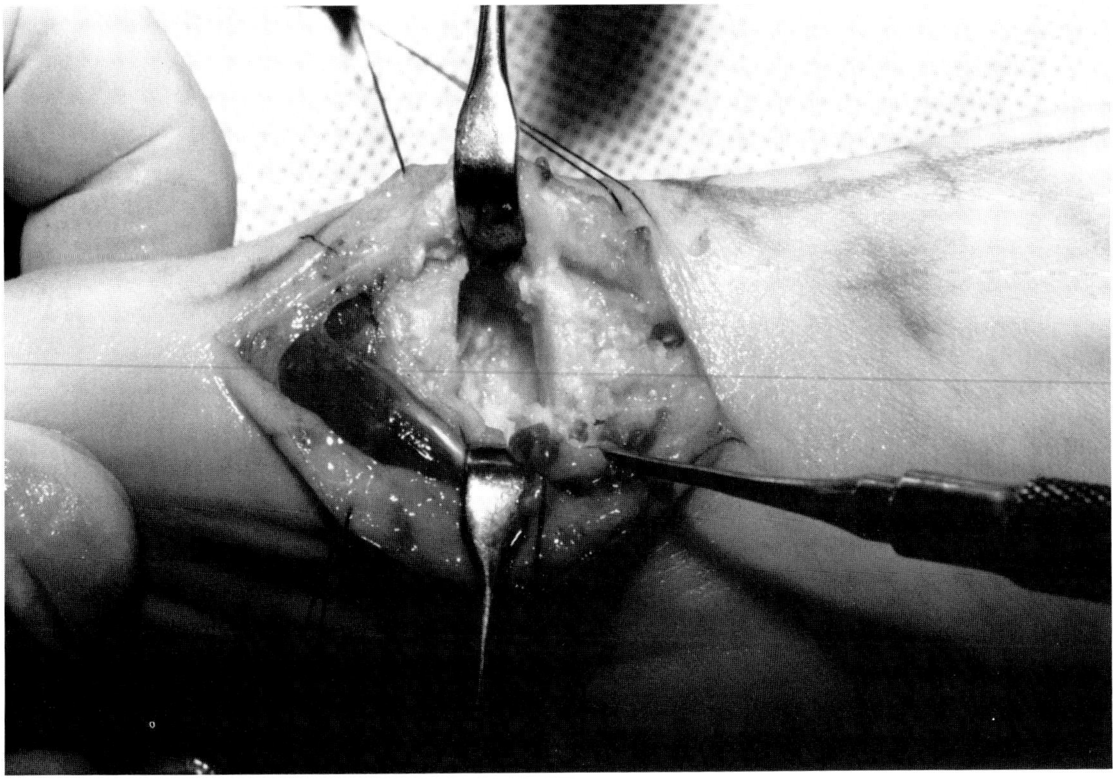

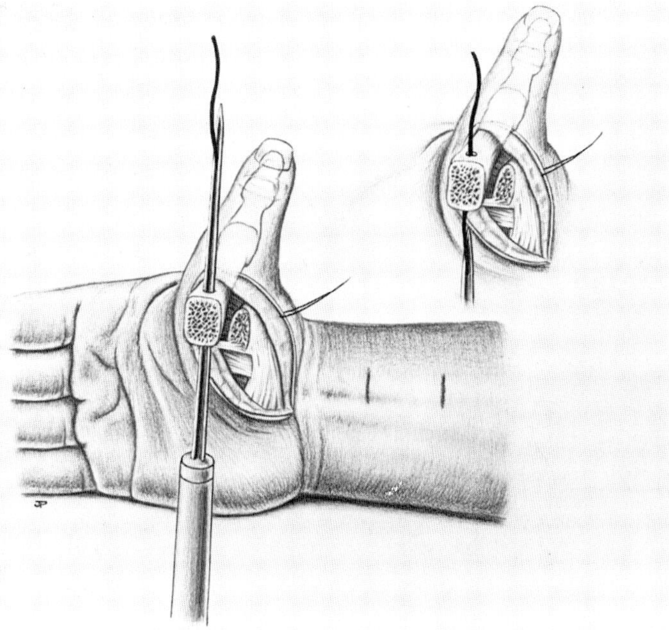

**Fig. 4-22** Gouges of increasing size are used to create a tract through the volar metacarpal base and out the dorsum. This tract must be perpendicular to the long axis of the metacarpal and to the plane of the fingernail. The largest gouge has a groove which allows a No. 30 wire to be passed dorsal to volar; the wire will be used to guide the flexor tendon through the metacarpal.

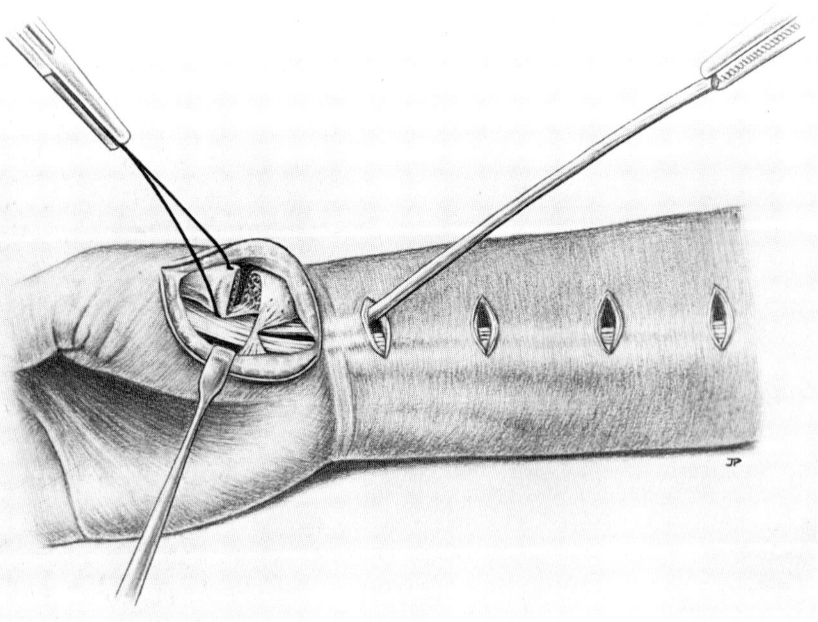

**Fig. 4-23** The radial half of the flexor carpi radialis tendon is divided from its proximal attachment and freed along its length. It must be freed distally to the point where it begins to head dorsally under the crest of the trapezium. The tendon is withdrawn into the distalmost incision.

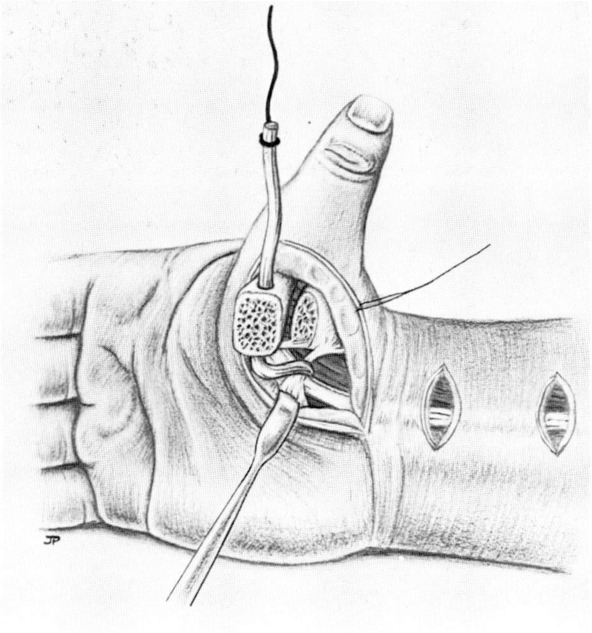

**Fig. 4-24** The wire suture is tied around the cut end of the tendon, and both are withdrawn through the metacarpal. At this point, a Kirschner wire may be threaded retrograde through the metacarpal base, being careful not to impale the flexor tendon. The wire will stabilize the basal joint in its new position when the ligament reconstruction is complete.

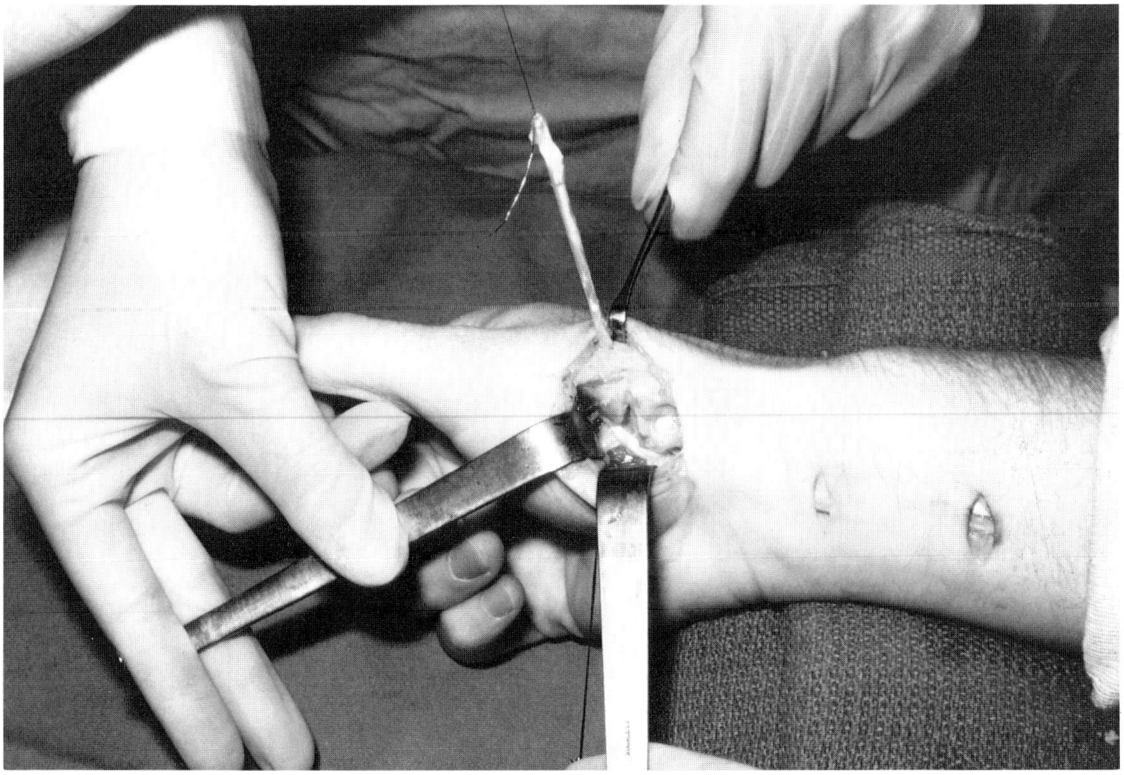

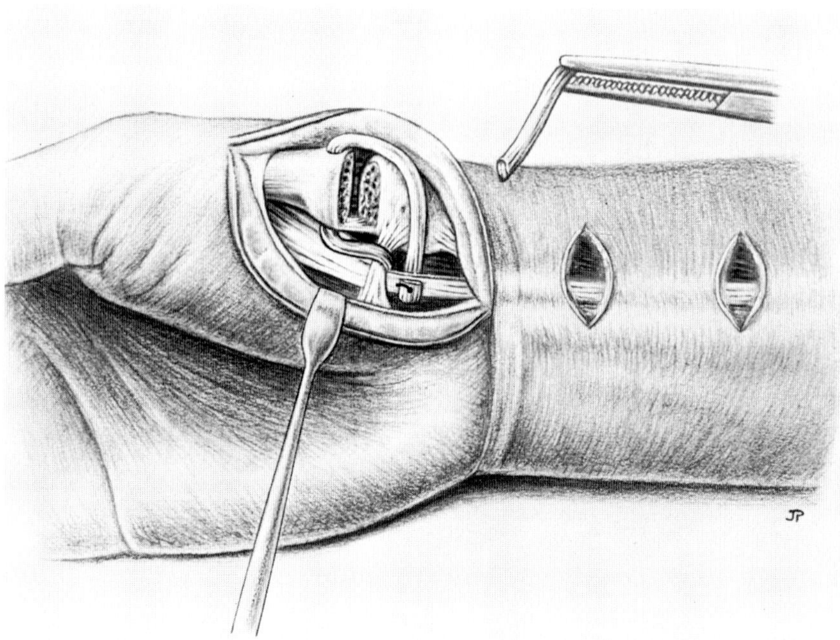

**Fig. 4-25** The tendon is brought volarly and sutured to the intact flexor carpi radialis tendon, with the excess tendon trimmed, folded, sutured, and interposed into the space. A small plain suture may be used to fix the interposition securely in place.

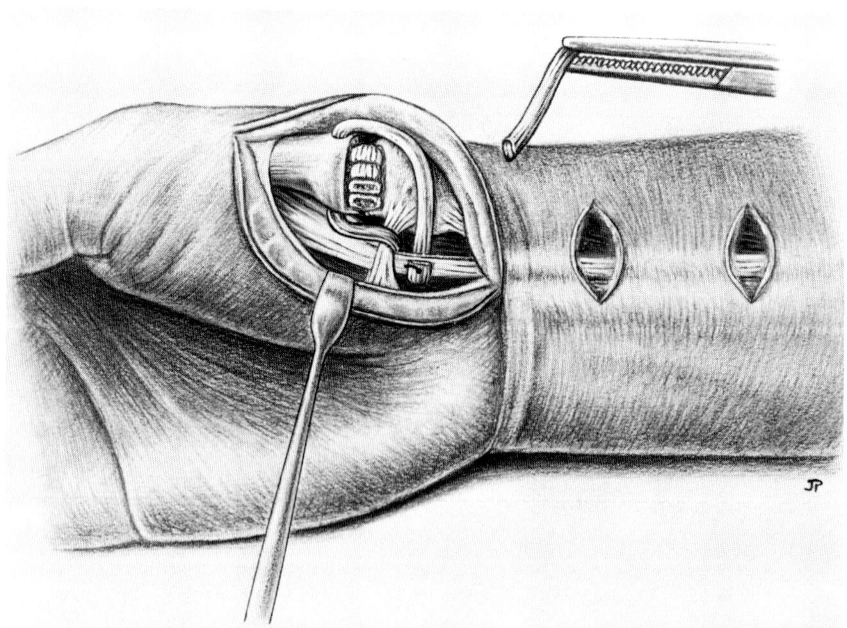

**Fig. 4-26** Tension is set with the metacarpal base snug against the interposed cushion; the ligament reconstruction is fixed with a permanent suture at the point where it emerges dorsally from the metacarpal, and again where it folds back on the intact flexor tendon. The Kirschner wire is then driven across the reconstructed joint, and the capsule is closed.

# Arthroplasty of the Hip

# 5

Michael J. Bronson
W. Norman Scott
Richard D. Scott
William Thomas Stillwell

## Historical Considerations

Total hip arthroplasty has been considered by many as one of the most significant medical breakthroughs in the last 50 years. It has been estimated that between 60,000 and 80,000 hip replacements are performed annually in the United States, and possibly 250,000 are performed worldwide. Although initial success in almost all series of hip replacements approaches 90%, all new developments attempt to address the permanence of the arthroplasty.

The evolution of our current technique, which is in itself still rapidly evolving, began in the early 1800s. In 1826, Barton osteotomized an ankylosed hip with the resultant pseudoarthrosis yielding a satisfactory result. Although the use of osteotomy to change the biomechanical stresses around the hip led to a completely separate evolutionary school, the concept of maintaining pain free movement was furthered by the work of Verneuil in France utilizing the interposition of biological materials such as fat, fascia, and muscle. In the United States, Baer (1918) inserted chromicized pig bladder, whereas other investigators used inert substances such as zinc. These techniques were remarkably successful in maintaining motion after osteotomy. Rapid advancements began in 1923 when Smith-Peterson introduced the concept of covering a carefully reamed femoral head and acetabulum with a nonbiological material. Although initially fraught with breakage of the glass, and later Bakelite, Venable and Stuck achieved success with Vitallium in 1930. This material was strong while eliciting a low level of reactivity. The melding of the techniques of the Smith-Peterson cup with the material properties of Vitallium gave excellent function to many destroyed hips, many of these patients still enjoying this success after 25 years.

At the same time, the interest in replacing the diseased femoral head was furthered by the efforts of Bohlman utilizing custom stainless steel prosthetics and later through the work of the Judets in France utilizing an acrylic femoral head component. Although restoring motion, material properties were still not ideal. Fixation of metallic femoral components was improved by Thompson and Moore, who used long stem components to take advantage of the cancellous bone in the proximal femur. The self-locking Austin Moore prosthesis still enjoys widespread and satisfactory use.

Efforts at total replacement of the hip joint were pioneered in 1951 by Haboush in the United States and McKee and Watson-Farrar in England. Their attempts to resurface both sides of the joint with metal alloy were frought with problems of fixation and wear: the metallic acetabulum that was secured with screws exhibited rapid loosening, while the high friction arthroplasty resulted in excessive wear. Undoubtedly, the greatest contribution to our present day success came through the work at Wrightington by Sir John Charnley. Although early attempts at acetabular replacement using Teflon polymer were unsuccessful, the introduction of ultrahigh molecular weight polyethylene acetabular components, with fixation provided by poly(methyl methacrylate) was historic and serves as the basis for all of our present research.

## Prosthetic Selection

With the rapid evolution in total hip replacement, the selection of suitable components becomes extremely difficult. Part of this difficulty comes from the attempt of the orthopaedic surgeon to separate biomechanical fact from the overenthusiastic literature supplied by the orthopaedic companies. Although considerable controversy exists as to the ideal hip implant, there are certain facts that are incontrovertable. The most important of these is that, with the evolution of orthopaedic design away from those complicated by high early failure rates, the designs available today and their selection is less important than the surgical technique used to implant them. The second factor is that the early success reported with surface replacement has been unable to be reproduced in most surgical reports and for the most part occupies no place in the selection of prosthetics for the average patient.

Metallurgical considerations are of considerable import. Although the ideal implant material has yet to be found, the work of the metallurgist in choosing and fabricating higher strength alloys has eliminated the early problems of late stem fracture. The ideal material must approach the properties of bone both in strength and, more importantly, in approaching a reasonable compatible elastic modulus. Titanium, for instance, has a lower modulus than chrome cobalt, yet it is still a power of magnitude greater than bone. The debate over collar versus collarless may well not see a resolution in this century. From a theoretical point of view, the collar acts to increase the stress transmission through the proximal femur and thus avoid a late bone resorption secondary to stress shielding. This, however, has been substantiated in vitro only. This theoretical concern has effected many design considerations, yet unequivocable answers are awaited. Attempts to improve component fixation have included coating the femoral stems (pre and porous) and have to be evaluated in conjunction with the effects of specific metal alloys.

Femoral head sizes are currently available in 22, 26, 28, and 32 mm components. Although the early 22 mm design of Charnley had the lowest frictional coefficient, it had the lowest inherent stability. The 32 mm prosthesis had the highest stability from dislocation, but it had a higher rate of socket loosening in long term retrievals. Most agree that, at least for cemented arthroplasty, a 26 or 28 mm head would seem optimal.

Femoral stems have evolved from the early sharp-cornered, curve design to the straighter stems with round edges and larger diameters. These modifications attempt to diminish stress on the composite bone cement prosthesis interface. Some recent designs, especially in the porous coated prostheses, have attempted to achieve an anatomical configuration by mimicking the physiological curves of the proximal femur.

The most difficult and yet the most important choice lies in the type of fixation. Whether to use PMMA or to rely upon the newer techniques of cementless arthroplasty will be proven over the next 5–10 years. In addition, the type of cementless fixation to be used varies from attempts at true bone ingrowth to an interference fit.

Adequate three-dimensional finite element analysis studies have been done to substantiate the need to back polyethylene with metal in an attempt to eliminate the detrimental effects of cold flow. Although the metal backing seems to have less importance in cups whose diameter is greater than 10 mm, it is extremely important in the smaller diameters. Not only is cold flow limited by metal backing, but the finite element studies show a more normal stress distribution in the pelvis.

## Indications

The indications for total hip arthroplasty, surprisingly, have not changed substantially from those recommended by Charnley in the early 70s.

The patient subjected to hip replacement must meet the criteria of moderate to severe pain that is unresponsive to conservative modalities of antiinflammatories or to such weight-relieving devices as canes. Disability encompasses loss of motion, function, and decreased ambulation. Age limitations are, by necessity, somewhat arbitrary, but in general with a diagnosis of osteoarthritis the patient should be at least 50 years of age. The disease state may be primary or secondary to arthritis, congenital hip dysplasia, or congenital maladies. Attempts to apply a successor of this technique to younger osteoarthritic patients, i.e., less than 40, have shown higher rates of loosening than in an older population. Rather than arbitrarily deciding on a definitive chronological age, most physicians consider the physiological factors and expectations of the patient prior to recommending a procedure. Although the age limitation for osteoarthritis is significant, it does not apply to the other inflammatory arthritidies. In addition, all patients with a diagnosis of avascular necrosis, regardless of the etiology, nonunited fractures, previous arthrodesis, or failed reconstructions are also potential candidates for a hip arthroplasty. As long as the bone stock is adequate and the technique is feasible based on roentgenographic analysis, these patients represent potential candidates who remain a growing challenge for the orthopaedic community.

## Contraindications

While sepsis in its fulminant form remains a contraindication to hip replacement, recent successes with low grade gram positive infections combined with meticulous debridement and carefully monitored postoperative antibiotics, with or without antibiotic-impregnated cement, have expanded the indications to those patients previously or currently infected. Any successful arthroplasty requires a functioning musculature, and, thus, patients in whom there is a neuromuscular impairment about the hip represent relative contraindications to surgery. Similarly, a biomechanical assessment regarding gait and multiple joint disease must determine the advisability of another replacement.

## Present and Future Research

Current research efforts and those of the future hopefully will make available to us a method to replace the diseased hip of all age groups with a technique that allows a person a lifetime worth of function, with the functional limits of the "prosthesis" mimicking the biological hip. If loosening can be eliminated through better fixation techniques and material properties improved allowing a better composite, then this goal will be realized.

Current research efforts seem to be in two directions. The first is to enhance the methods of total hip replacement using the current design and materials available with the principles of Charnley still present. The major problem in this regard is, of course, cement fixation. Some regard poly(methyl methacrylate) as the cause of loosening and the reason for the histicocytic membrane that is seen in very aseptic loosening, whereas most feel it is the lack of proper available techniques that leads to failure. In an effort to reinforce the strength of the cement, work is being done with carbon fiber-reinforced PMMA, with bench tests showing increased resistance to fatigue. Techniques of cement handling are in constant flux, with methods of cement pressurization, cement restriction, and lowering of the cement viscosity under research, especially as applicable to acetabular fixation, where long term loosening seems to reside. It has been shown early on that admixture of blood to polymerizing cement significantly decreases strength. It has recently been demonstrated that admixture of air has the same result. In an attempt to "purify" the cement, techniques such as cement centrifugation to eliminate air bubbles has been recently introduced.

The second path that current research efforts have taken is to introduce the concept of biological fixation. On a theoretical basis, biological fixation would seem, if indeed it is achievable, to answer the problem of long term loosening. For a while a cemented hip would have its greatest fixation to loosening at the time of surgery; a biologically fixated hip would theoretically grow stronger with time. Cementless hip replacement is certainly not new and has been commonplace in Europe for the past 10 years. This type of cementless fixation, however, must be distinguished from true biological or porous ingrowth. The interference fit of the European designs, although showing impressive long term results, may be different from biological ingrowth in the true sense of the term. It has been shown in vivo that the body is very selective in choosing to establish trabecular ingrowth into nonbiological substrates. The critical factors seem to be absolute initial rigidity and critical pore size, with 50–400 μm seeming to be the acceptable range of pore size. Whether these criteria can be fullfilled in the clinical setting remains to be seen. Certainly, initial success of designs instills a cautious option. We have, however, learned from early results with cemented arthroplasty that success is better defined by 10 year results. On the other hand, porous ingrowth arthroplasty has exhibited very early failure, i.e., the extremely young and the multiply operated patient have not shown the same tendency in early clinical trials.

Where the results of ongoing investigations in cartilage physiology will take us, in regard to cartilage pathology and osteoarthritis, is unknown. A better understanding of the pathophysiology of cartilage may have a profound effect on the manner in which we treat hip diseases, the vast majority of which start with cartilage insult.

The rapid sequence of new techniques, new methods and materials, and new concepts at the biological level make it difficult to write anything dogmatic regarding total hip replacement. A continuing appraisal of ongoing research efforts is mandatory for the clinician offering total joint replacement.

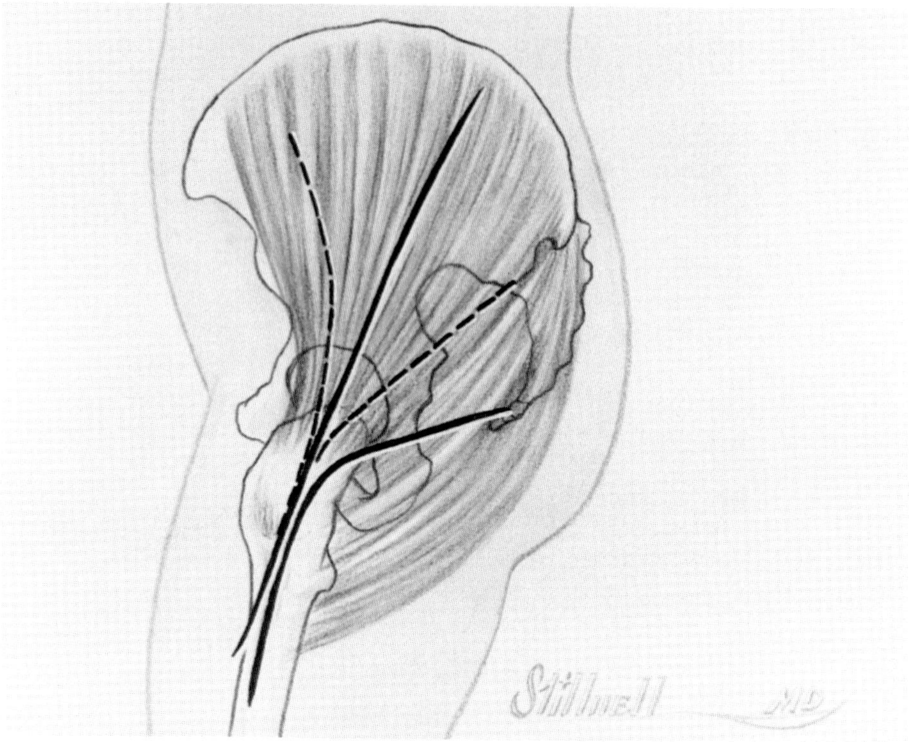

**Fig. 5-1** Various approaches about the hip.

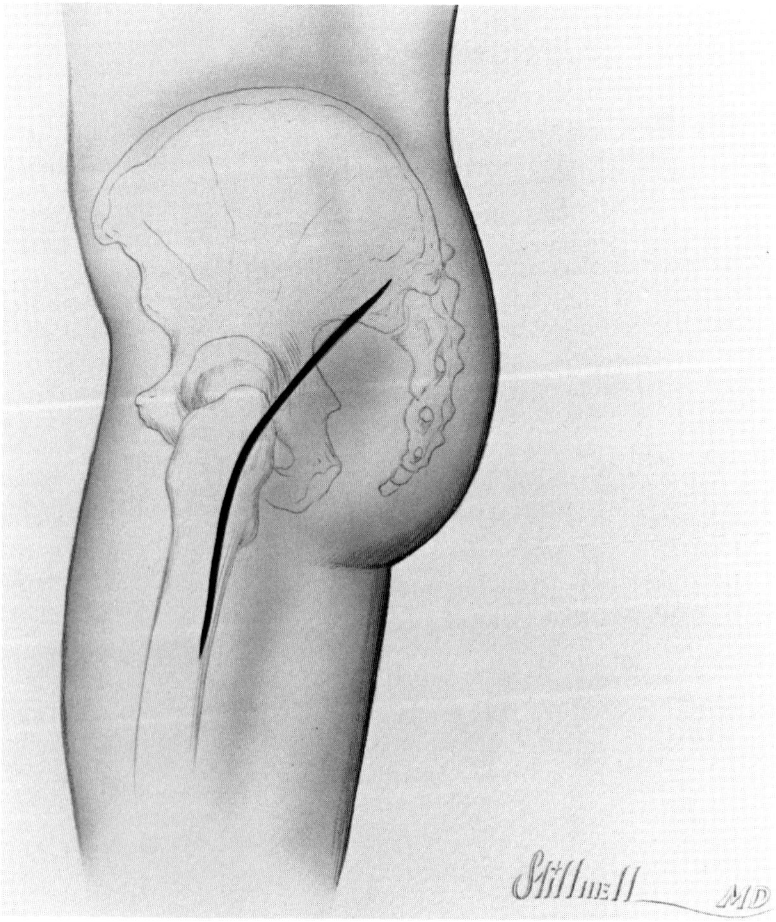

**Figs. 5-2 to 5-4** A Gibson or posterolateral approach. The skin incision is approximately 15 cm long. It is centered over the greater trochanter. Its distal extension is over the midshaft of the femur. Its proximal extension angles posteriorly approximately 30°.

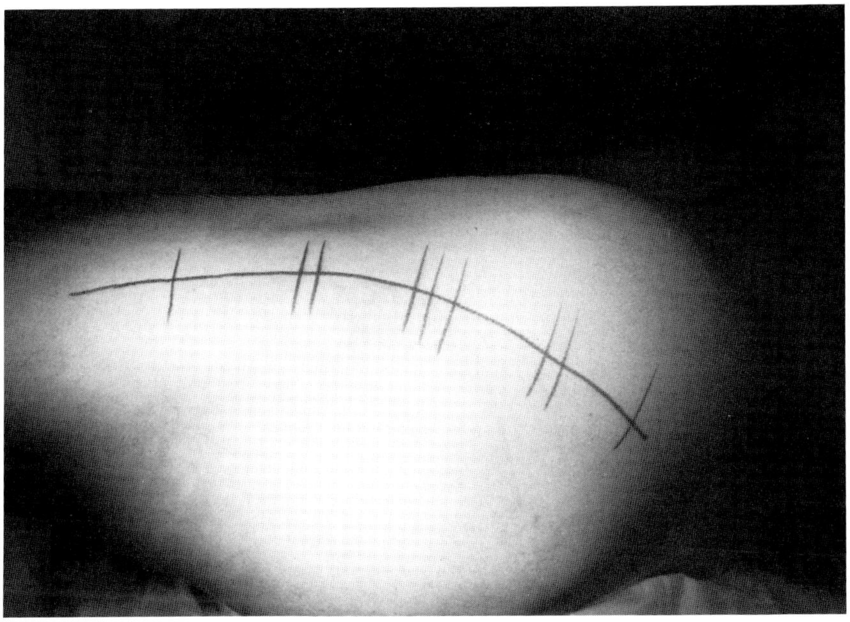

**Fig. 5-3**

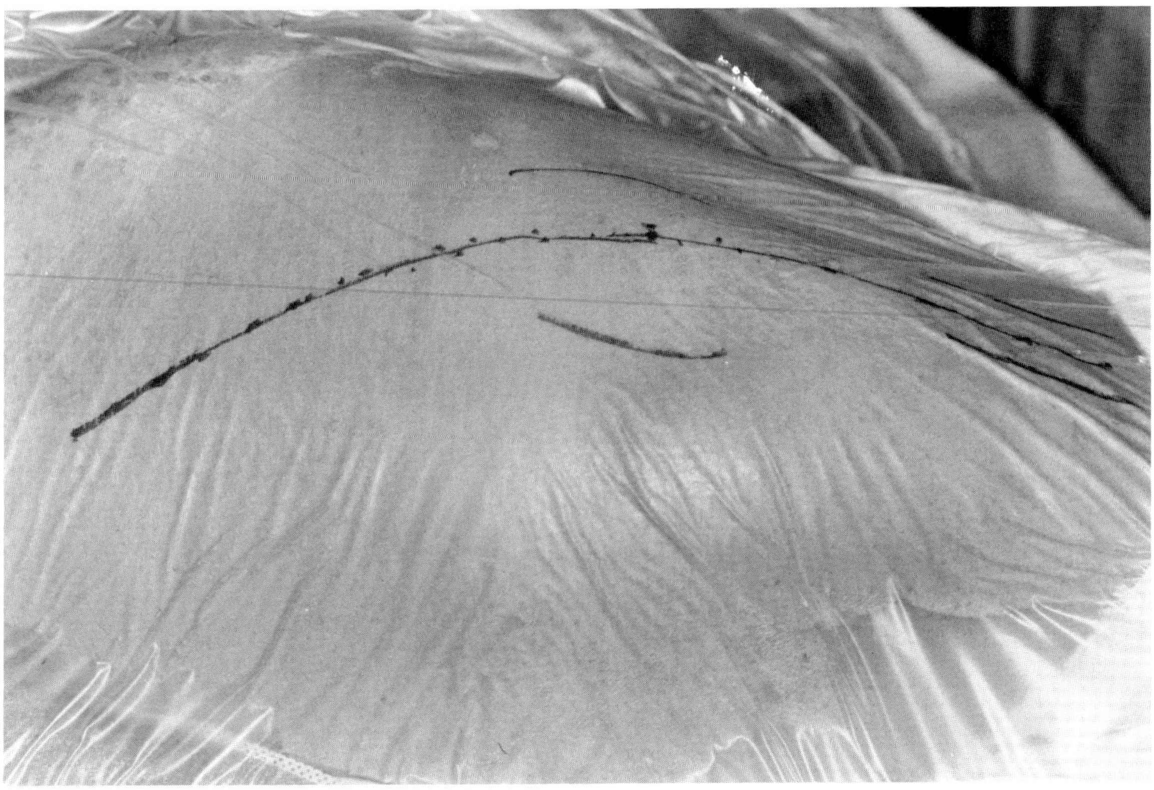

**Fig. 5-4**

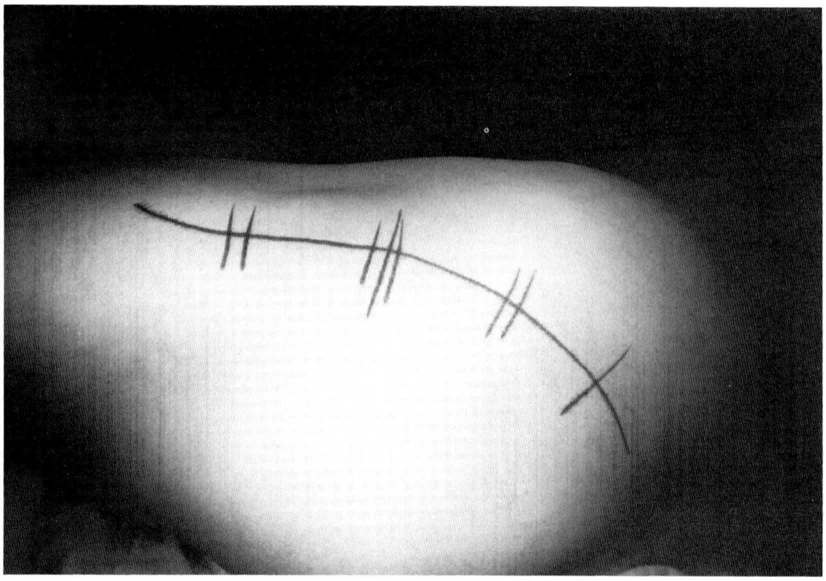

**Fig. 5-5** Modified posterolateral (Aufranc).

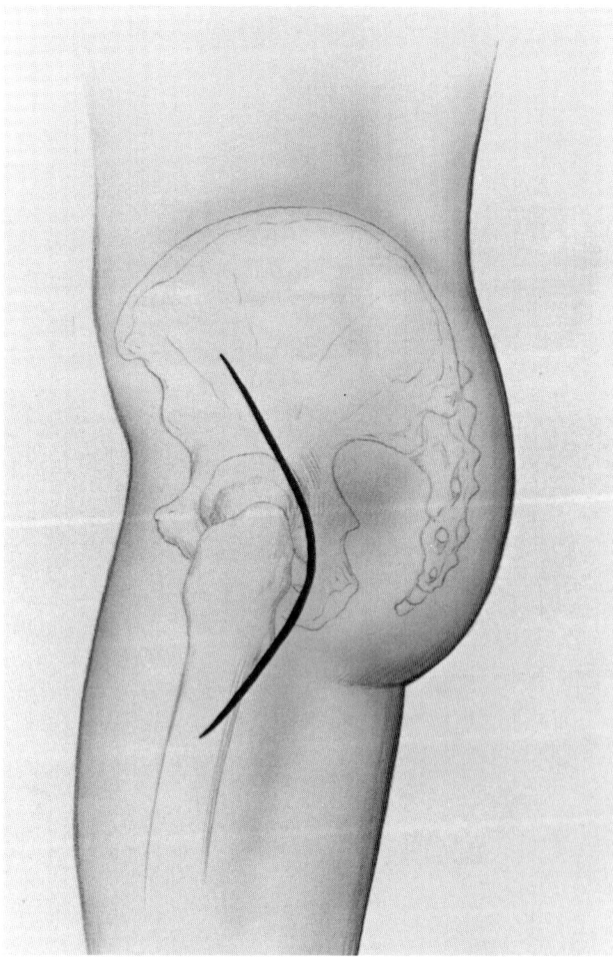

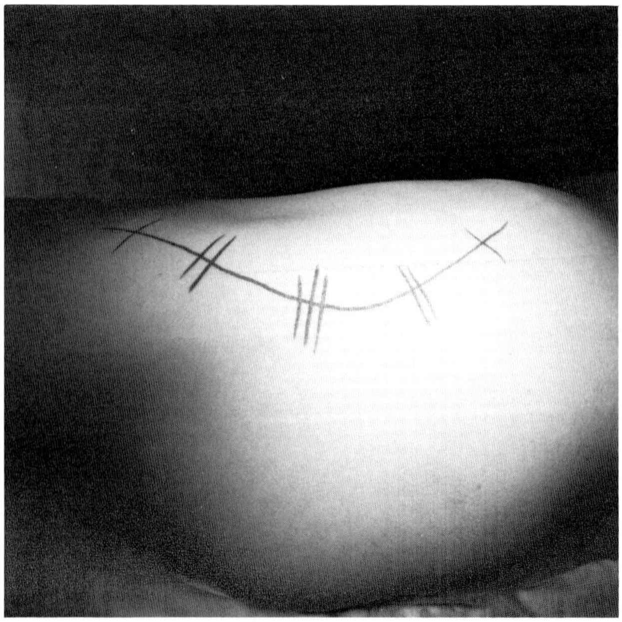

**Figs. 5-6 and 5-7** Watson-Jones or Harris approach.

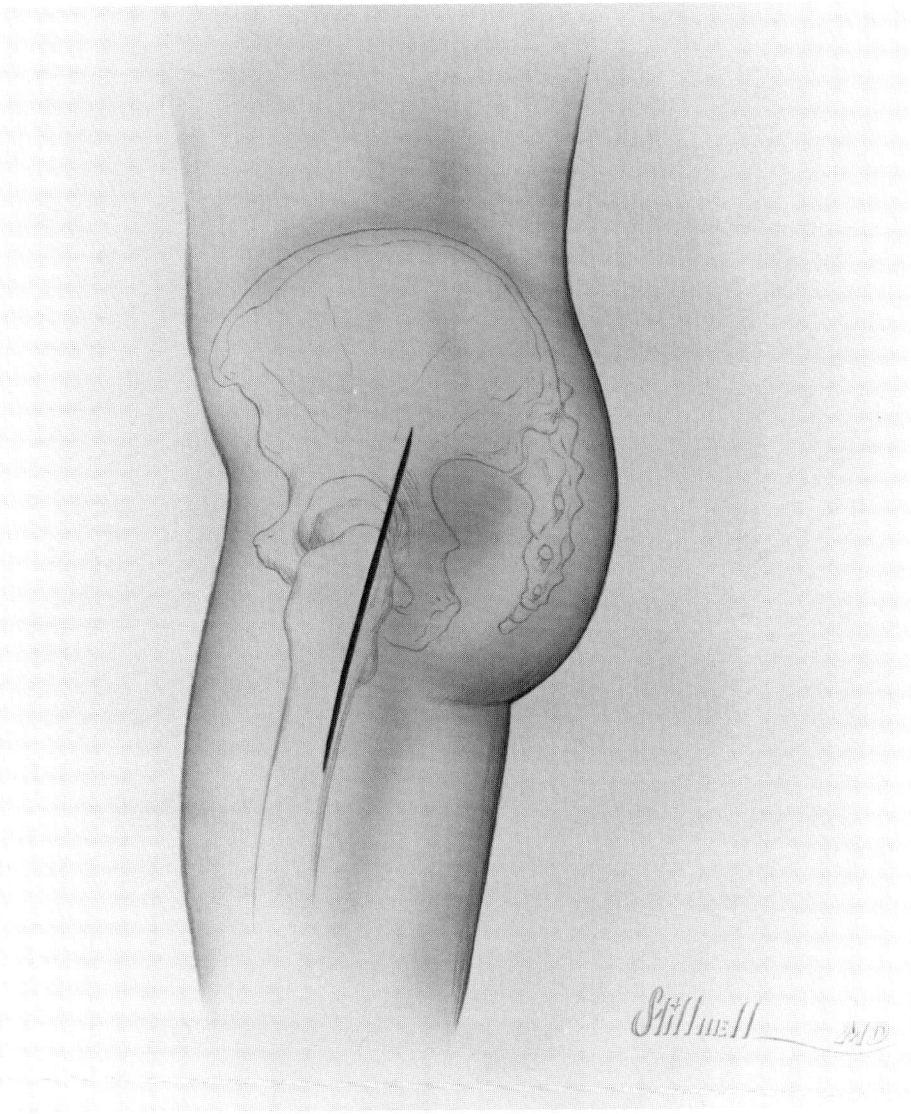

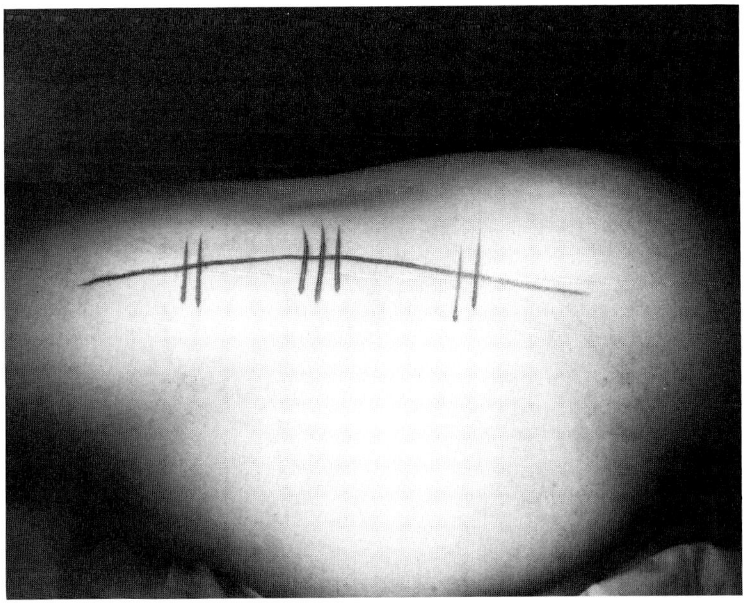

**Figs. 5-8 and 5-9** A straight lateral incision.

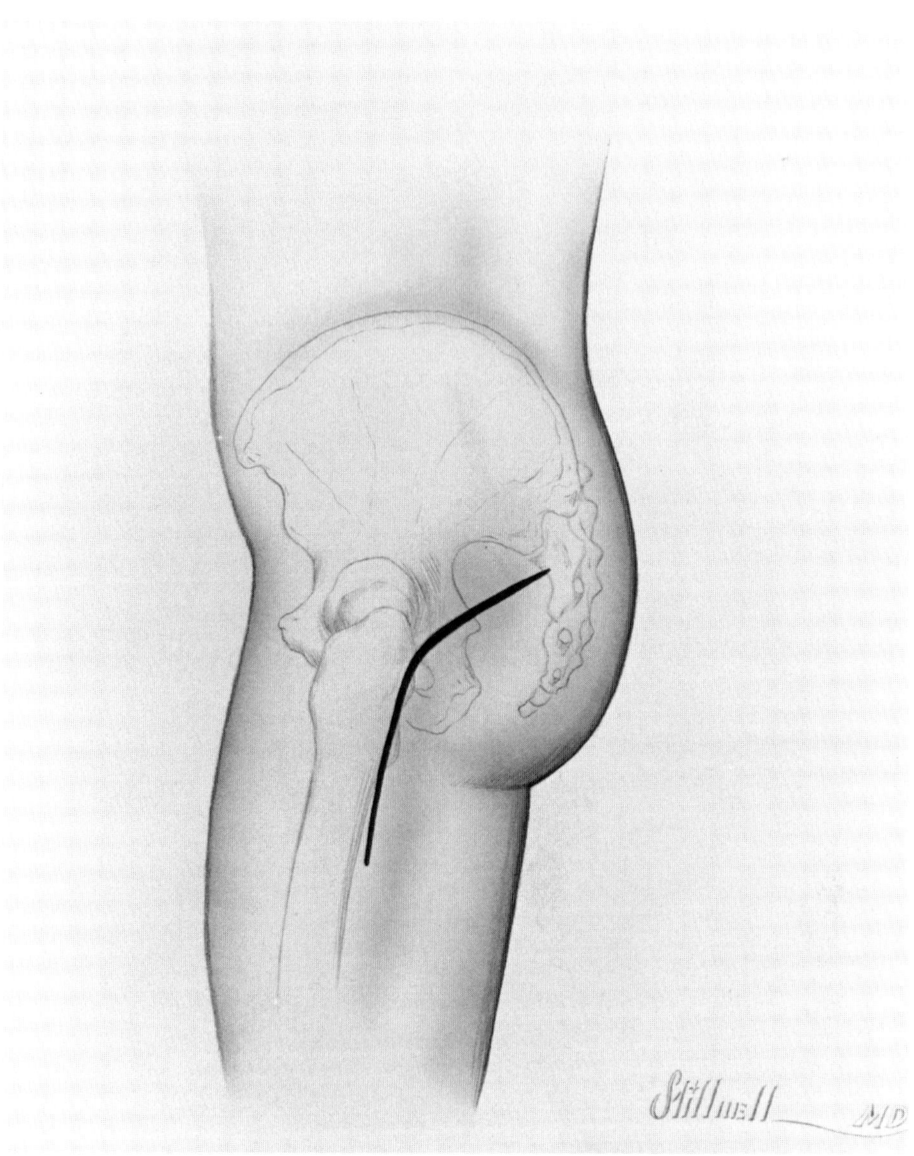

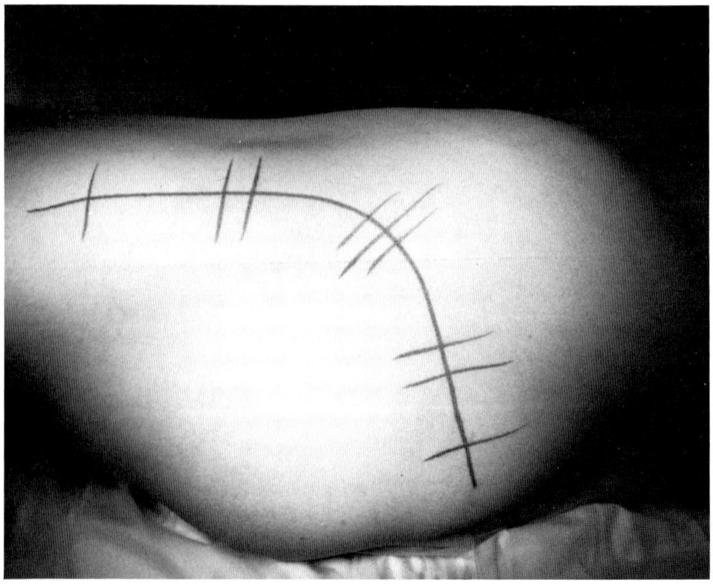

**Figs. 5-10 and 5-11** Moore or Southern approach.

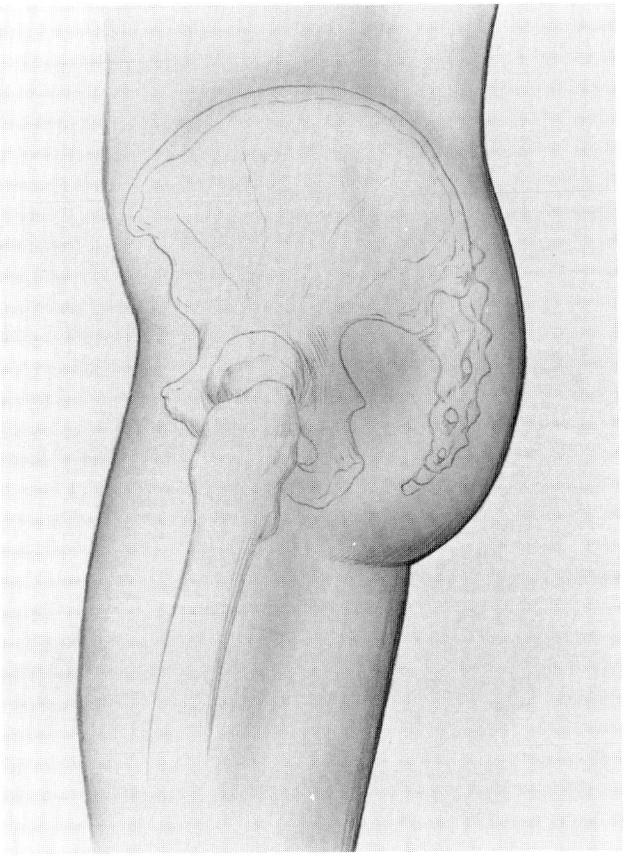
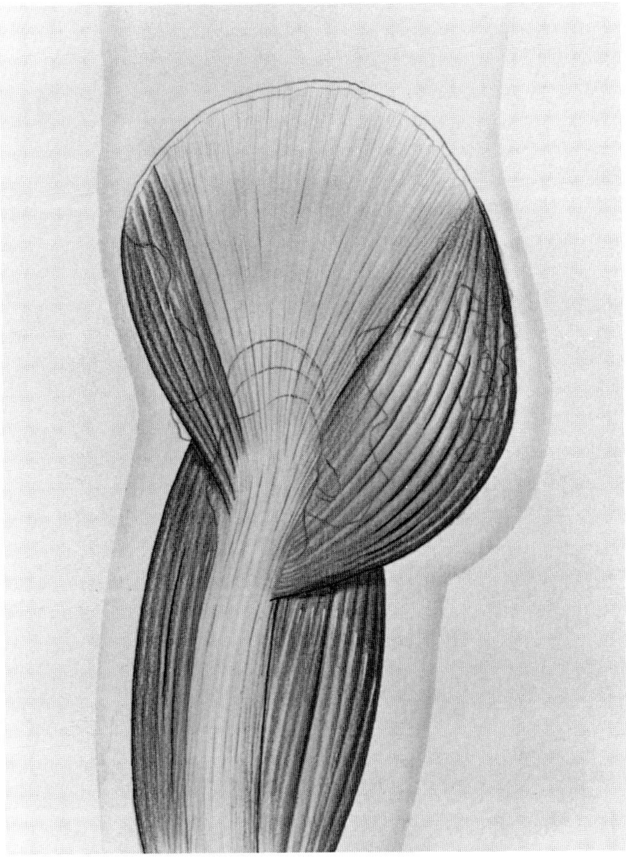

**Figs. 5-12 and 5-13** Relationship of bone landmarks to overlying fascial and muscular structures.

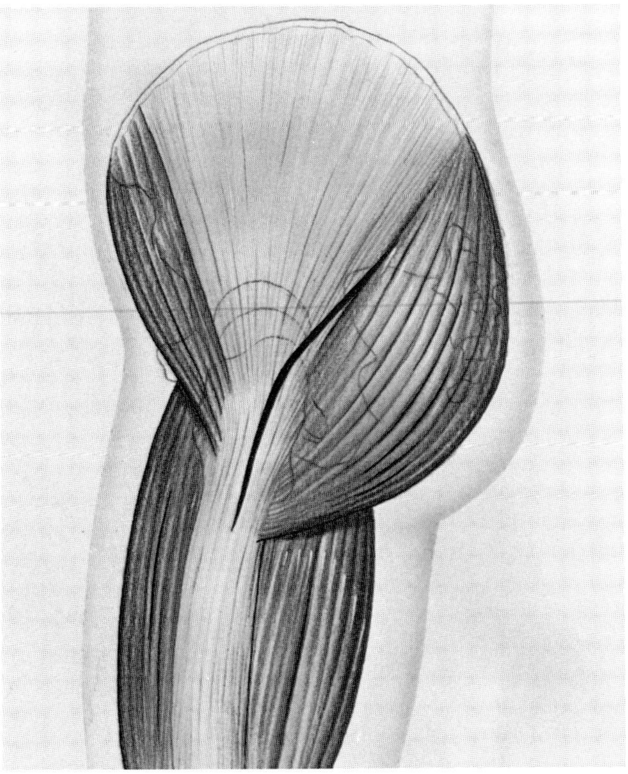

**Fig. 5-14** A posterolatral approach to the capsule.

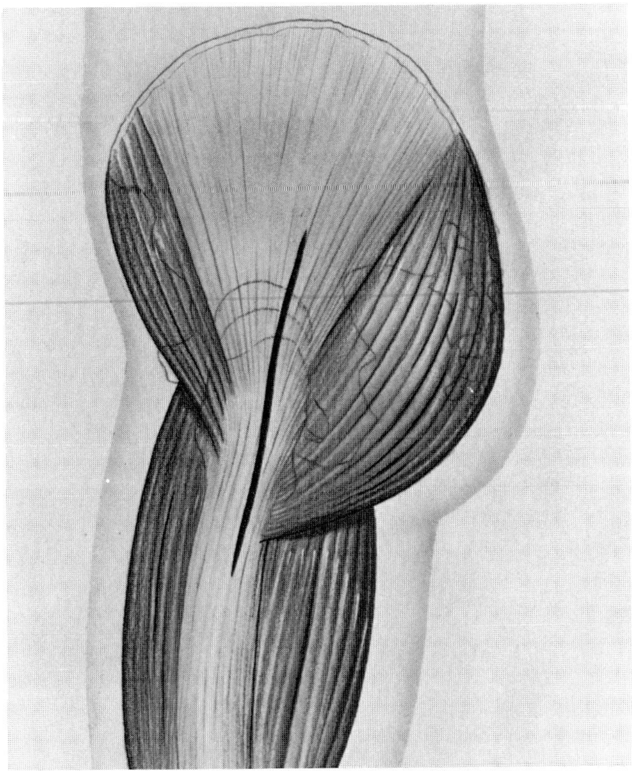

**Fig. 5-15** A straight lateral or gluteus-splitting incision.

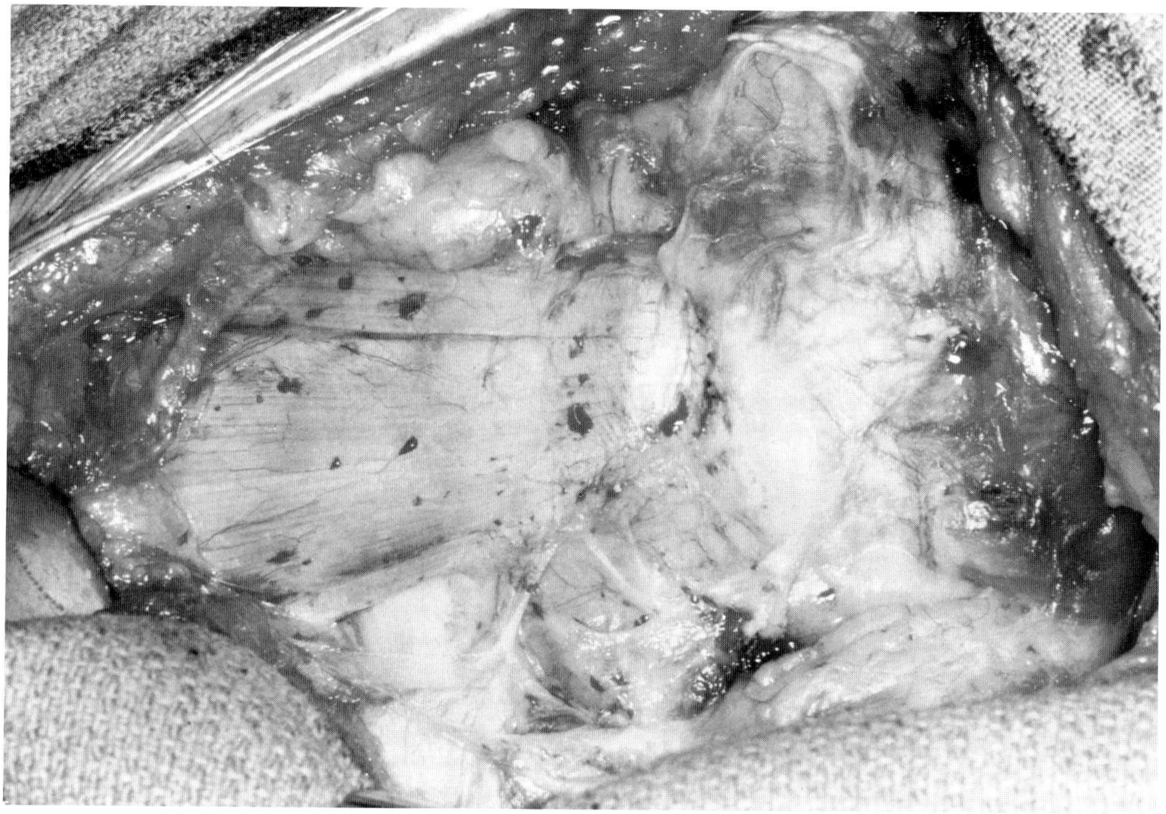

**Fig. 5-16** The relationship of greater trochanter, vastus lateralis, and insertion of gluteus maximus.

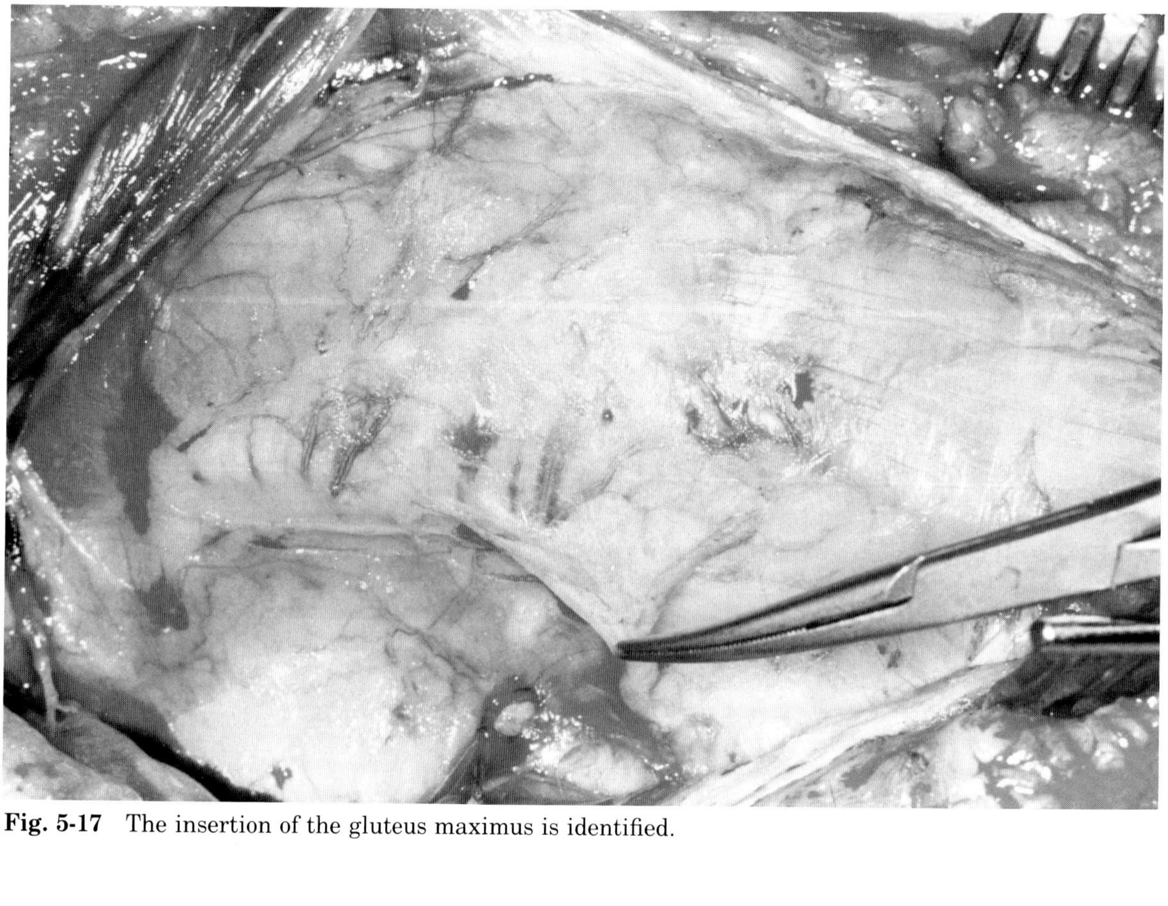

**Fig. 5-17** The insertion of the gluteus maximus is identified.

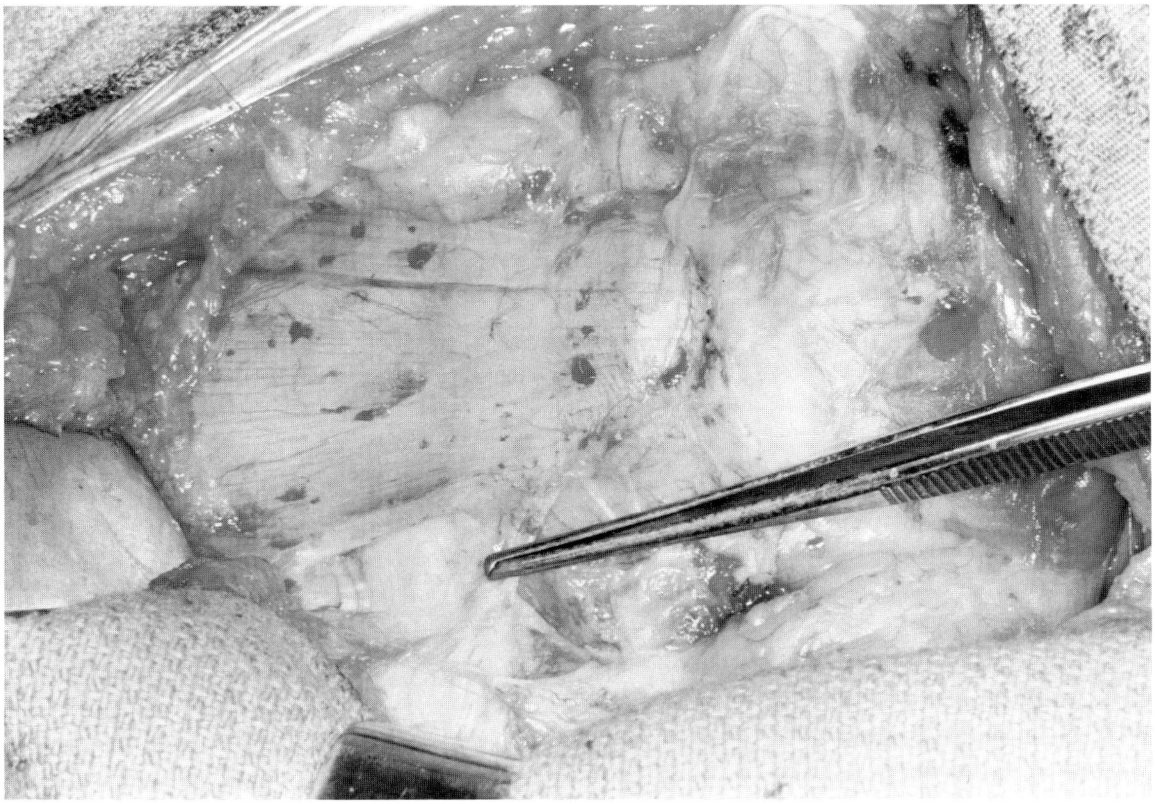

**Fig. 5-18** A posterolateral approach is utilized here, although almost any standard approach can be satisfactory. A transtrochanteric exposure is, however, not suggested.

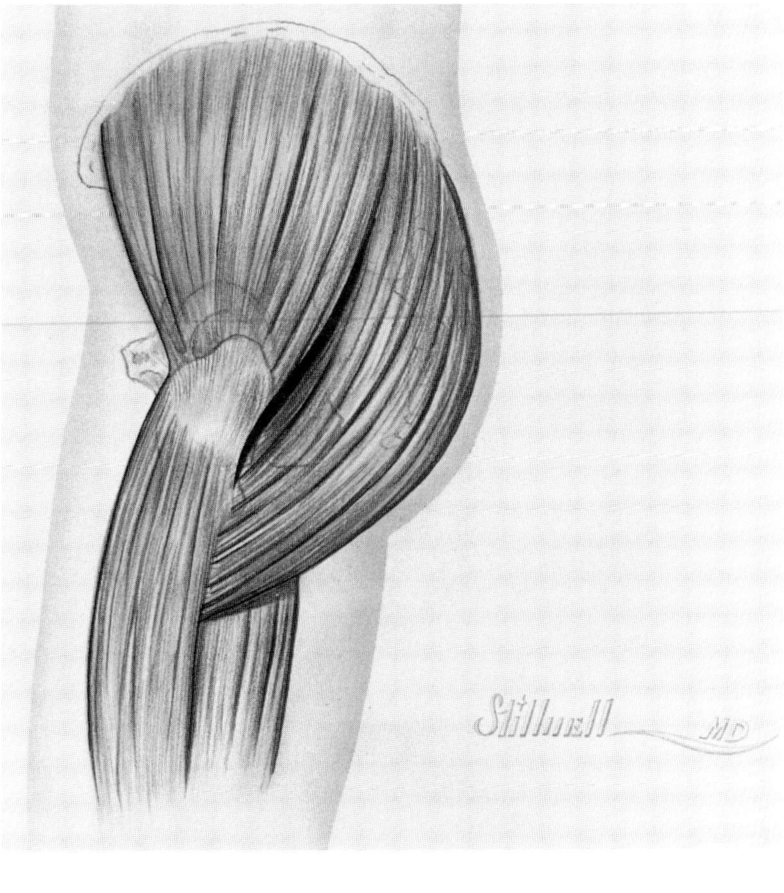


**Fig. 5-19** The relationship of the gluteus maximus and medius to the greater trochanter and femoral shaft.

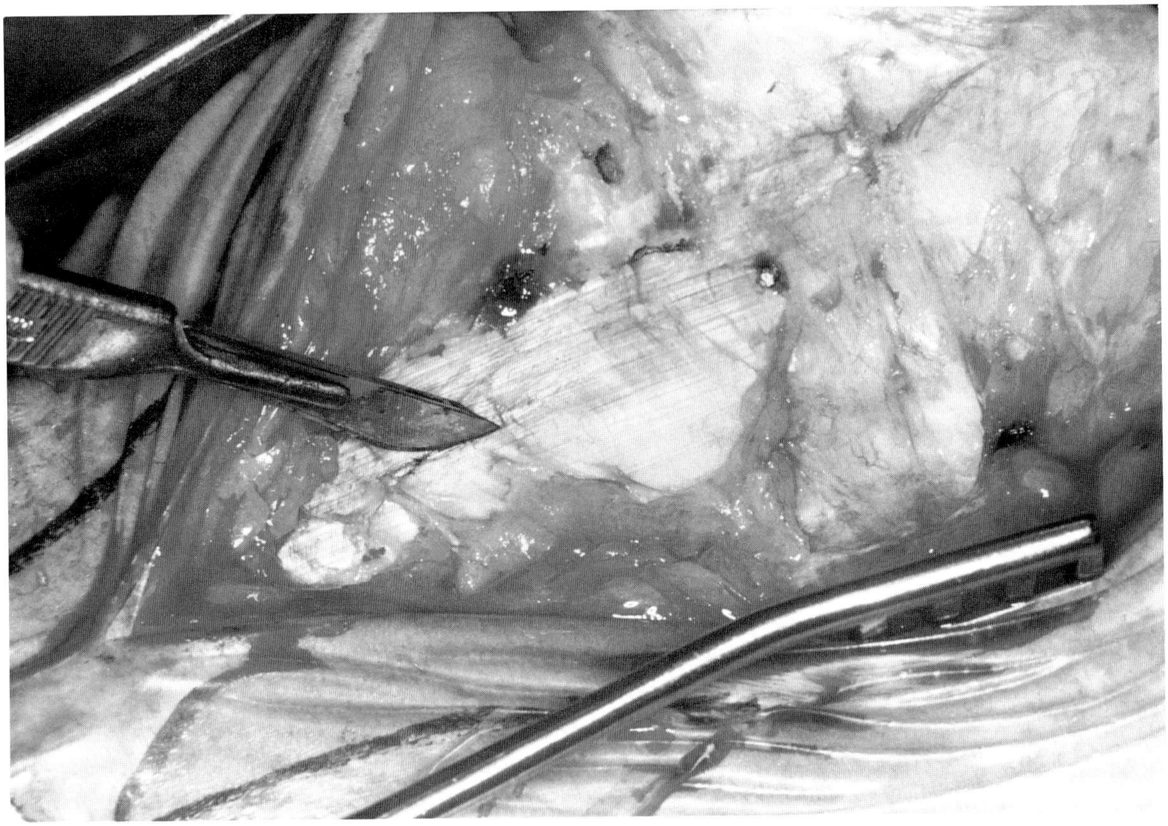

**Fig. 5-20** The fascia lata is incised longitudinally, usually in the same direction as the skin incision.

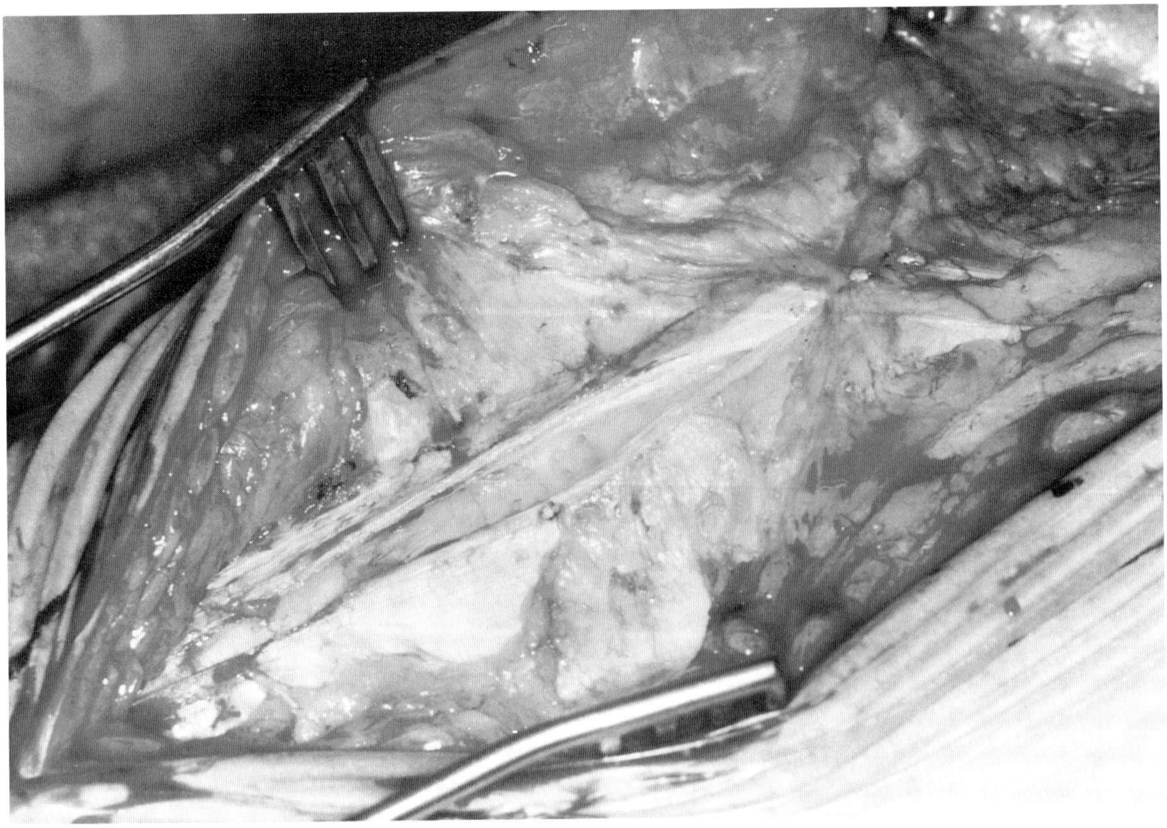

**Figs. 5-21 and 5-22** The gluteus fascia is split along the direction of its muscle fibers.

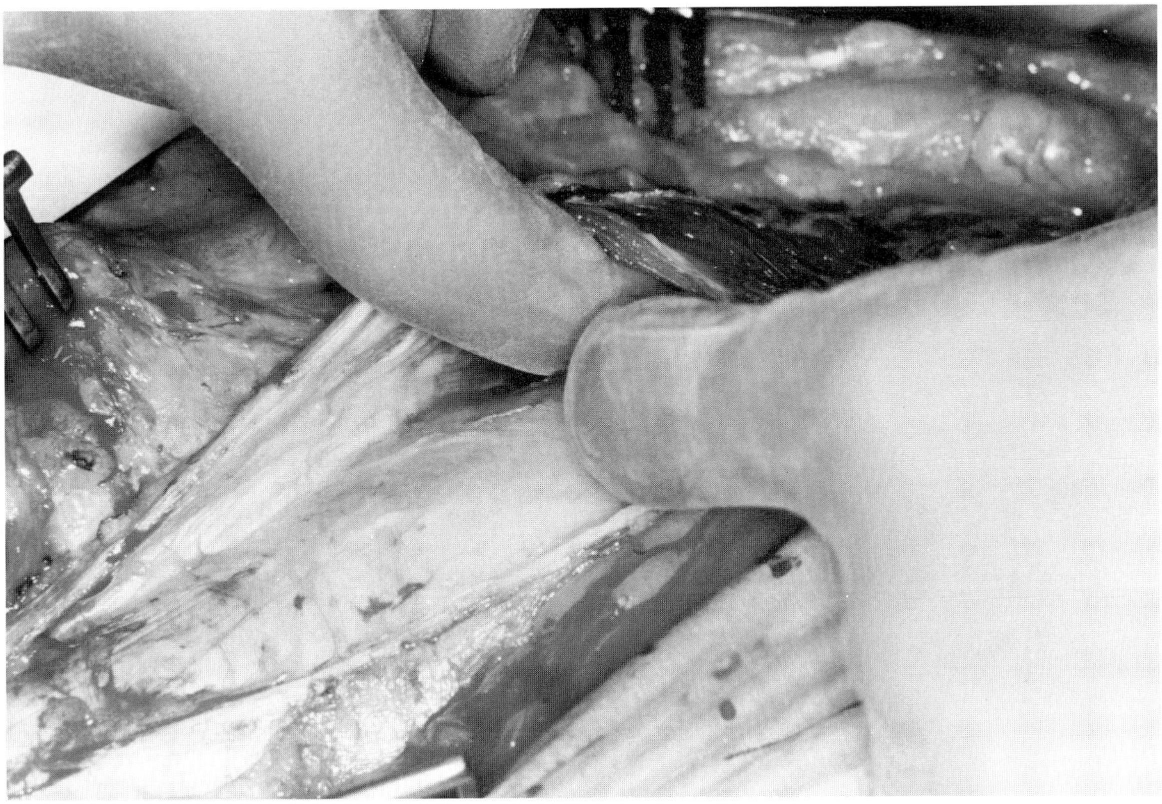

Fig. 5-22

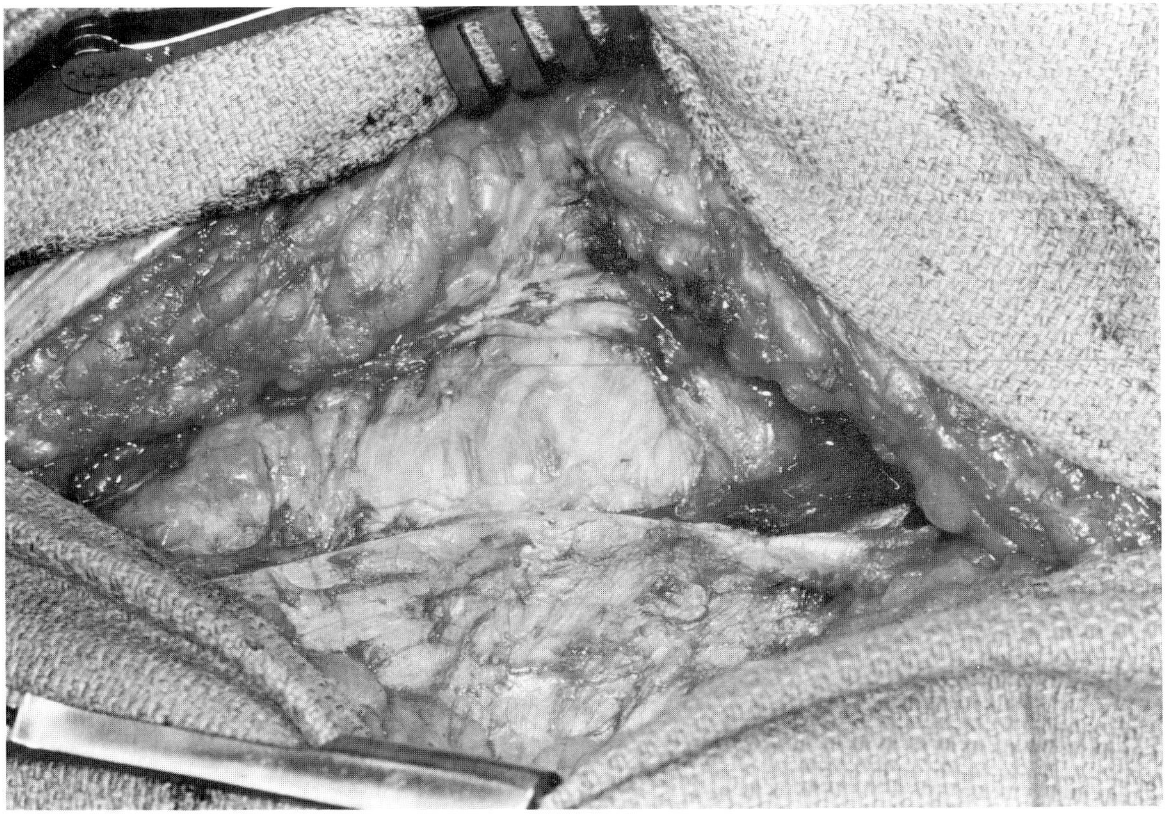

**Fig. 5-23** The fascia lata has been split in line with the incision and retracted, revealing the short external rotators. It is helpful in order to gain acetabular access to detach the tendon of the gluteus maximus.

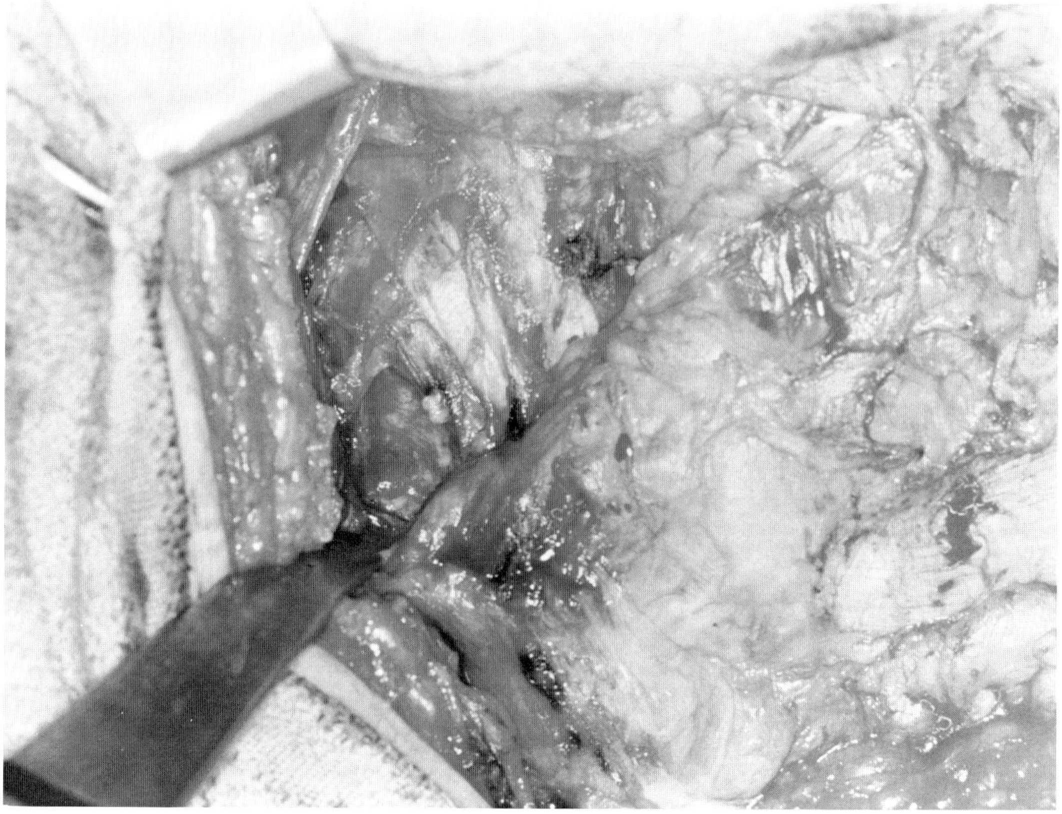

**Fig. 5-24** With the gluteus medius and minimus retracted anteriorly, the short rotators are detached from the greater trochanter. The capsule of the hip joint is opened with a T-shaped incision.

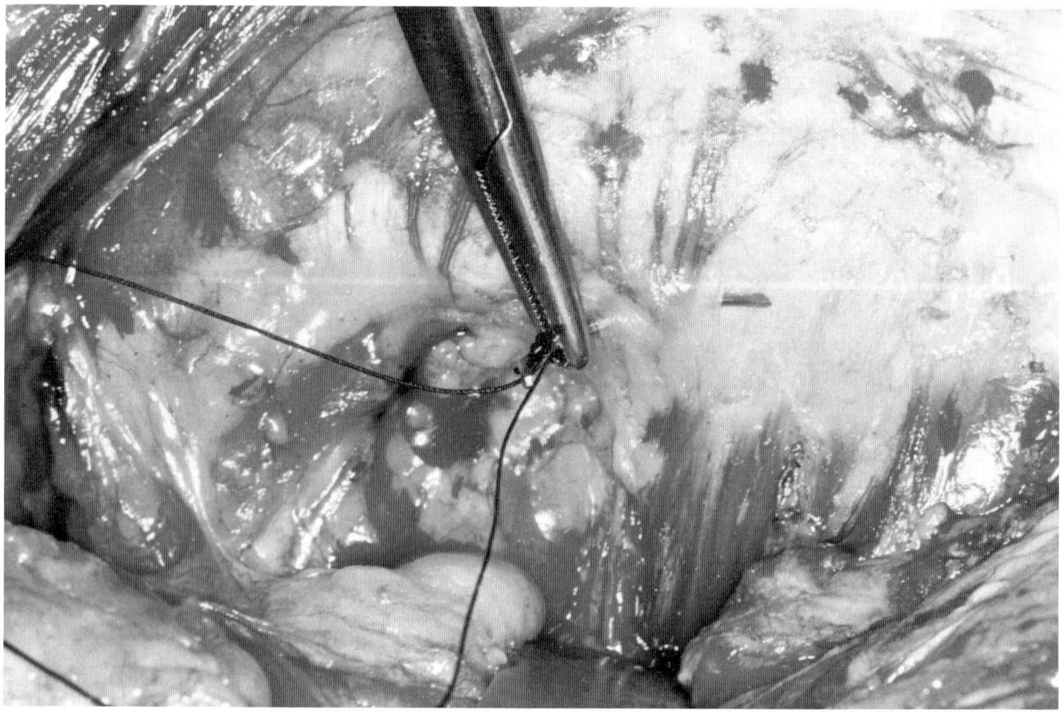

**Fig. 5-25** The posterior branch of the medial femoral circumflex artery is ligated just before it arborizes on the greater trochanter.

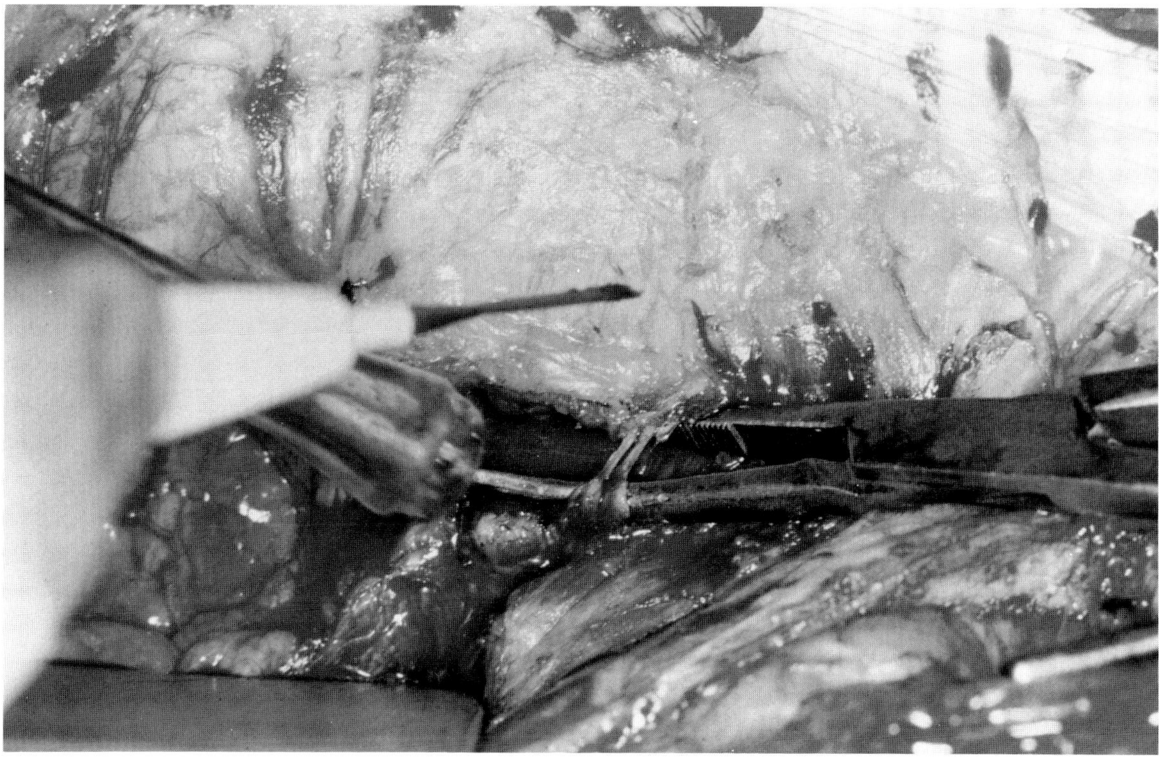

**Fig. 5-26** The quadratus femoris muscle is taken down with cutting cautery to expose the more proximal portion of the posterior branch of the medial femoral circumflex artery.

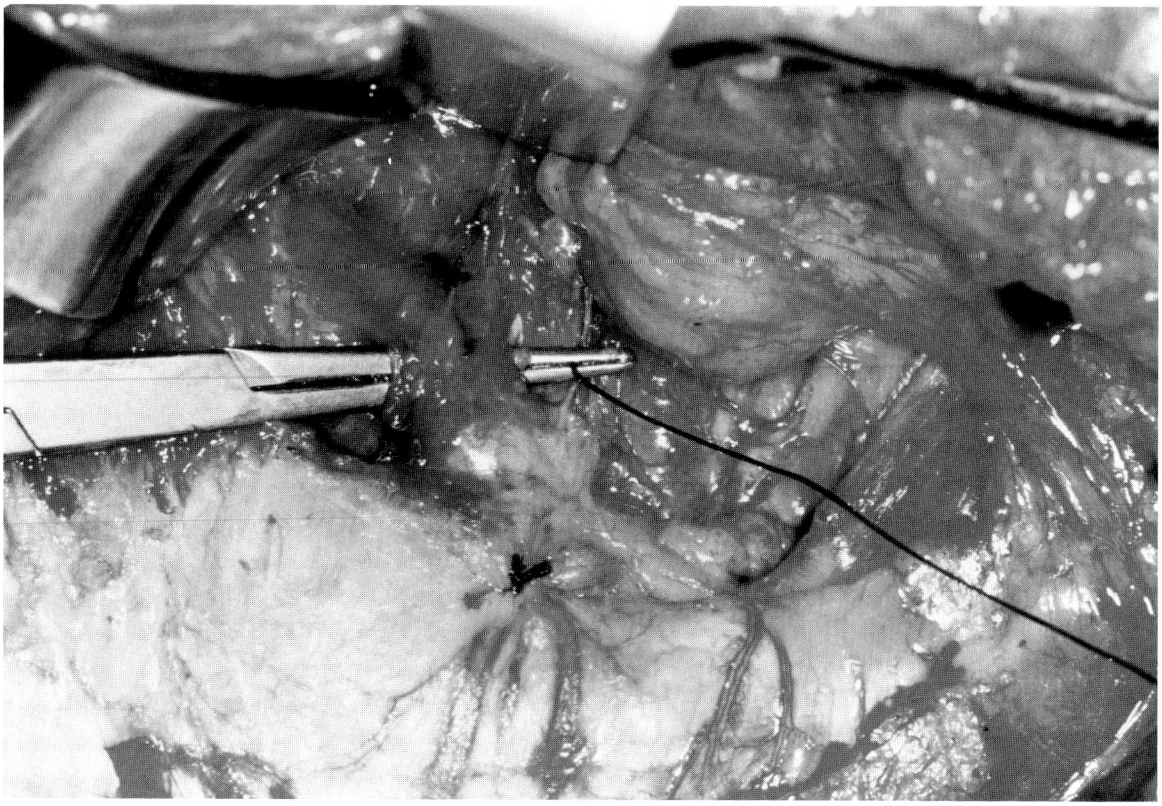

**Fig. 5-27** A suture is placed around the artery to ligate it. This important maneuver helps to minimize blood loss.

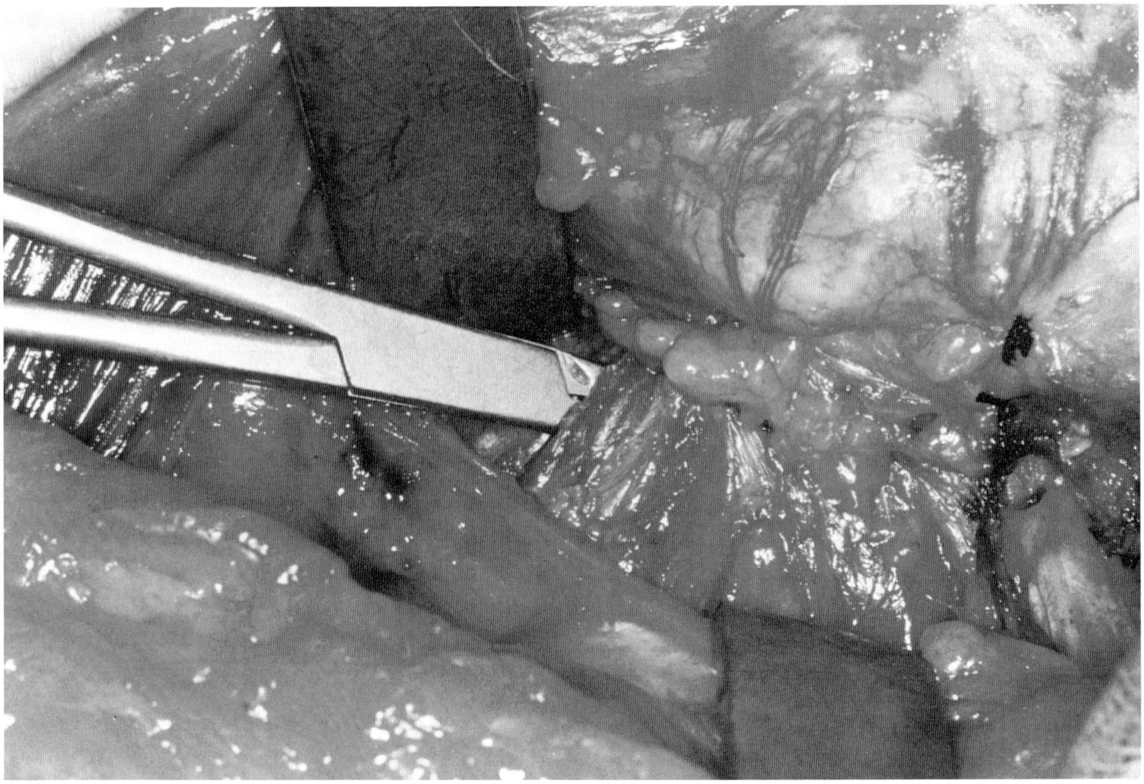

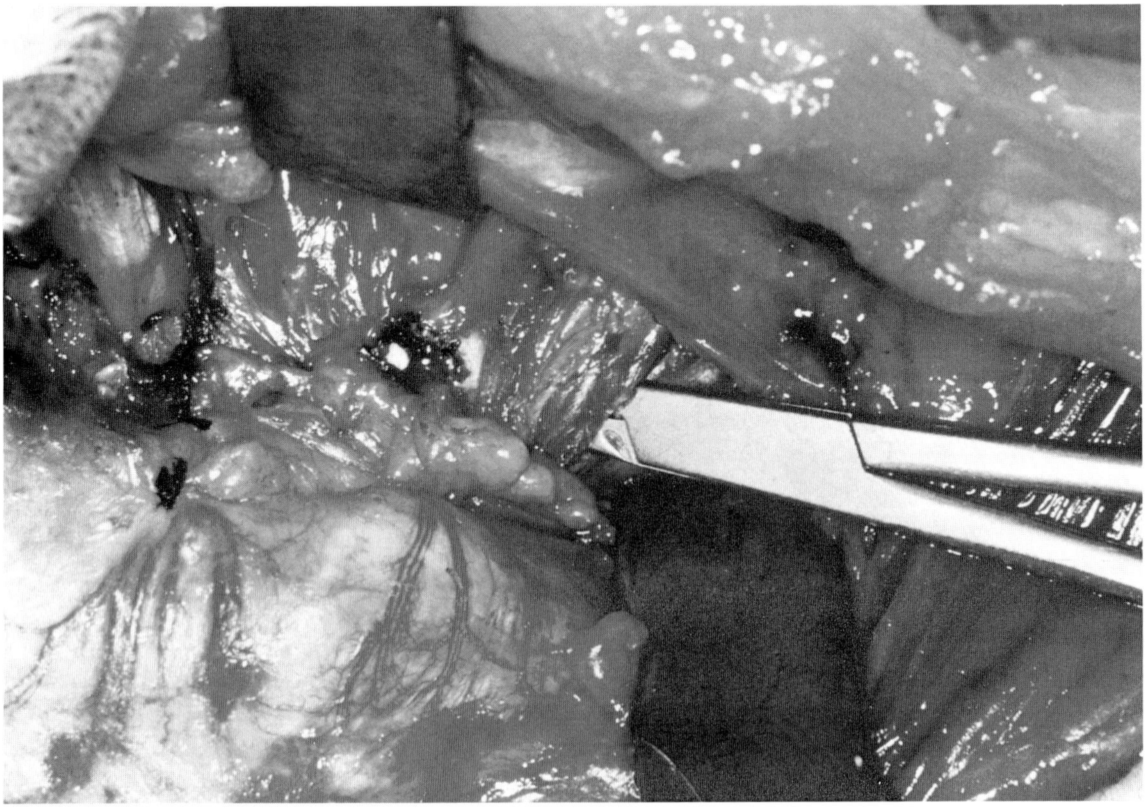

**Figs. 5-28 and 5-29** The piriformis, gamelli, and obturator internys attachments are taken down from the posterior border of the greater trochanter. At the discretion of the surgeon, they can be tagged and reattached at the end of the procedure.

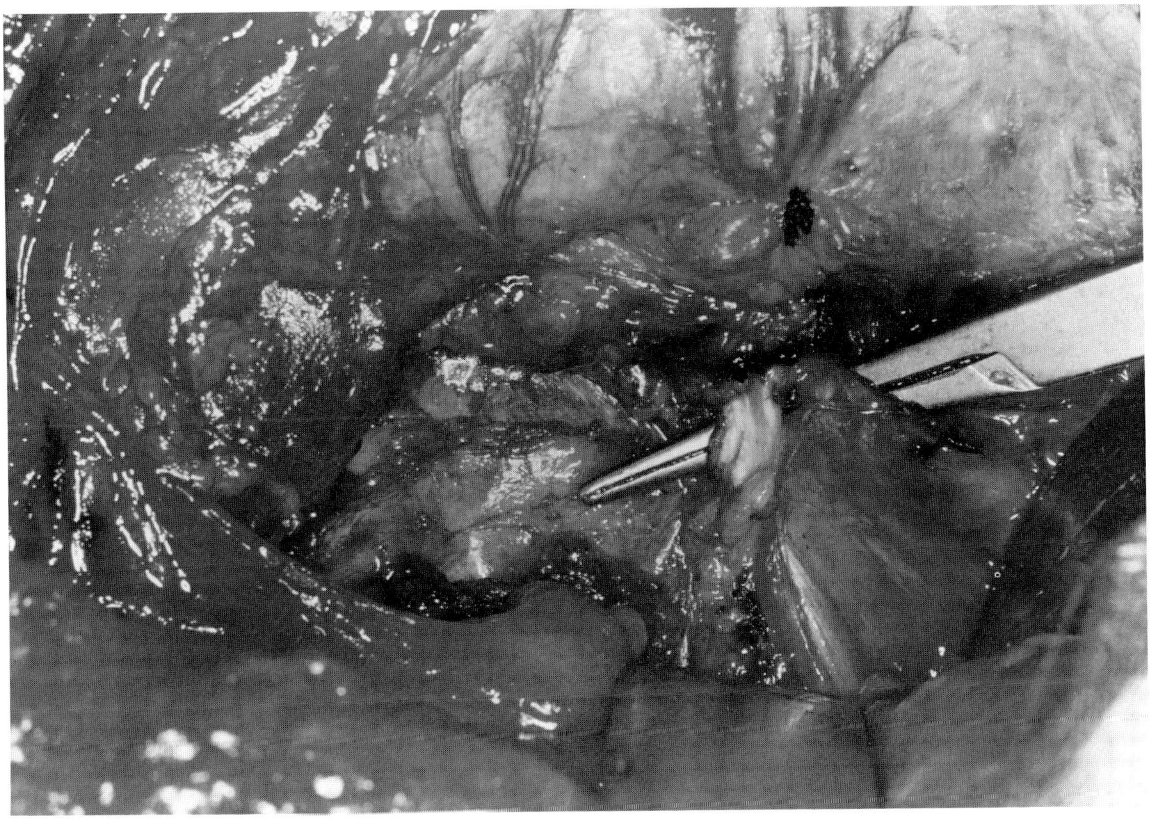

**Fig. 5-30** The obturator enternus tendon is isolated and detached. This is the key maneuver to allow adequate internal rotation and anterior displacement of the femur for exposure to both the acetabulum and proximal femoral canal.

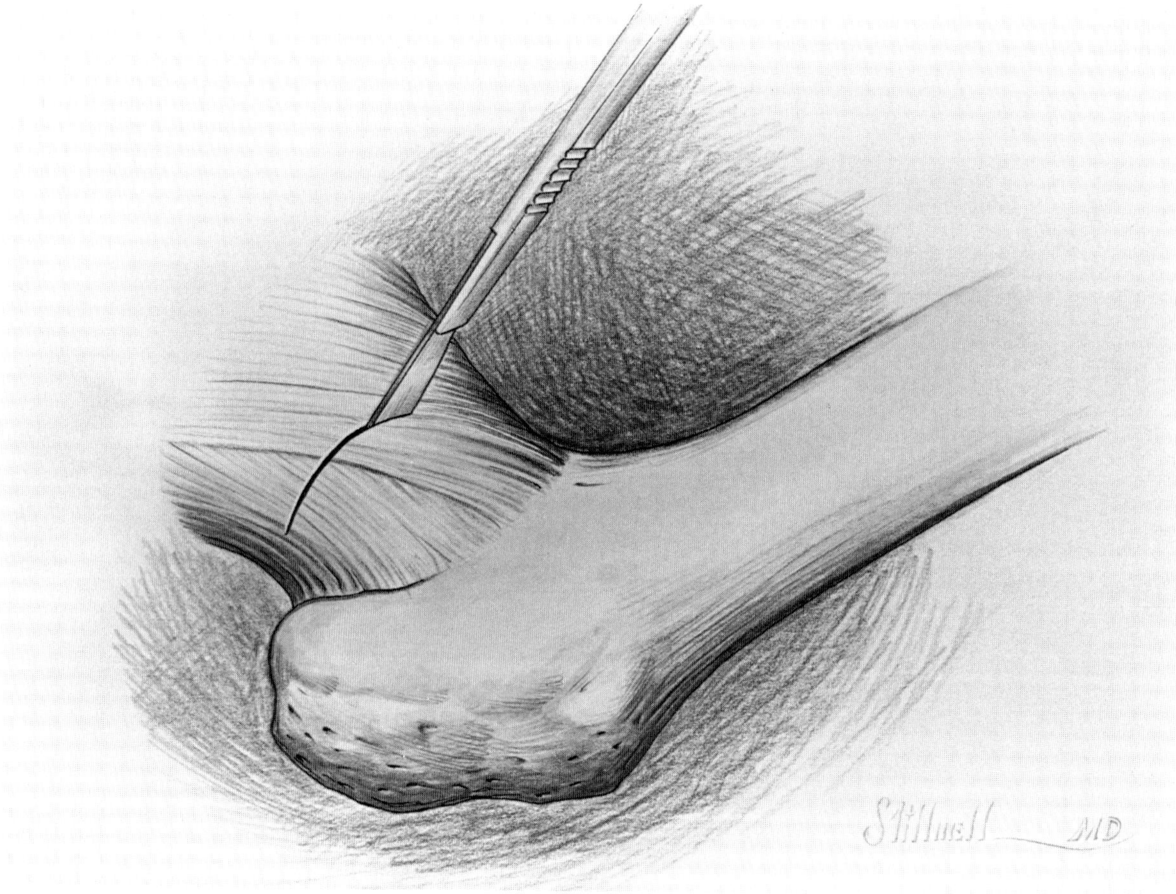

**Fig. 5-31** The capsule can be opened transversely or split as depicted in the following photographs.

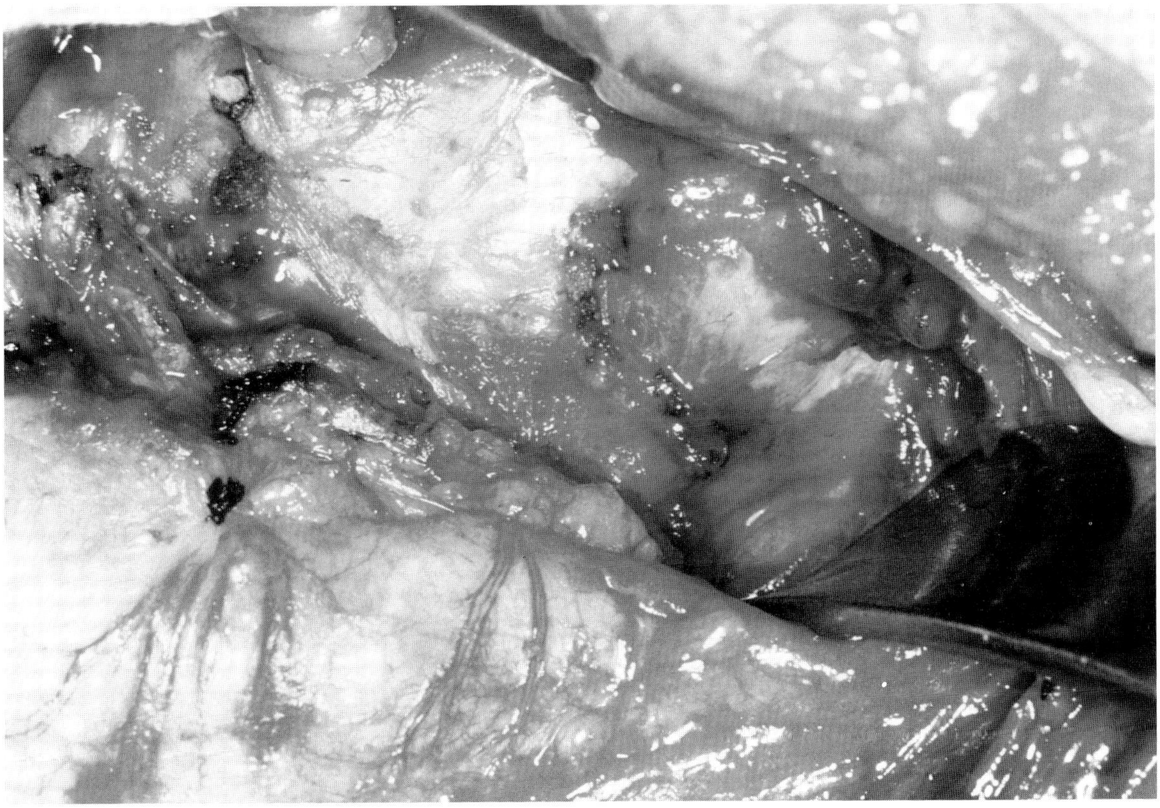

**Fig. 5-32** The joint capsule is exposed with small Hohmann retractors.

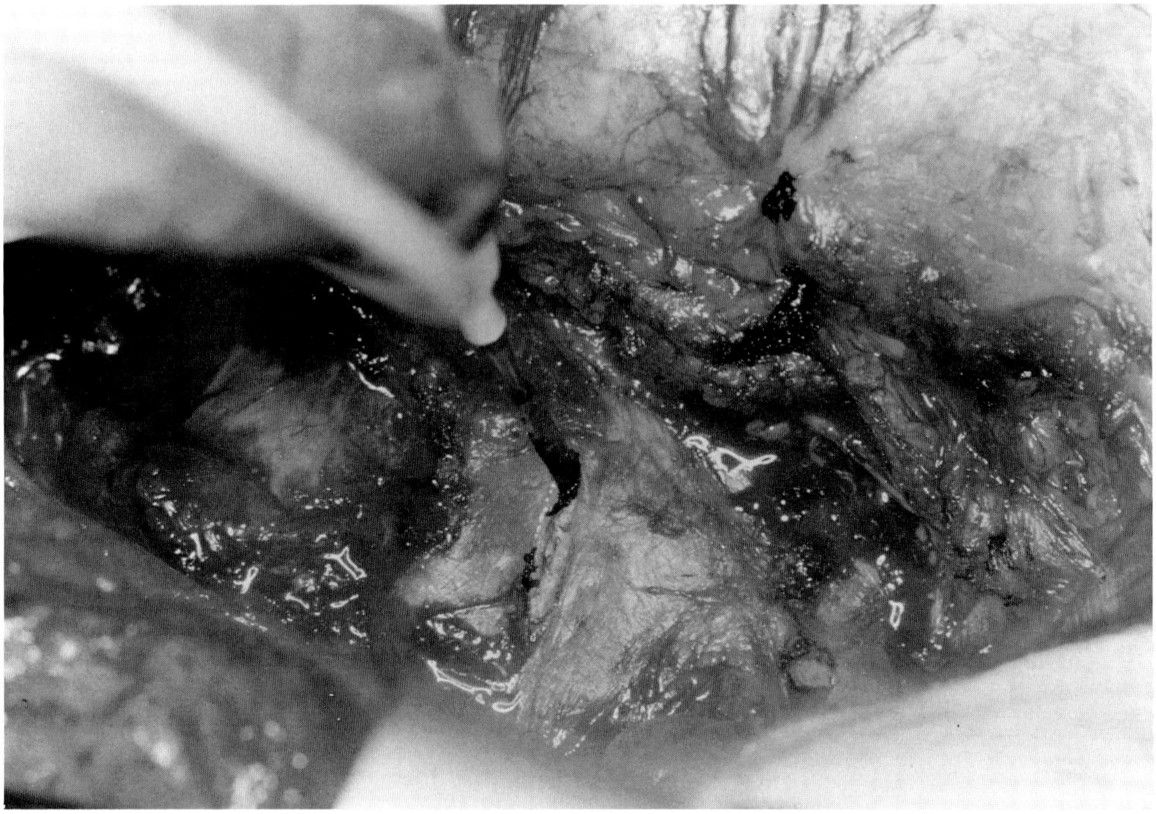

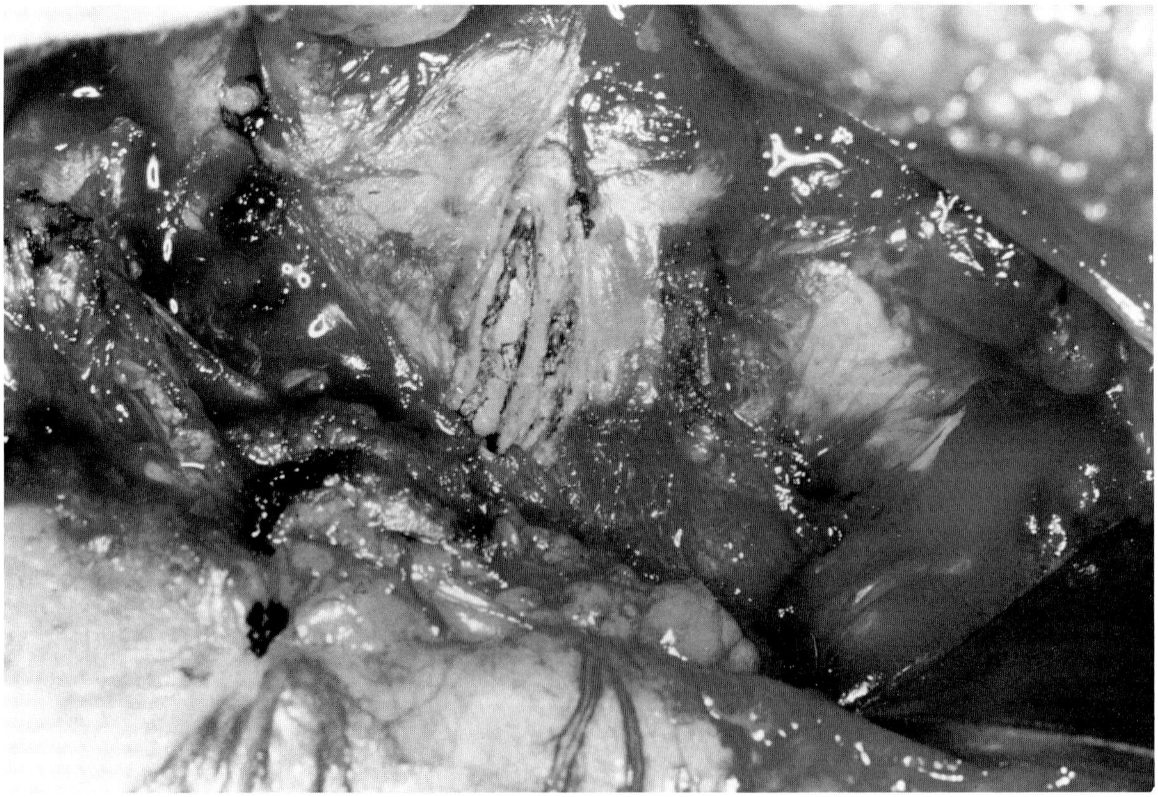

**Figs. 5-33 and 5-34** The superior, posterior, and inferior capsule is well exposed, and a radial cut is made in the posterior capsule.

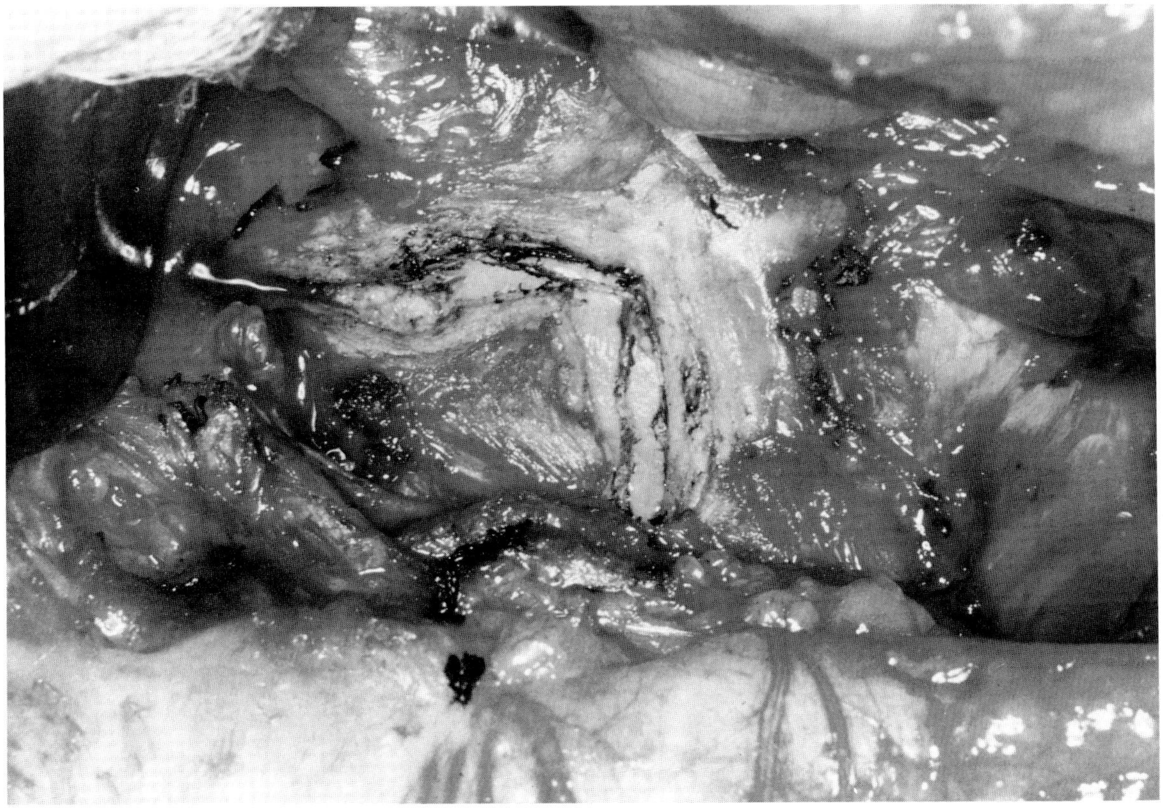

**Fig. 5-35** A triangular portion of inferior capsule is outlined and excised.

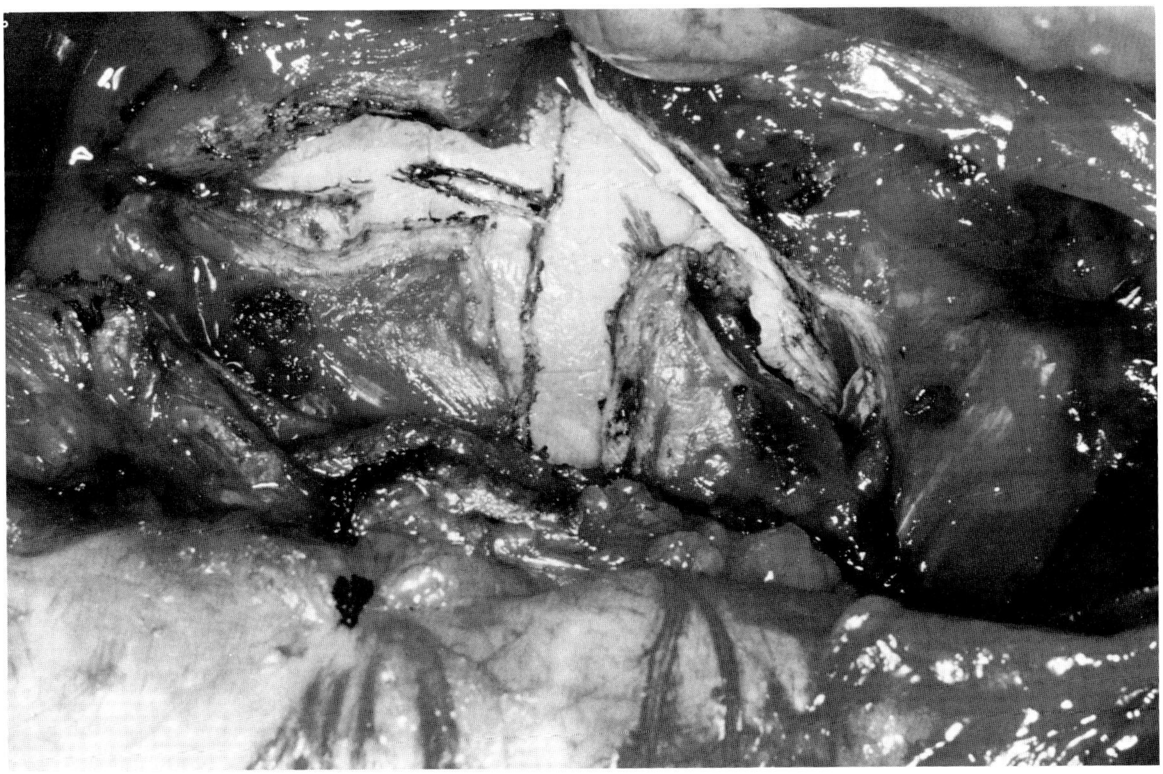

**Fig. 5-36** A triangular portion of superior capsule is outlined and excised.

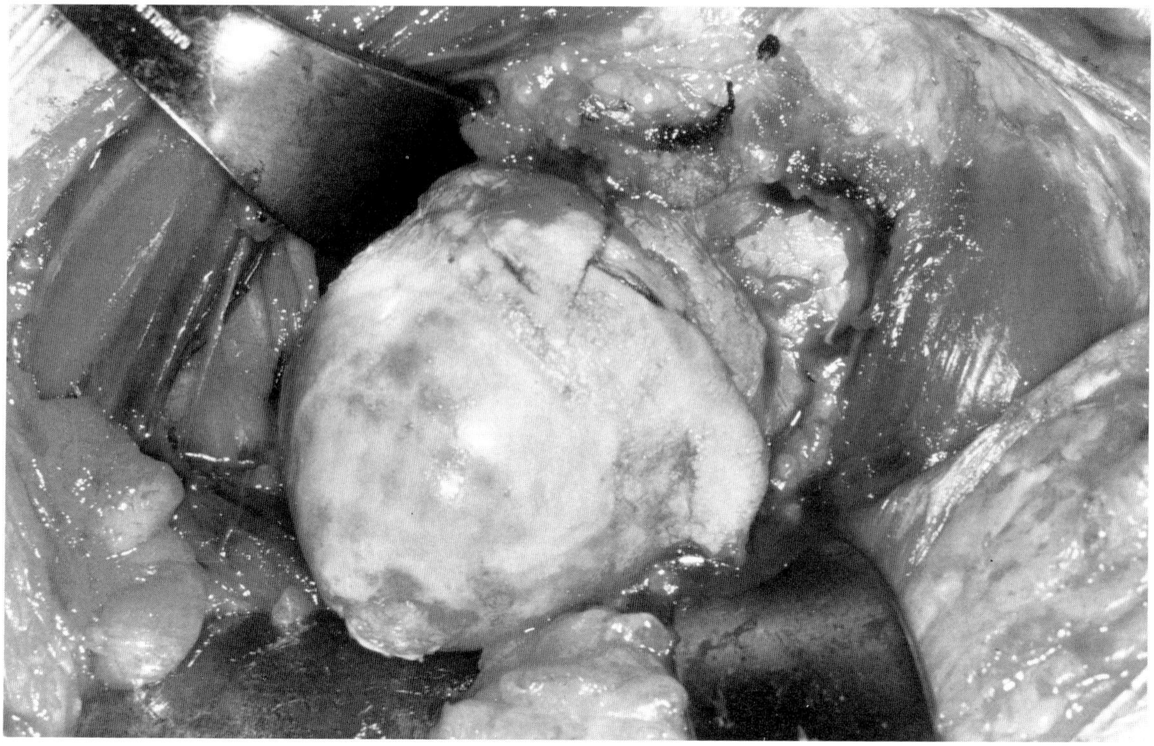

**Fig. 5-37** With flexion, adduction, and internal rotation of the femur, the femoral head is dislocated from the socket.

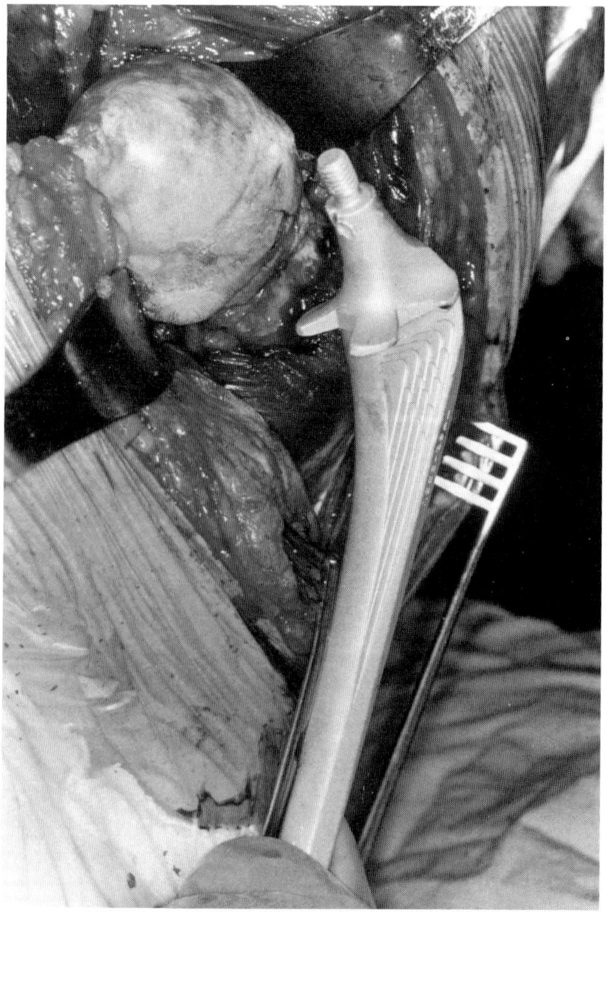

**Fig. 5-38** Using a trial component as a guide, the femoral neck is marked for a non–bridge-burning femoral head resection.

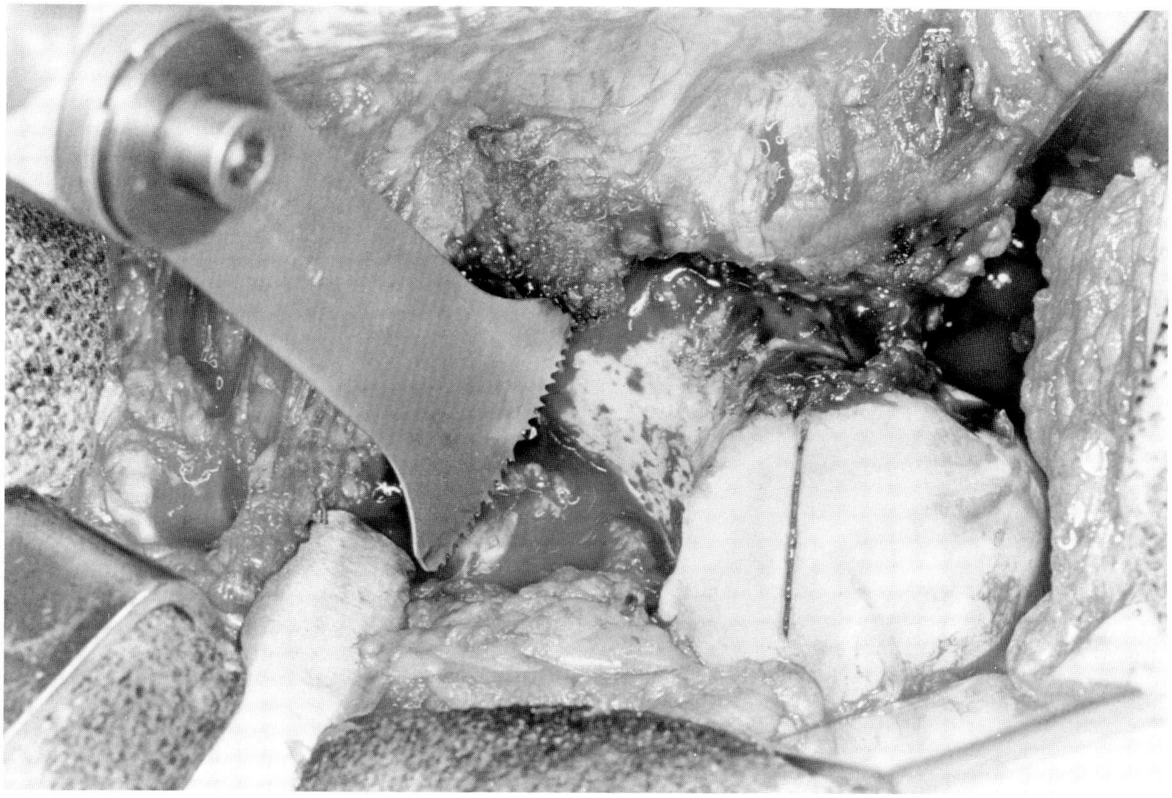

**Fig. 5-39** Having dislocated the hip with internal rotation, the neck is cleared of all capsular tissue to the intertrochanteric line. The neck is osteotomized, taking into account the line of osteotomy ascertained from prepoperative use of x-ray templates.

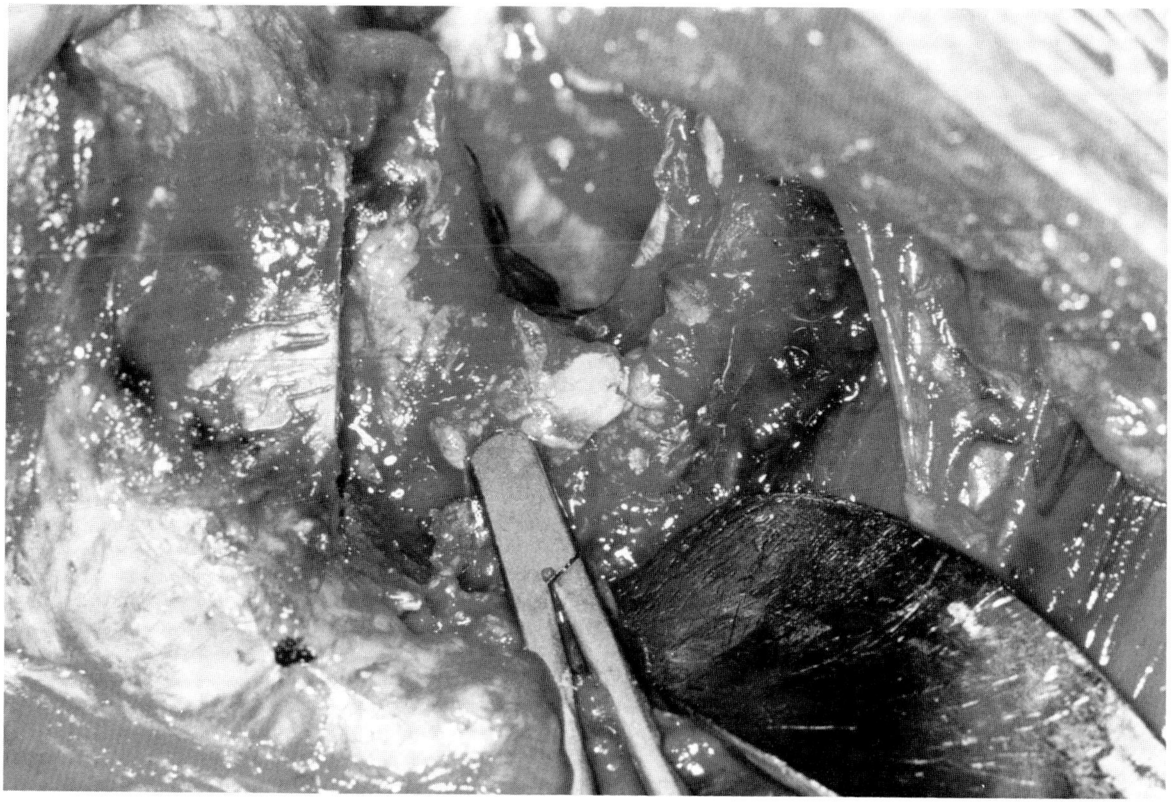

**Fig. 5-40** The anterior capsule is now isolated with a clamp passed outside the capsule from superior to inferior.

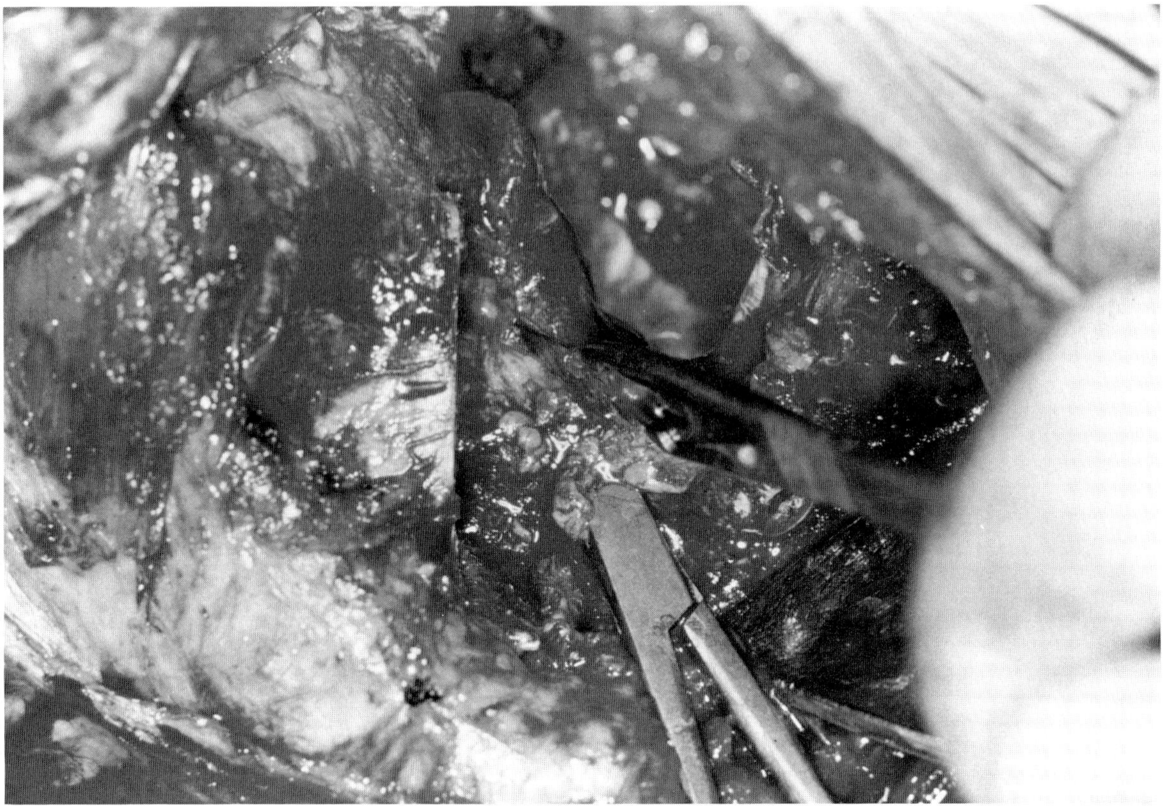

**Fig. 5-41** The anterior capsule is incised from inside the joint.

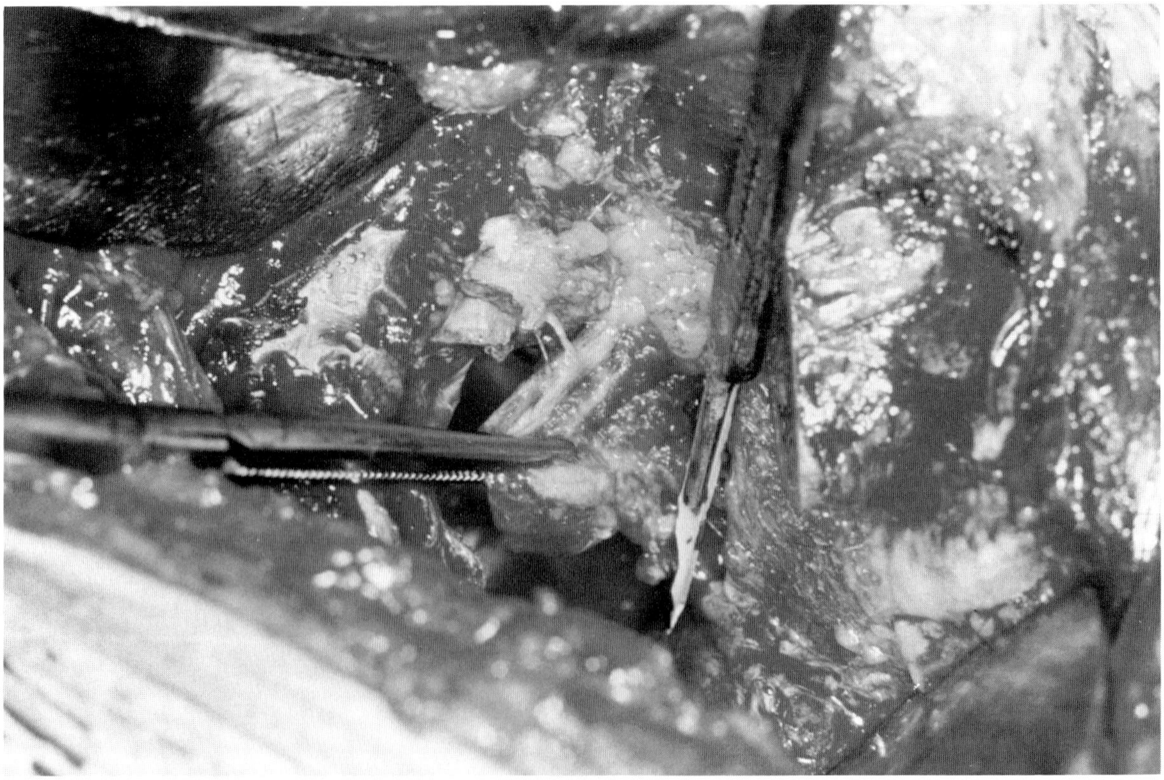

**Fig. 5-42** The incised anterior capsule is resected. This maneuver is also important for optimal exposure of both the acetabulum and proximal femoral canal.

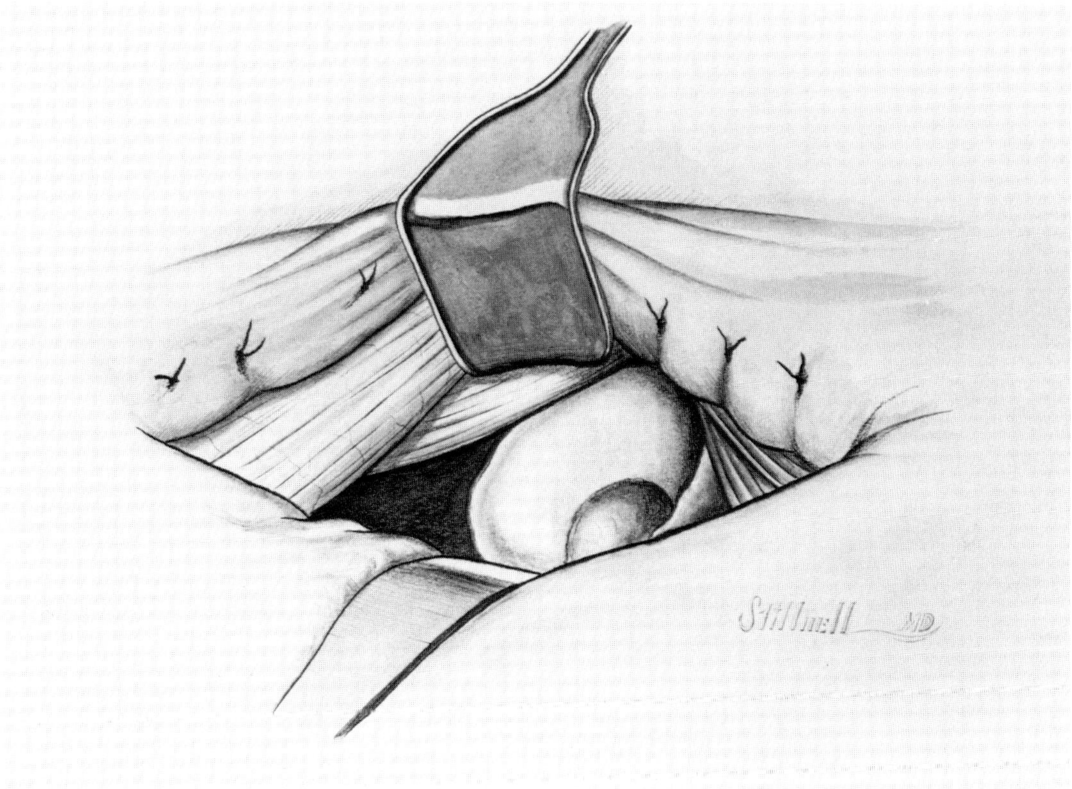

**Fig. 5-43** The acetabulum should now be exposed to allow correct orientation for anterior, posterior, superior, and inferior aspects.

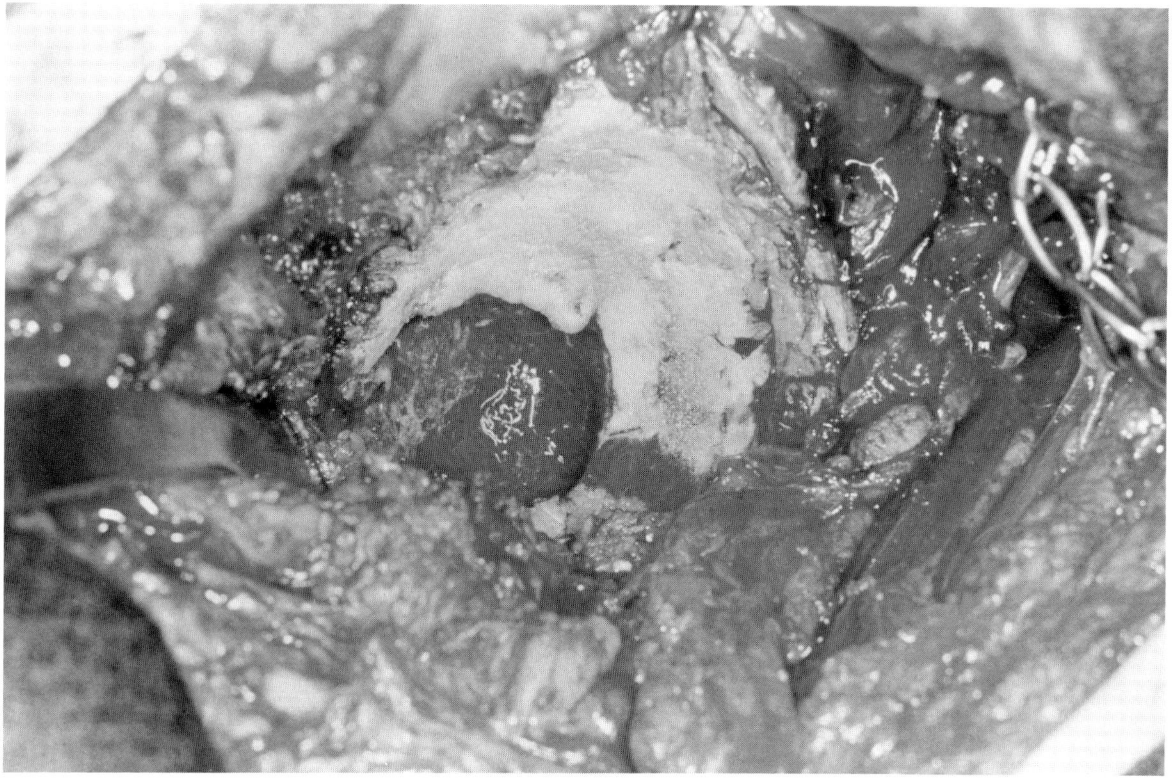

**Fig. 5-44** Acetabular exposure must be meticulous for proper reaming and seating, including a complete excision of the labrum and capsule.

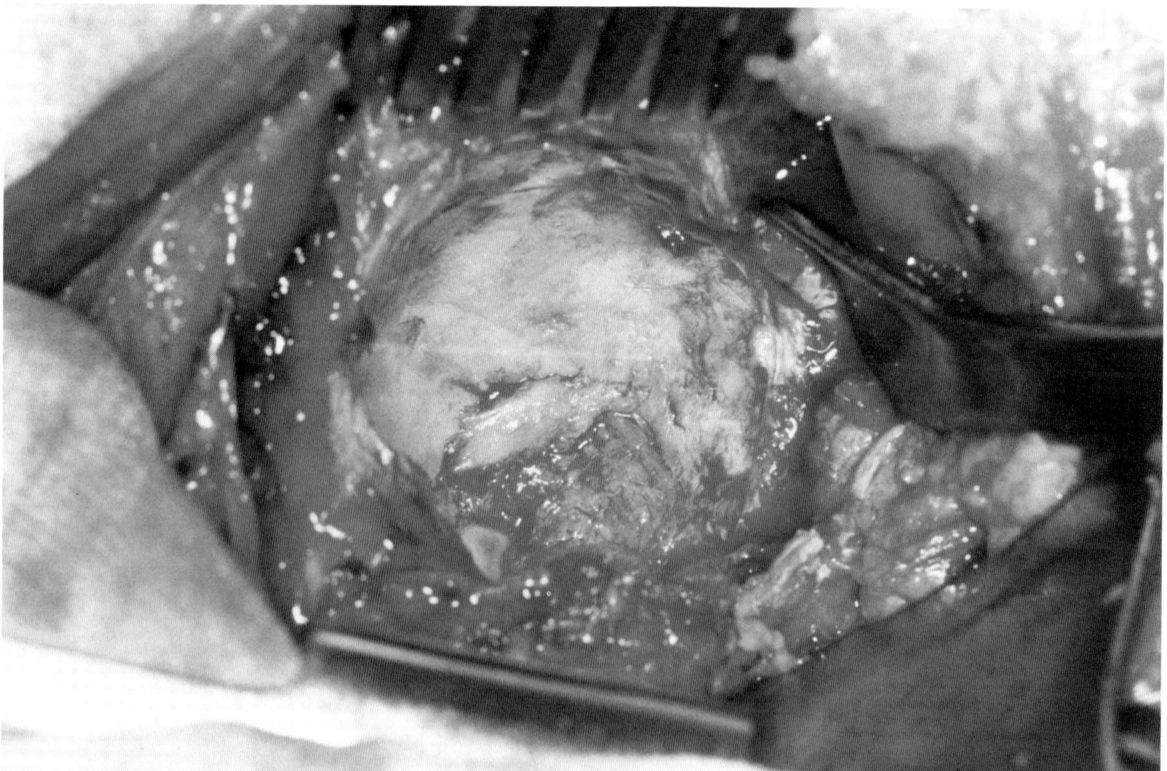

**Fig. 5-45** Excellent acetabular exposure is obtained using a cobra retractor in the acetabular notch, a cobra retractor anteriorly in the psoas sheath, and a self-retaining retractor in the gluteus.

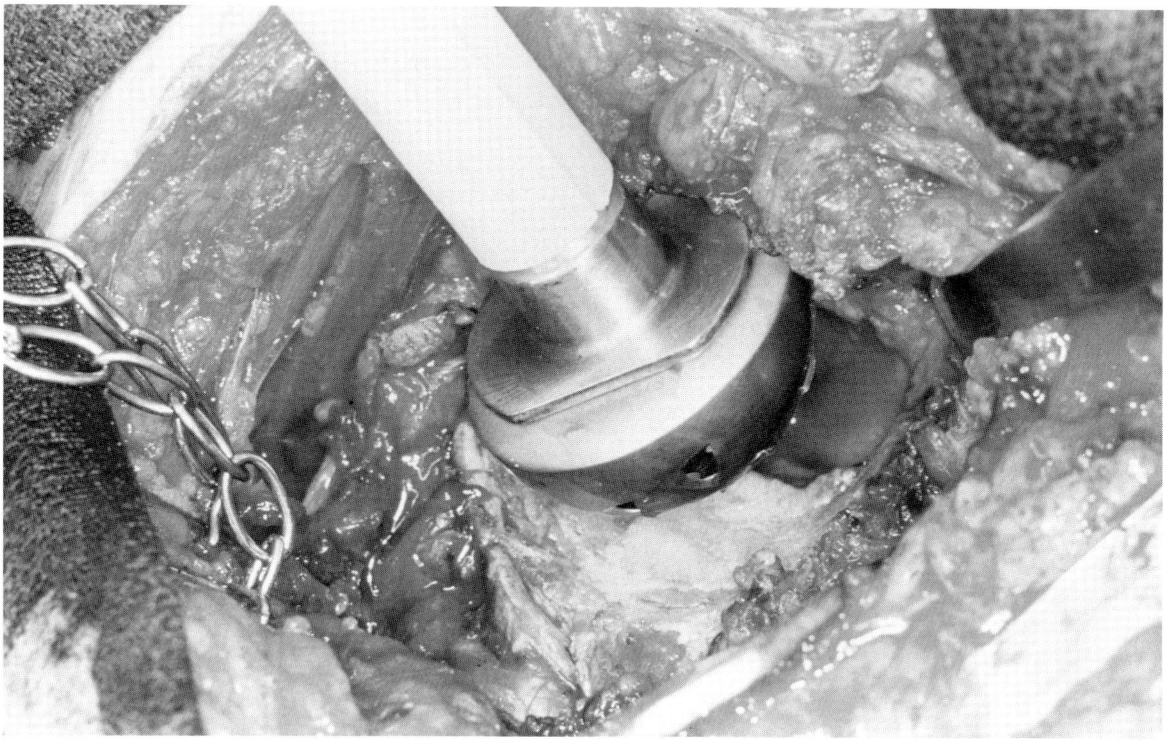

**Fig. 5-46** Acetabular reamers are exact size duplicates of the prosthesis. Thus, for an adequate press fit, reaming must be in the desired position of seating: 45° abduction and 20° flexion. Low profile and +5-mm-deep cups are used.

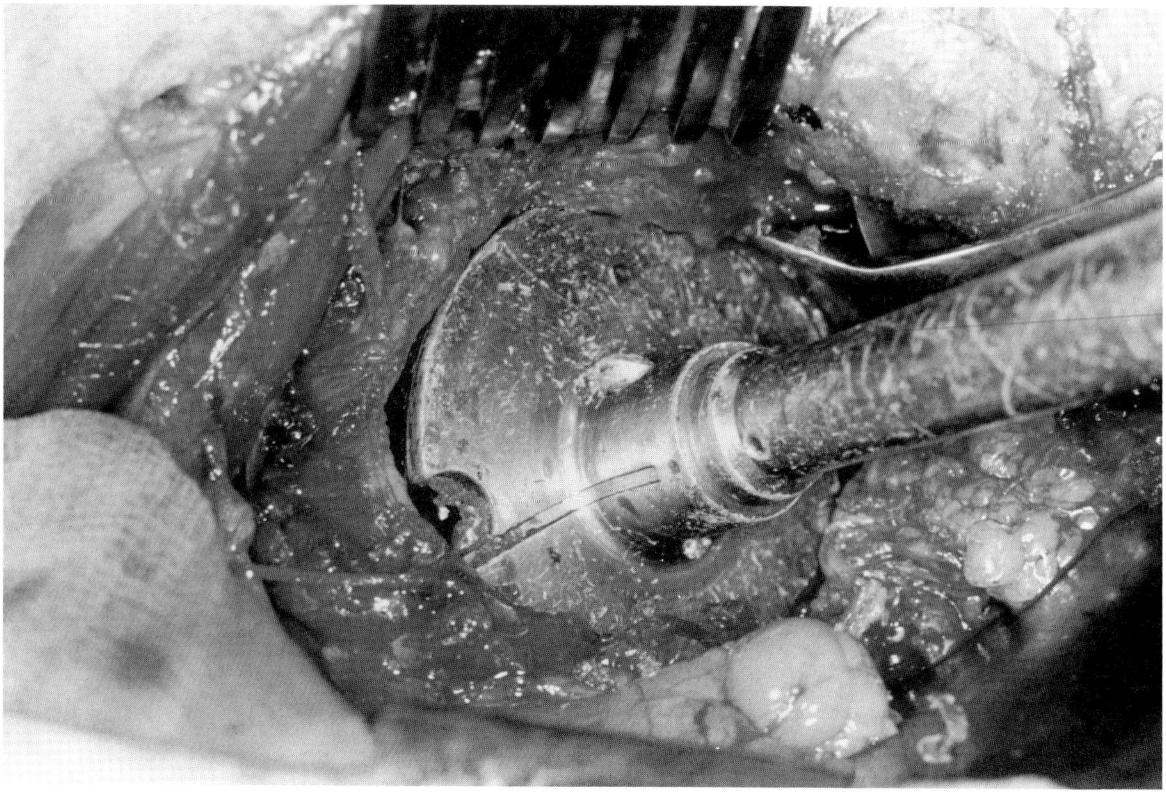

**Fig. 5-47** Acetabular reamers are introduced, starting with the diameter of the resected femoral head and progressing to larger sizes until a spherical ream is obtained.

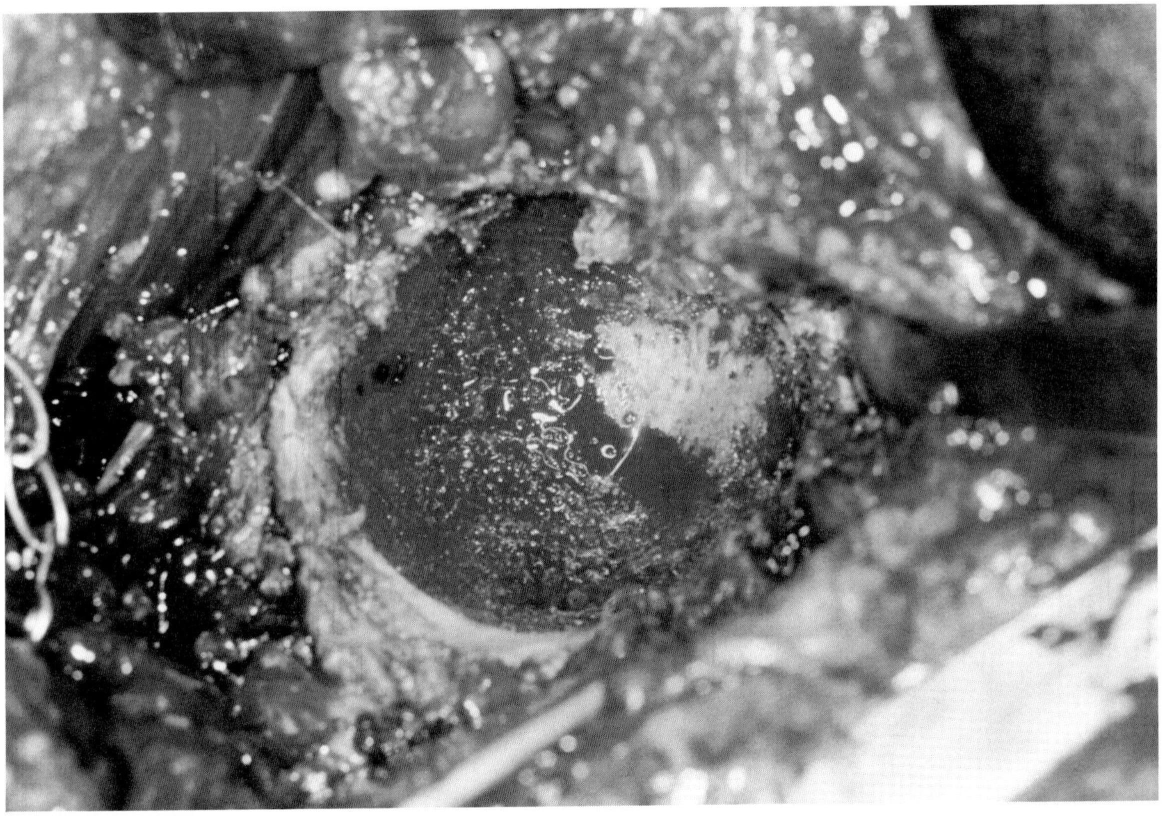

**Fig. 5-48** The appearance of a reamed acetabulum prior to lavage and implantation.

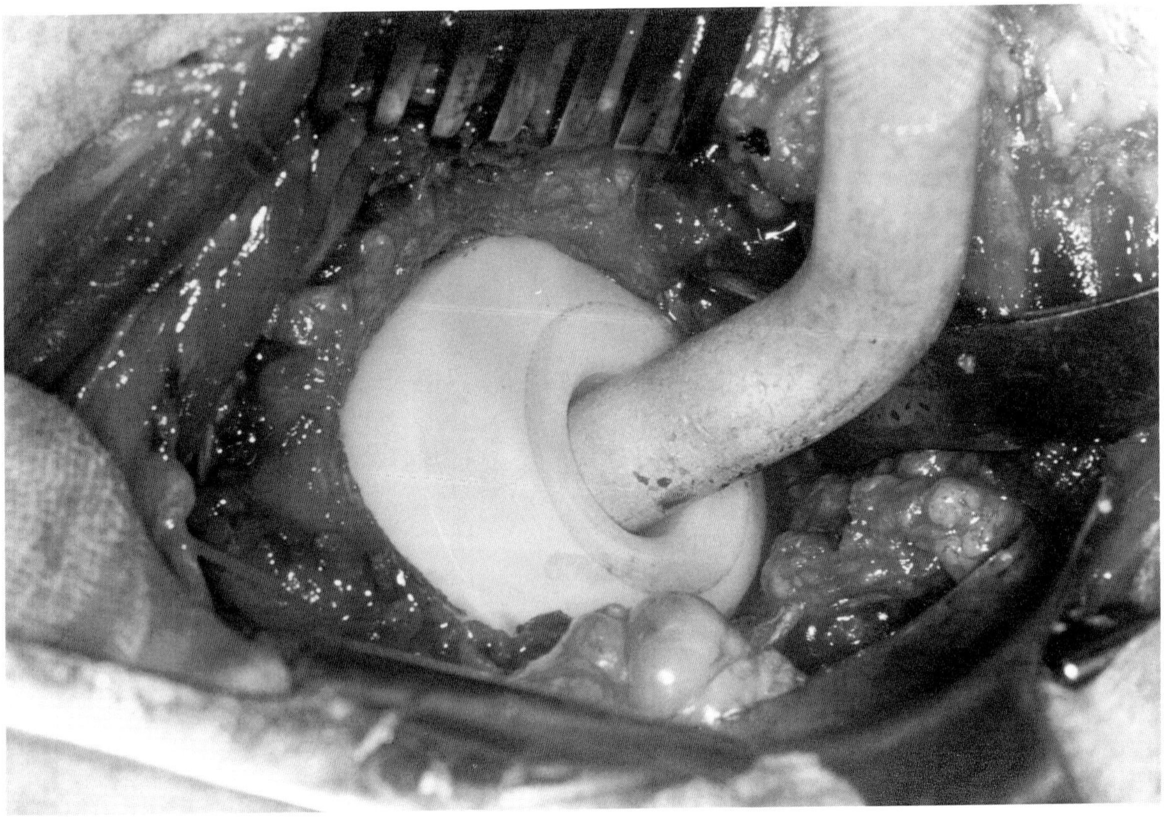

**Fig. 5-49** The trial bipolar sizer is inserted into the acetabulum.

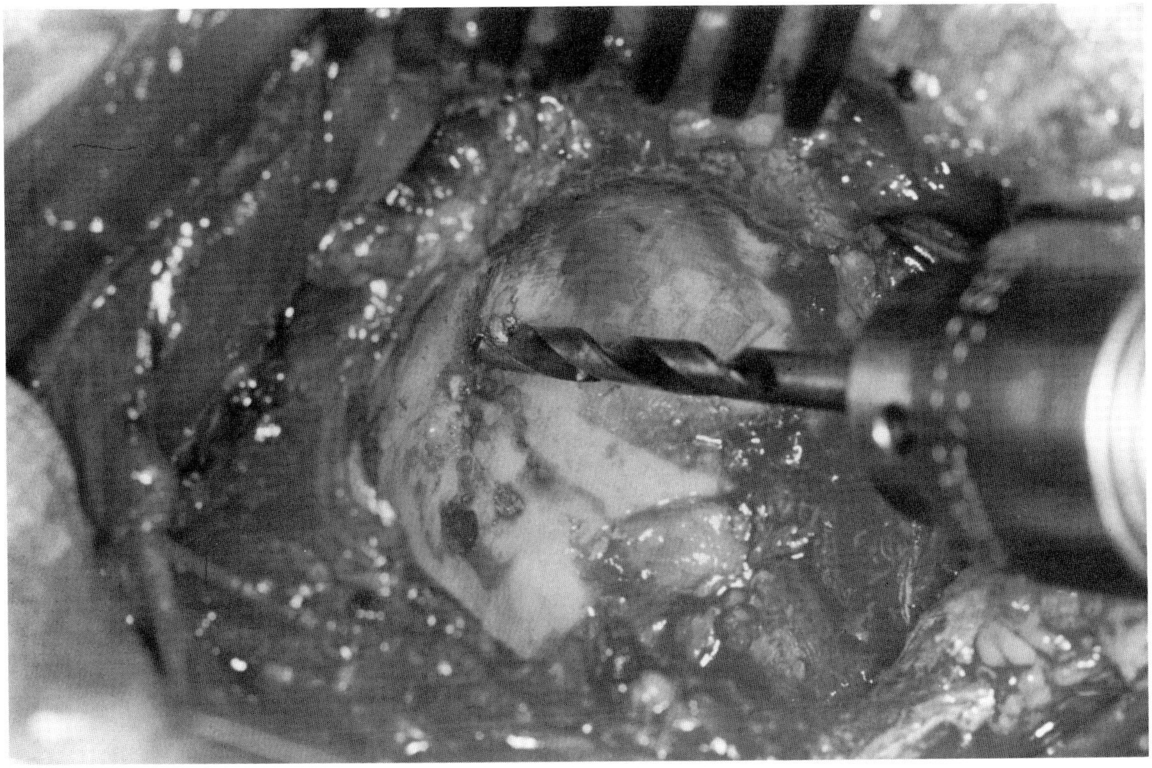

**Fig. 5-50** Multiple 3-mm drill holes are made into any residual areas of eburnated bone in the socket to stimulate bleeding and allow for the potential of fibrous metaplasia at the interface between the shell and the patient's socket.

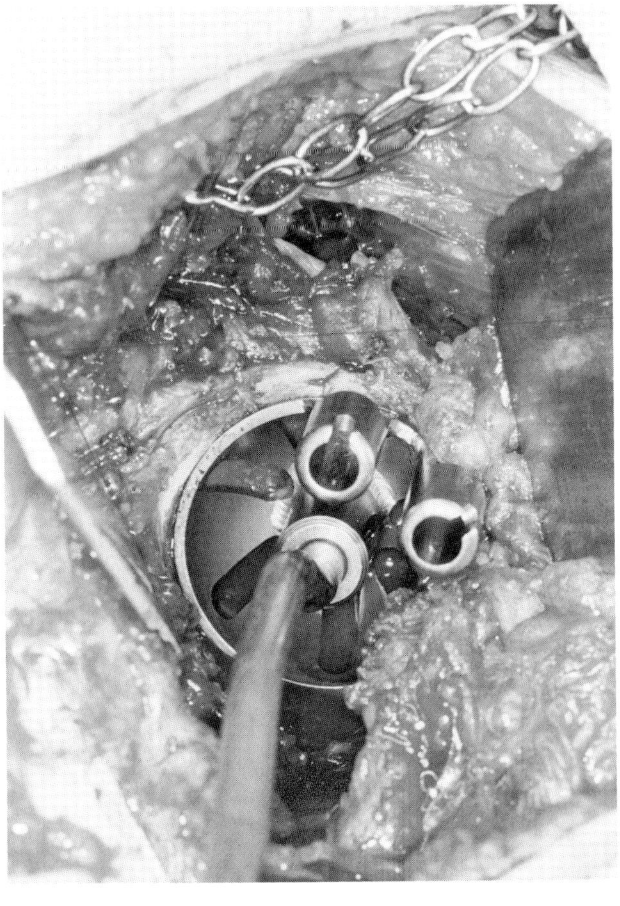

**Fig. 51** The drill guide is positioned in the reamed socket, and holes for the pegs are made where bone stock permits.

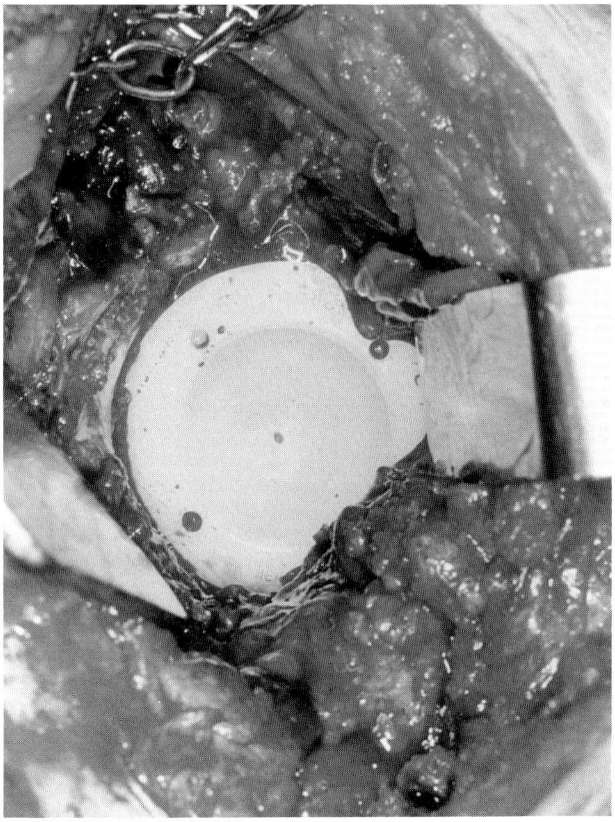

**Fig. 5-52** The seating of the acetabular component is accomplished with careful inspection as to the stability of the cup.

**Figs. 5-53 and 5-54** The gouge is inserted into the trochanteric bed to permit lateralization of the femoral reamers and rasps and to minimize the chance of varus placement of the femoral component.

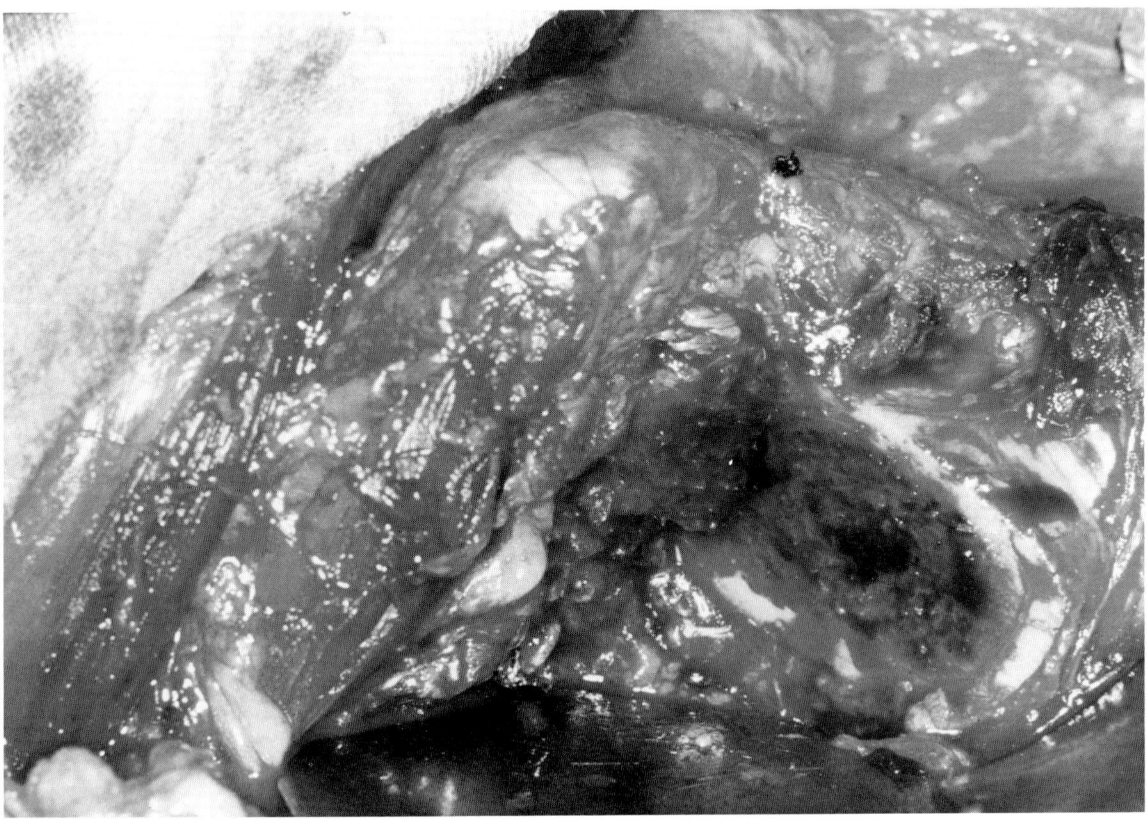

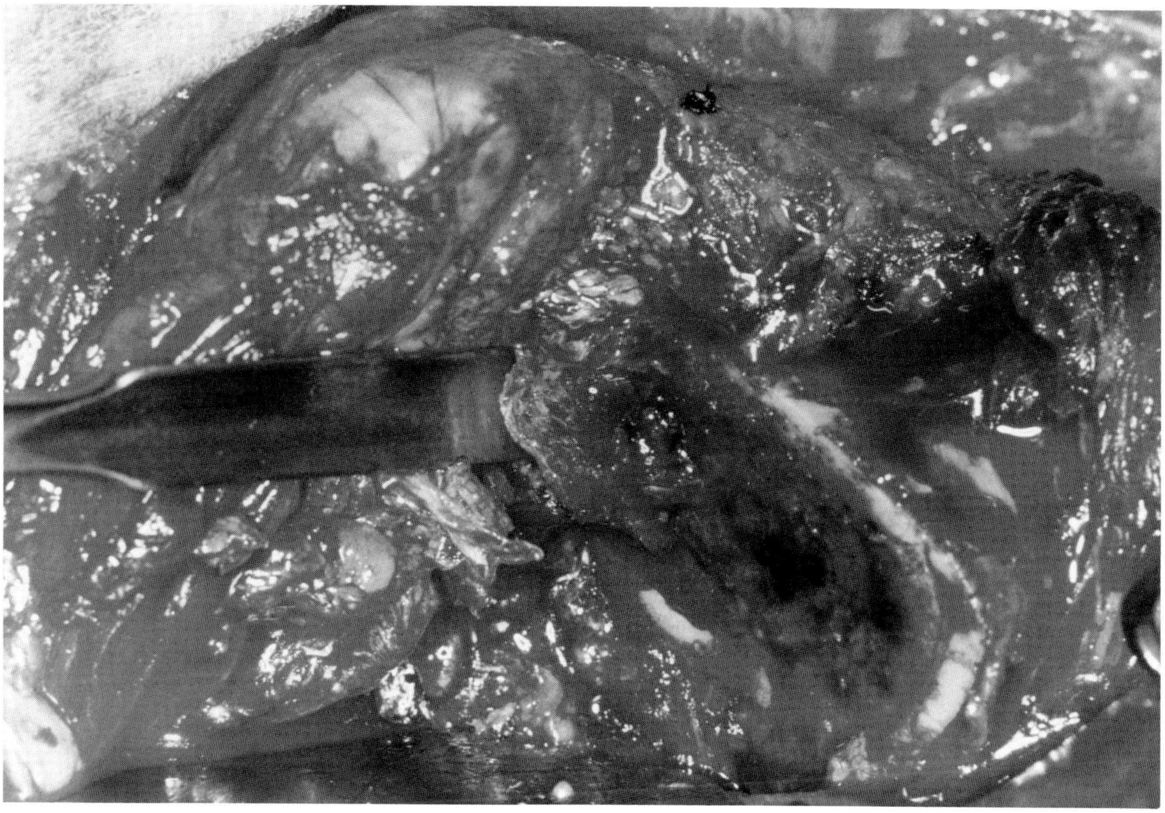

Fig. 5-54

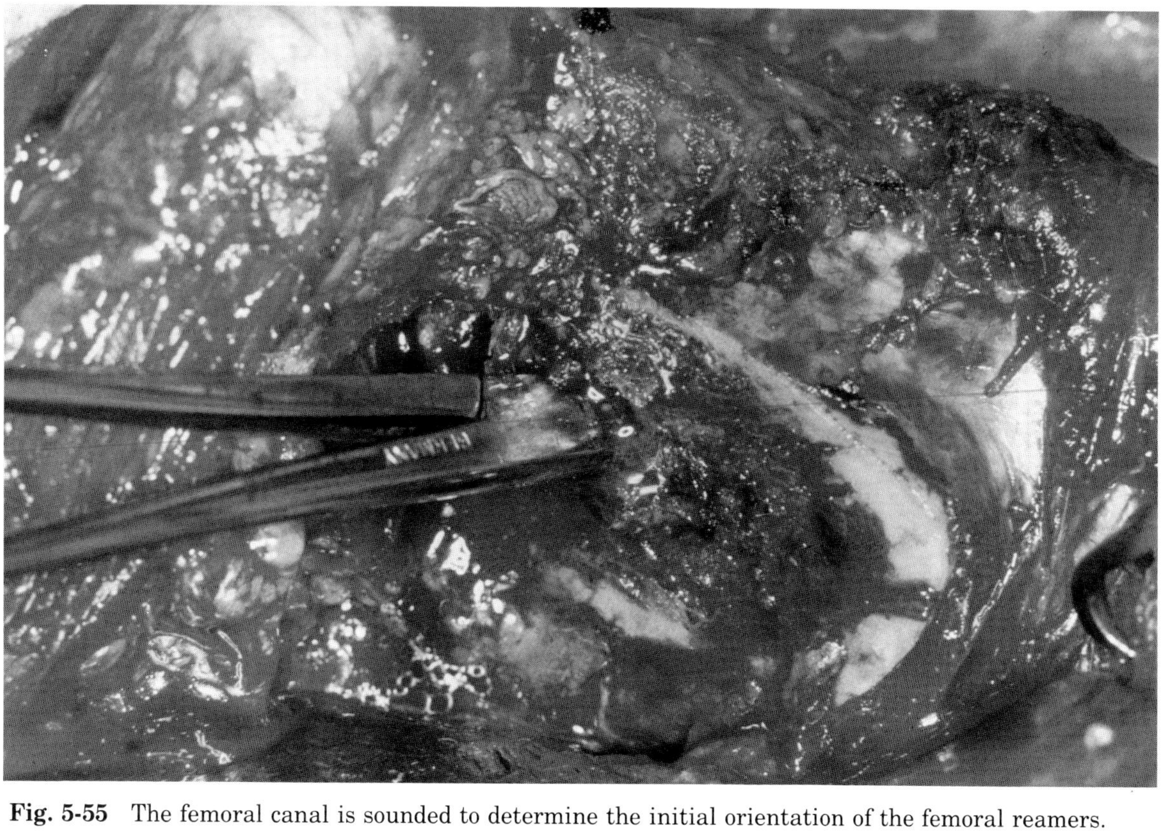

Fig. 5-55 The femoral canal is sounded to determine the initial orientation of the femoral reamers.

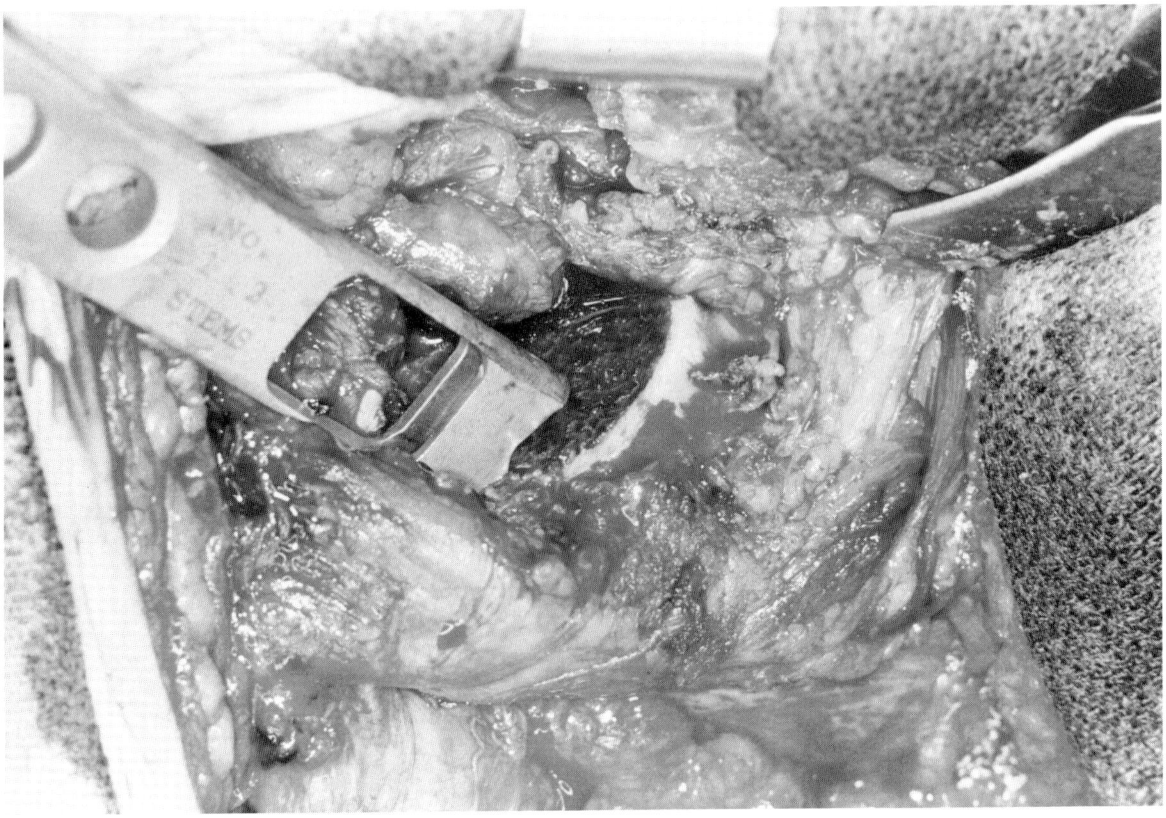

**Fig. 5-56** The width of the femoral canal having been sized with x-ray overlays, the appropriate box chisel is selected to open the neck of the femur into the greater trochanter.

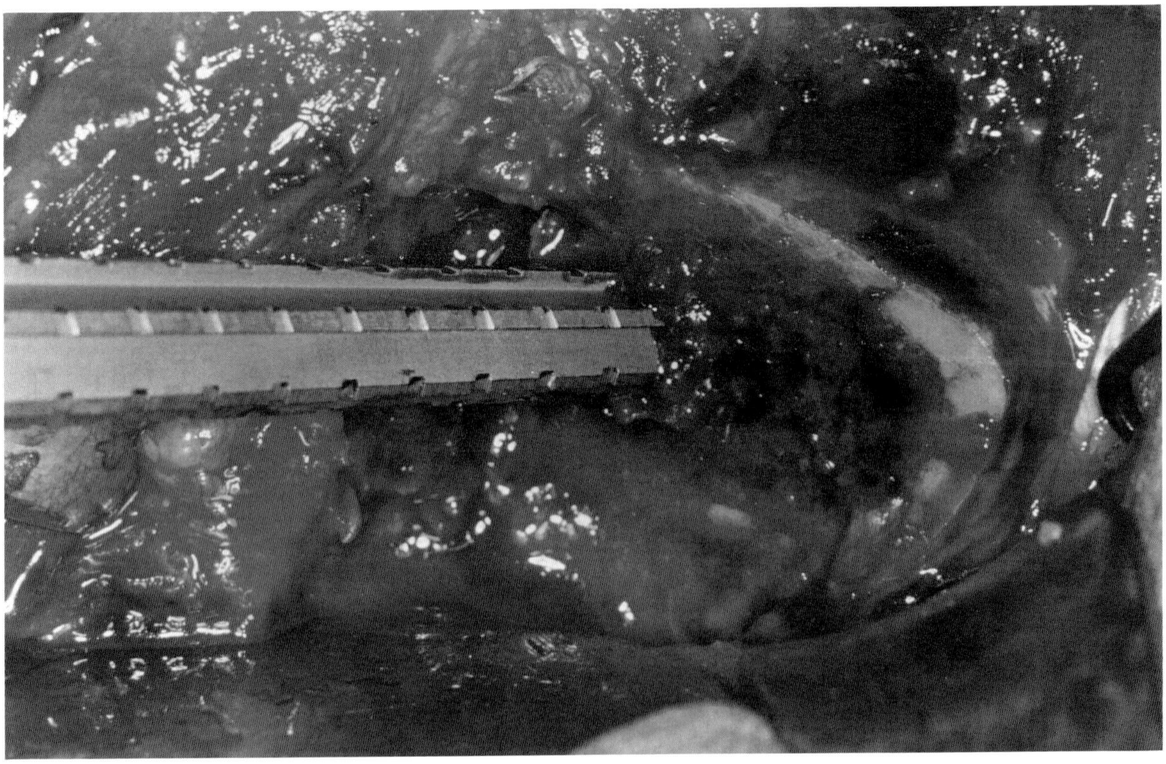

**Fig. 5-57** Sequential femoral reamers are introduced, starting with the smallest size and progressing to the size that corresponds to the diameter of the isthmus of the femoral canal.

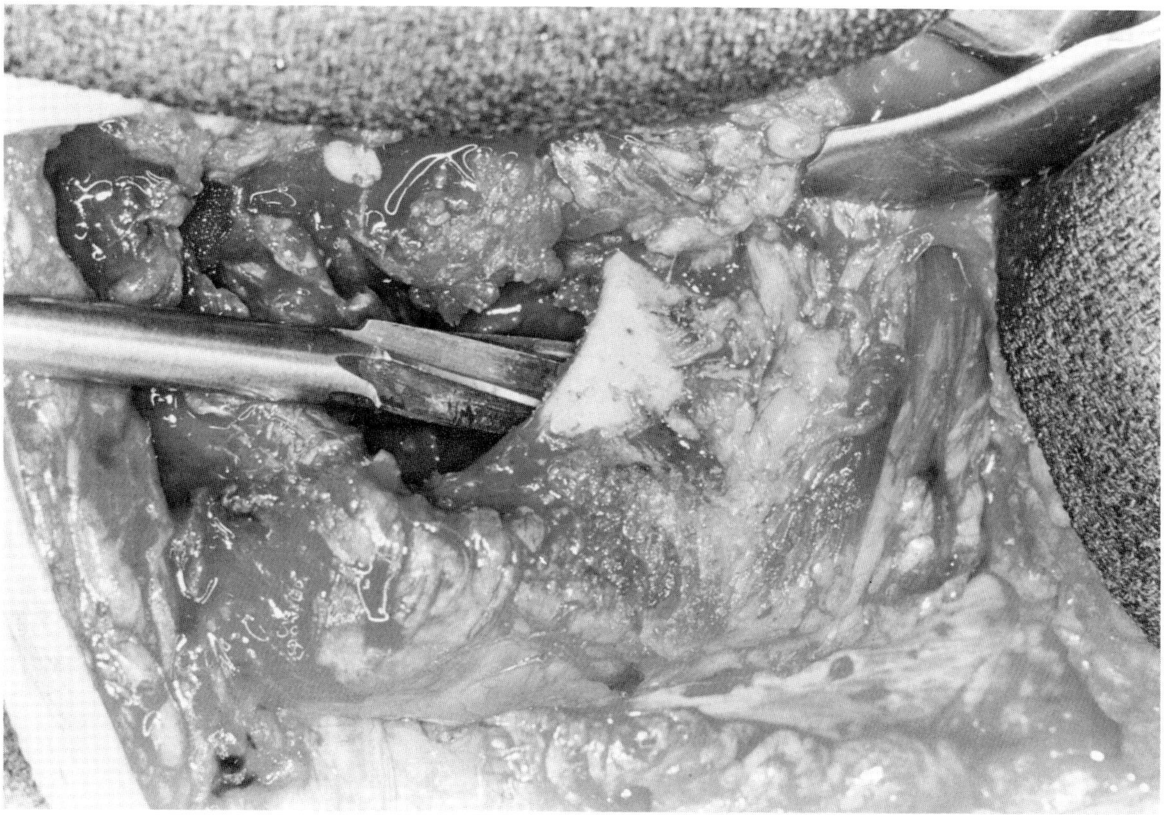

**Fig. 5-58** The rasp corresponding to the intended femoral component is attached to the inserting handle.

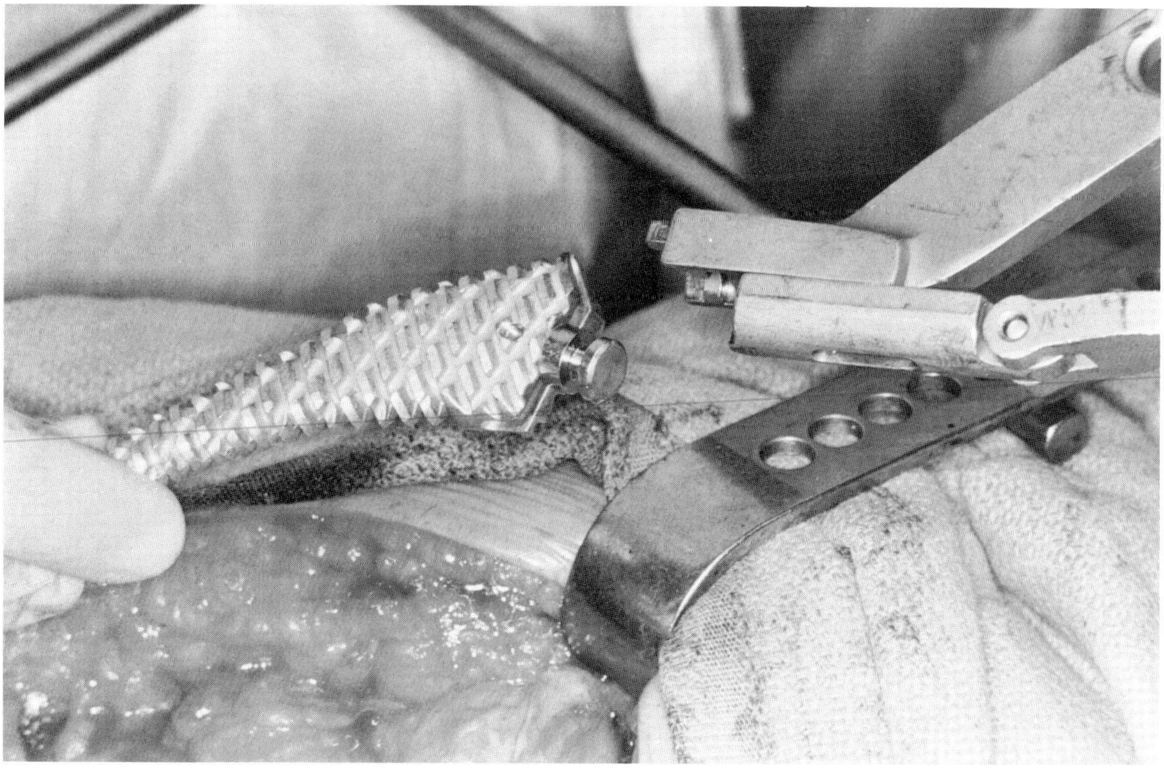

**Fig. 5-59** The femoral rasp is inserted straight down the shaft without the back and forth reaming utilized in cemented arthroplasty. Should the rasp enter too easily, the next size larger should be used until a tight fit of the rasp is achieved.

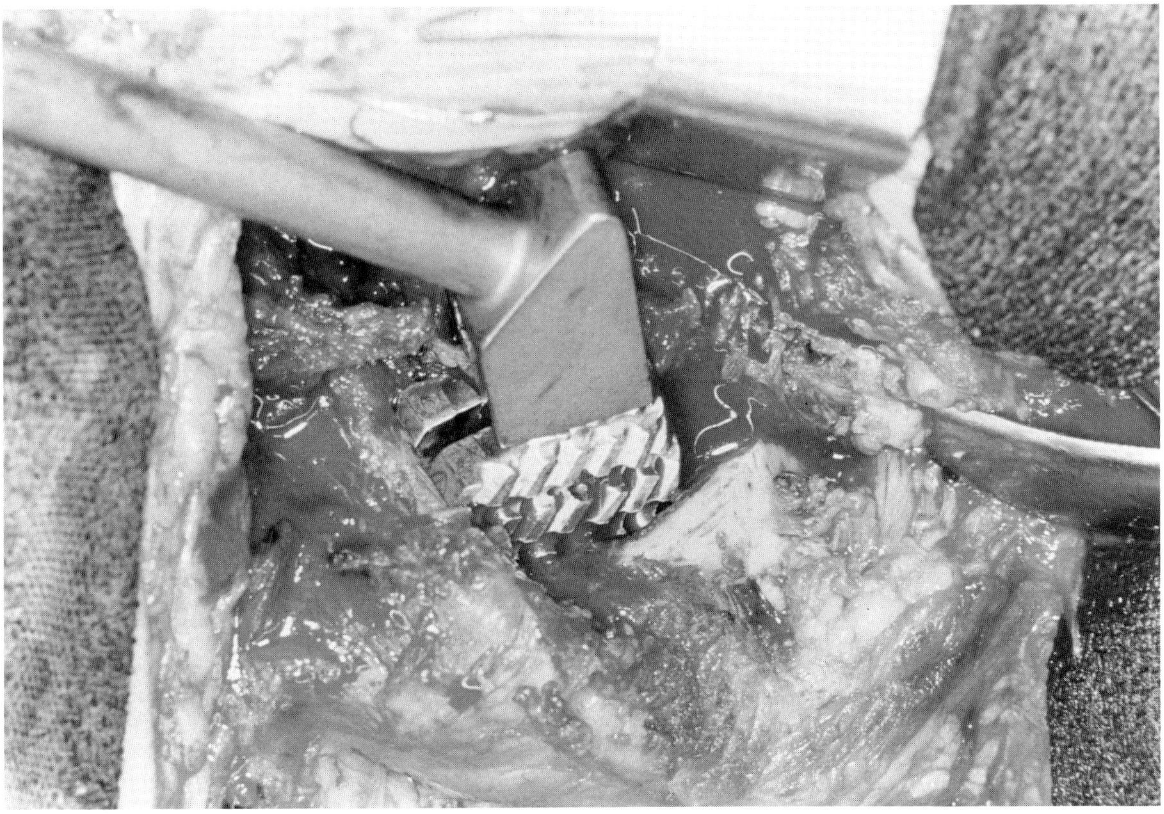

**Fig. 5-60** Should the femoral rasp not advance to the calcar, it is usually due to a narrow isthmus. Kuntscher reamers corresponding to the width of the tip of the femoral stem should be used freely to avoid iatrogenic femoral fracture.

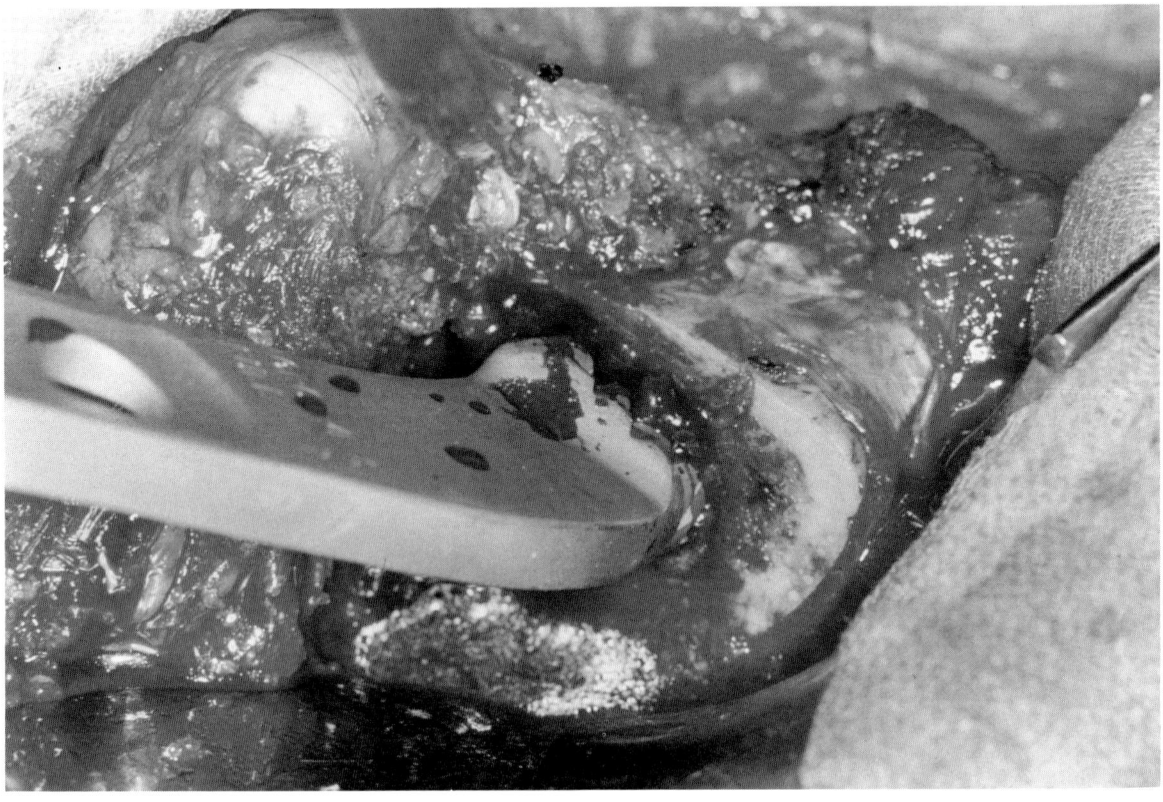

**Fig. 5-61** The femoral reamer is inserted to the position of the resected femoral neck.

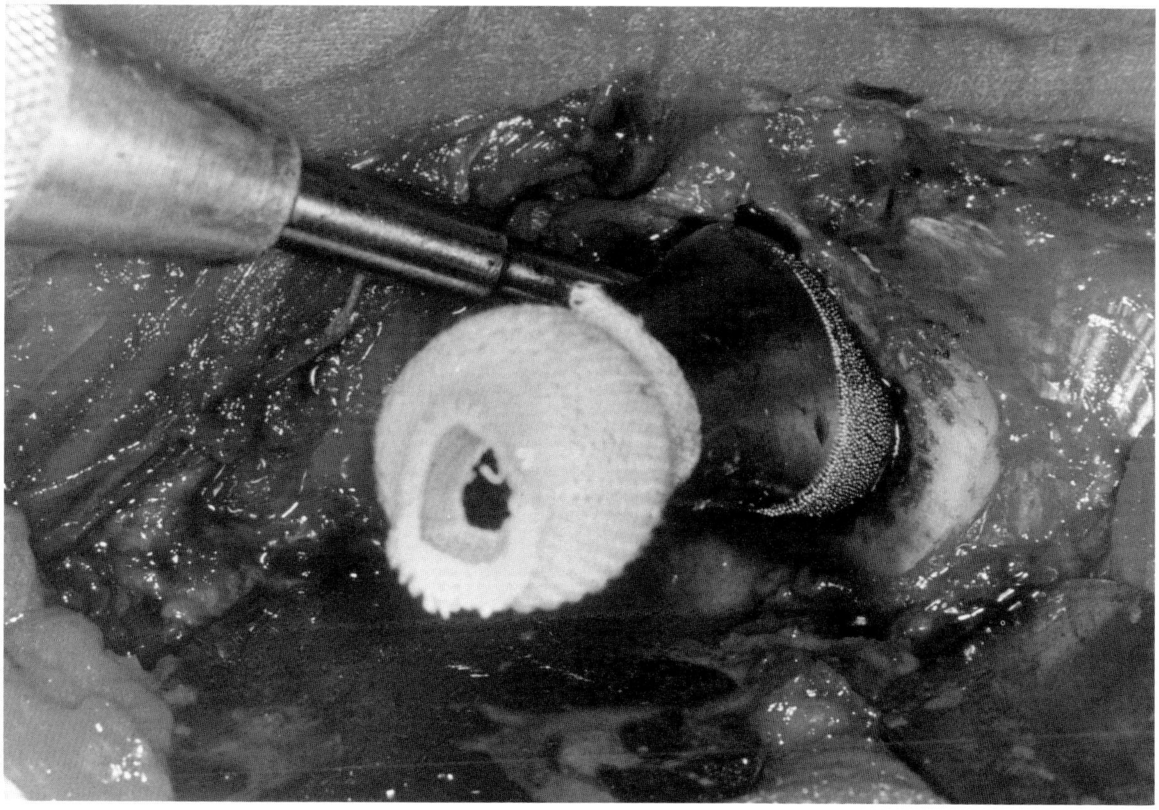

**Fig. 5-62** If a cementless press-fit prosthesis has been chosen, it is introduced after proper preparation of the femur according to the individual demands of the system being used.

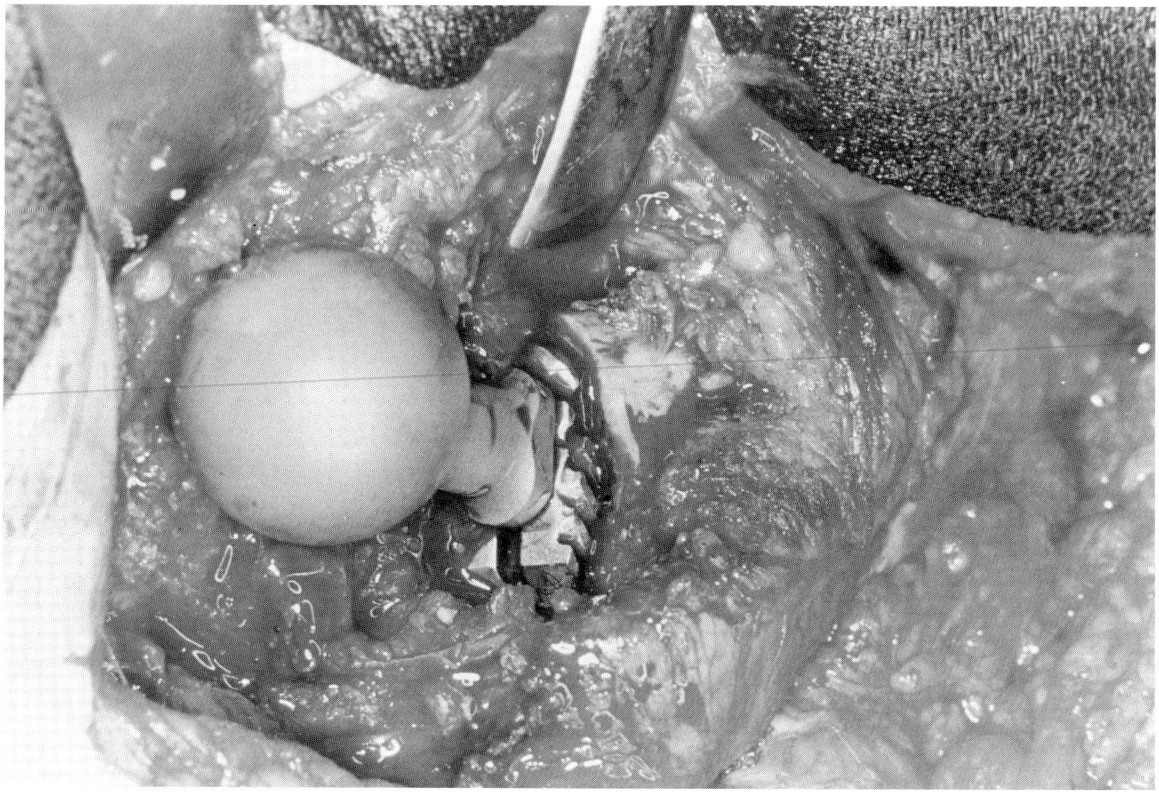

**Fig. 5-63** Femoral neck and head attach to the rasp for later trial reduction.

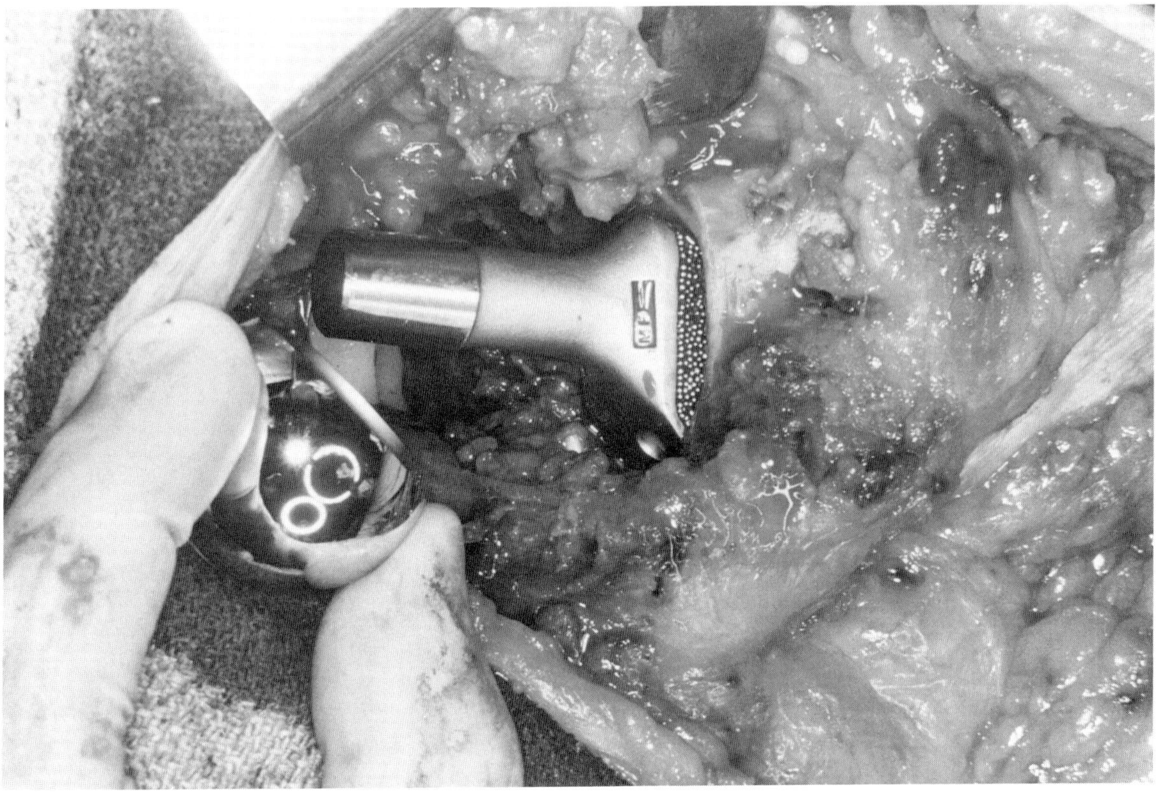

**Fig. 5-64** Depending on the stability of the trial reduction and correctness of the leg length, the standard or + 5 mm head component is impacted over the trunion bearing.

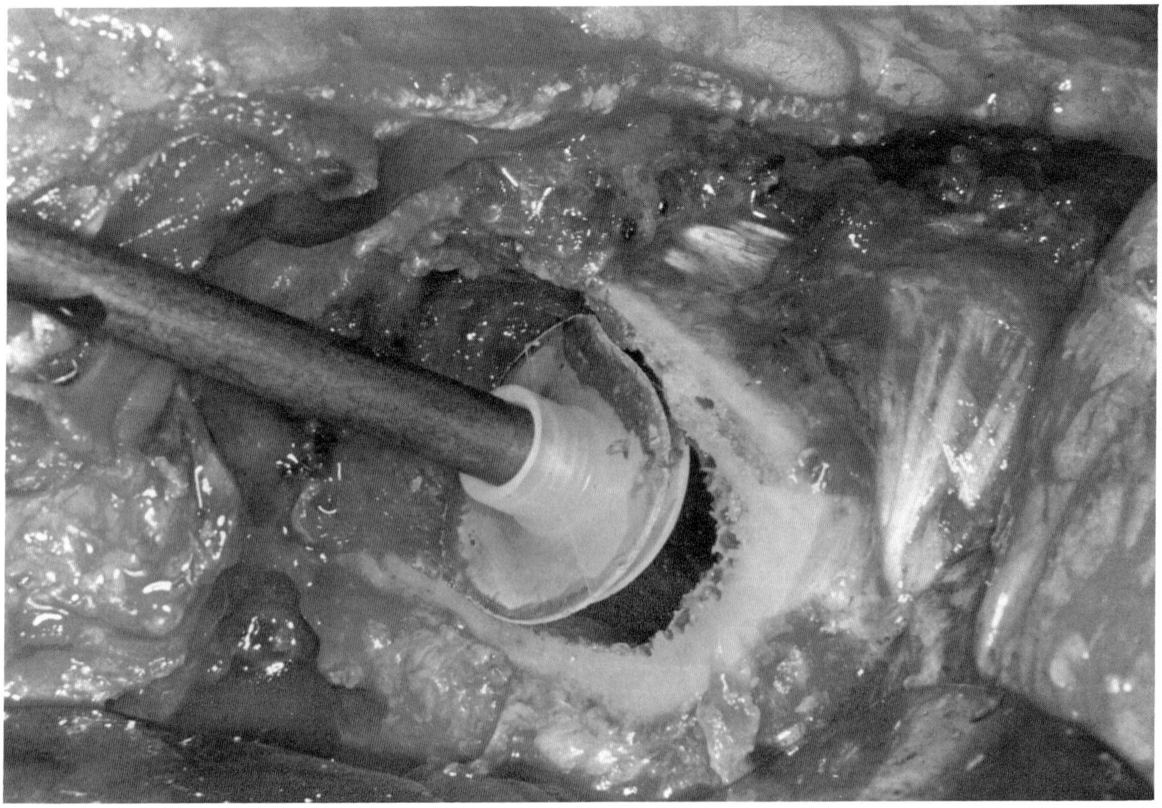

**Fig. 5-65** If a cemented prosthesis is being used, the femoral canal is plugged at the appropriate level.

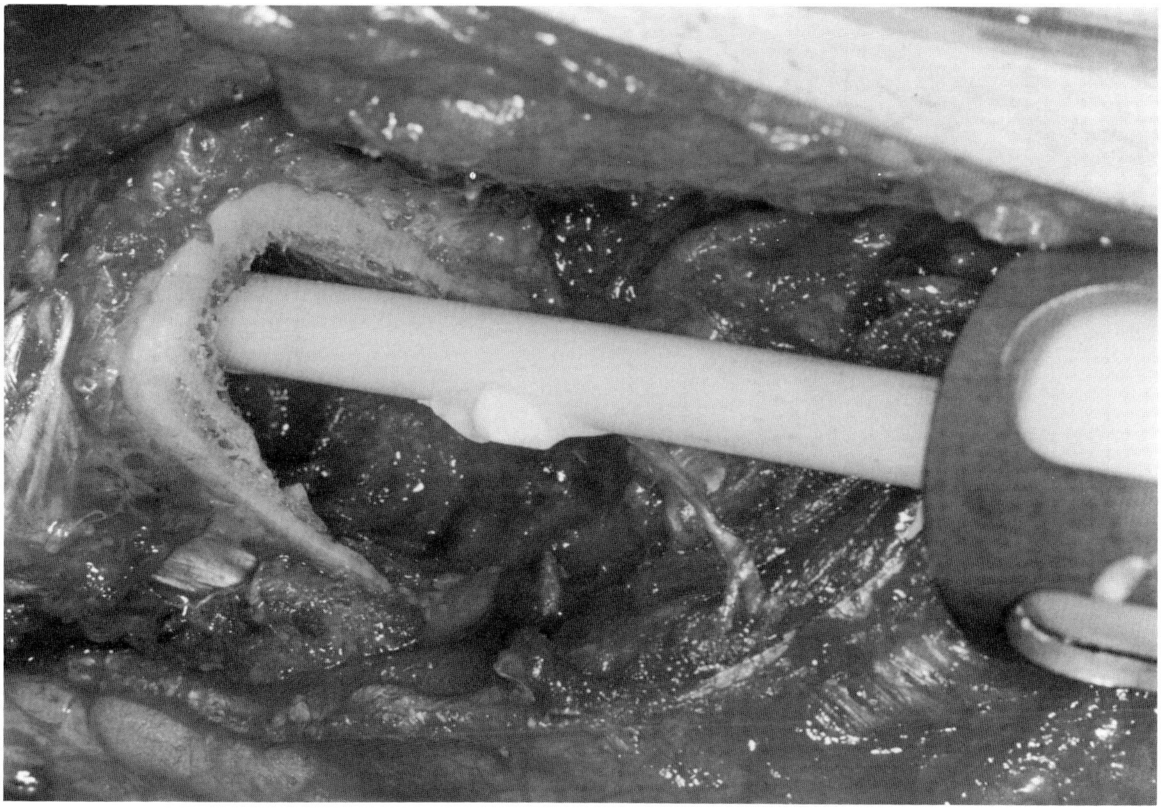

**Fig. 5-66** A cement gun is used to inject bone cement under pressure into the canal.

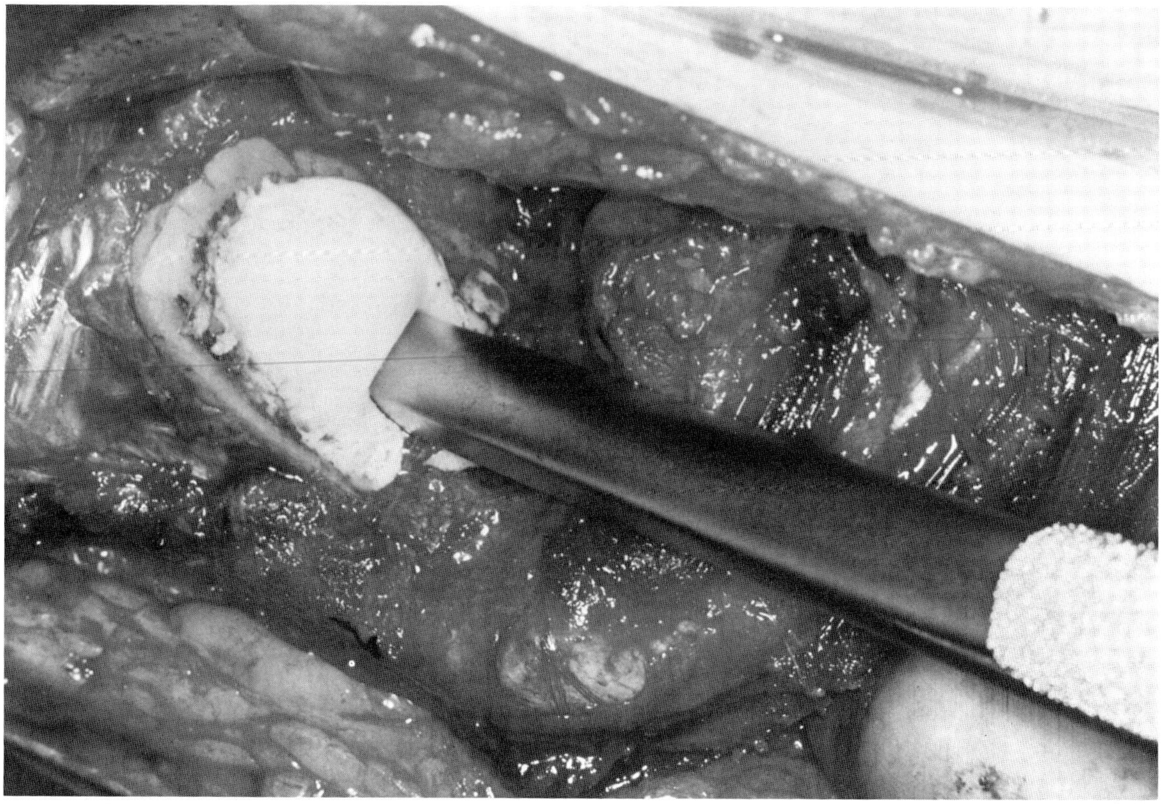

**Fig. 5-67** After the canal has been filled with pressurized cement, the prosthesis is inserted.

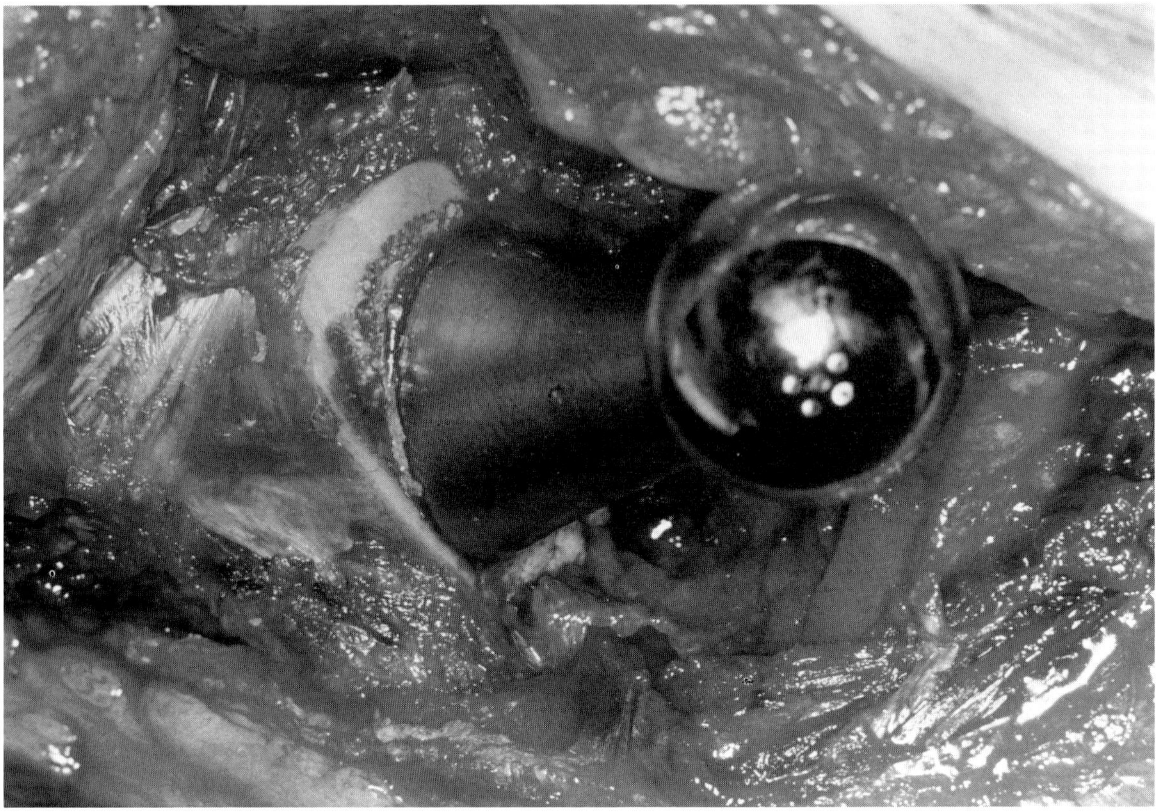

**Fig. 5-68** With the prosthesis in proper orientation, any excess cement is removed.

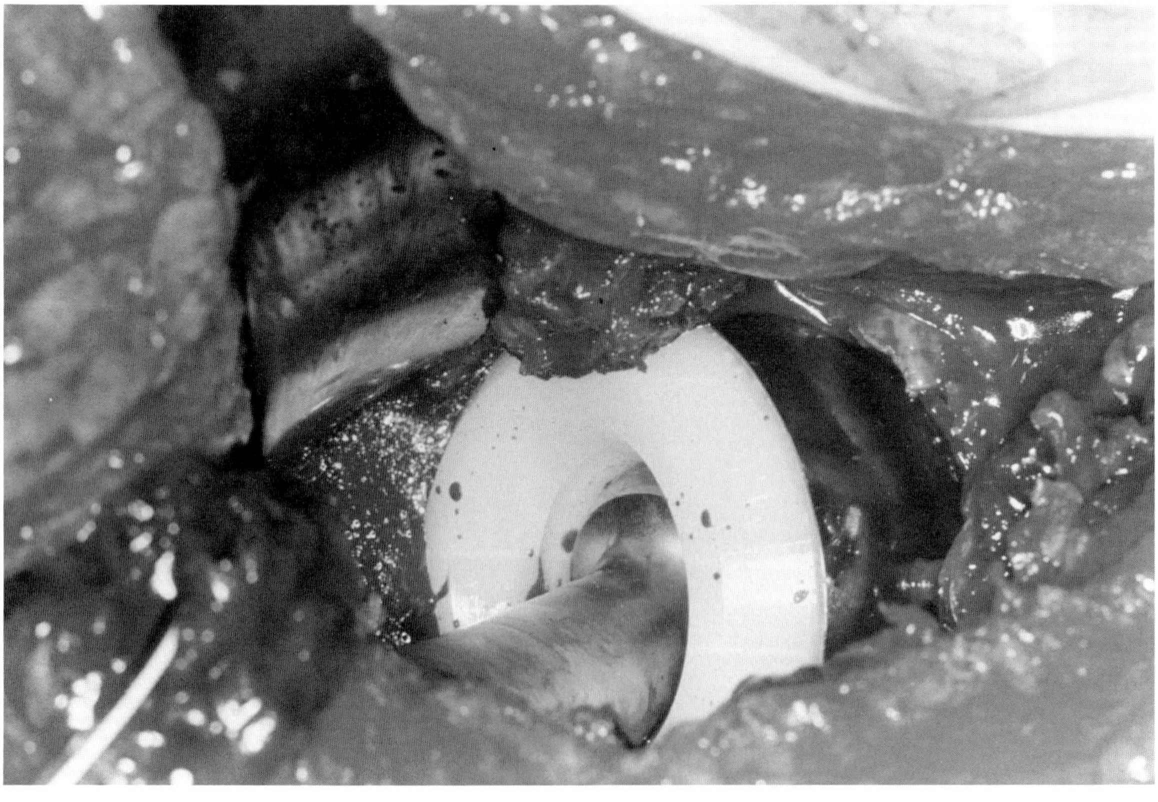

**Fig. 5-69** The assembled bipolar system is reduced and range of motion and stability are determined.

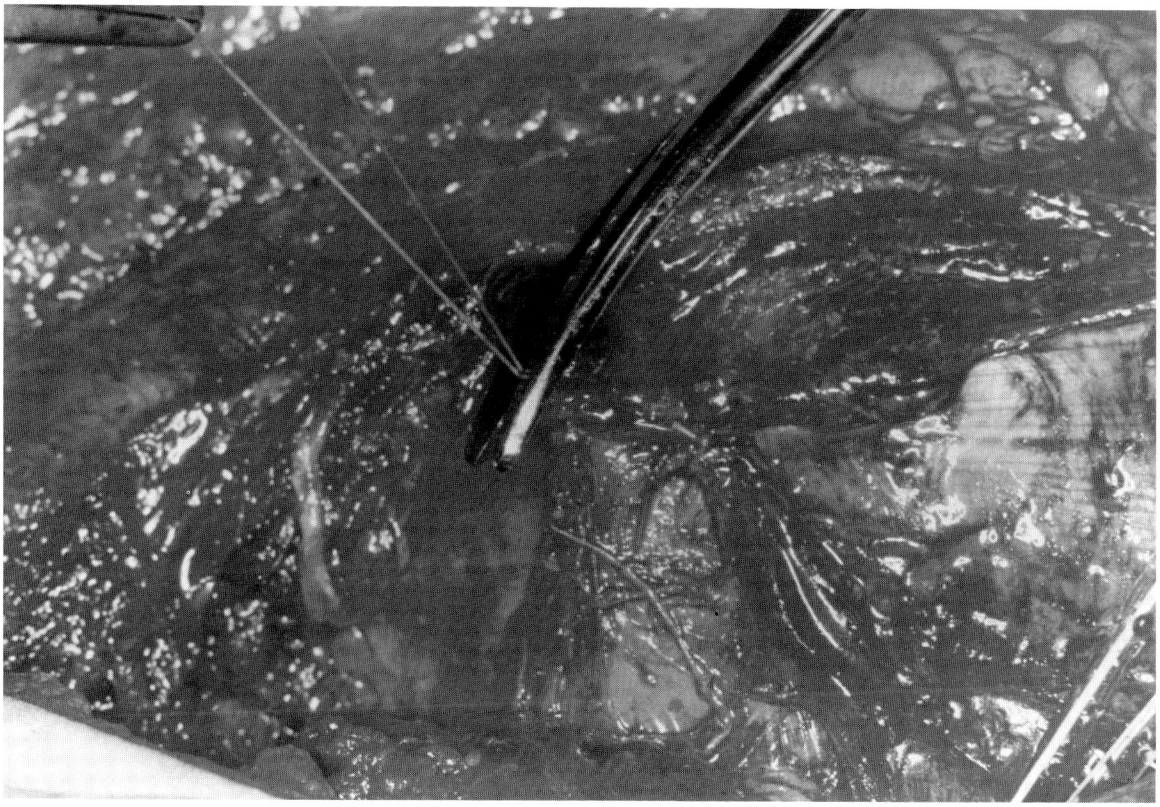

**Fig. 5-70** The trochanteric bursa is closed.

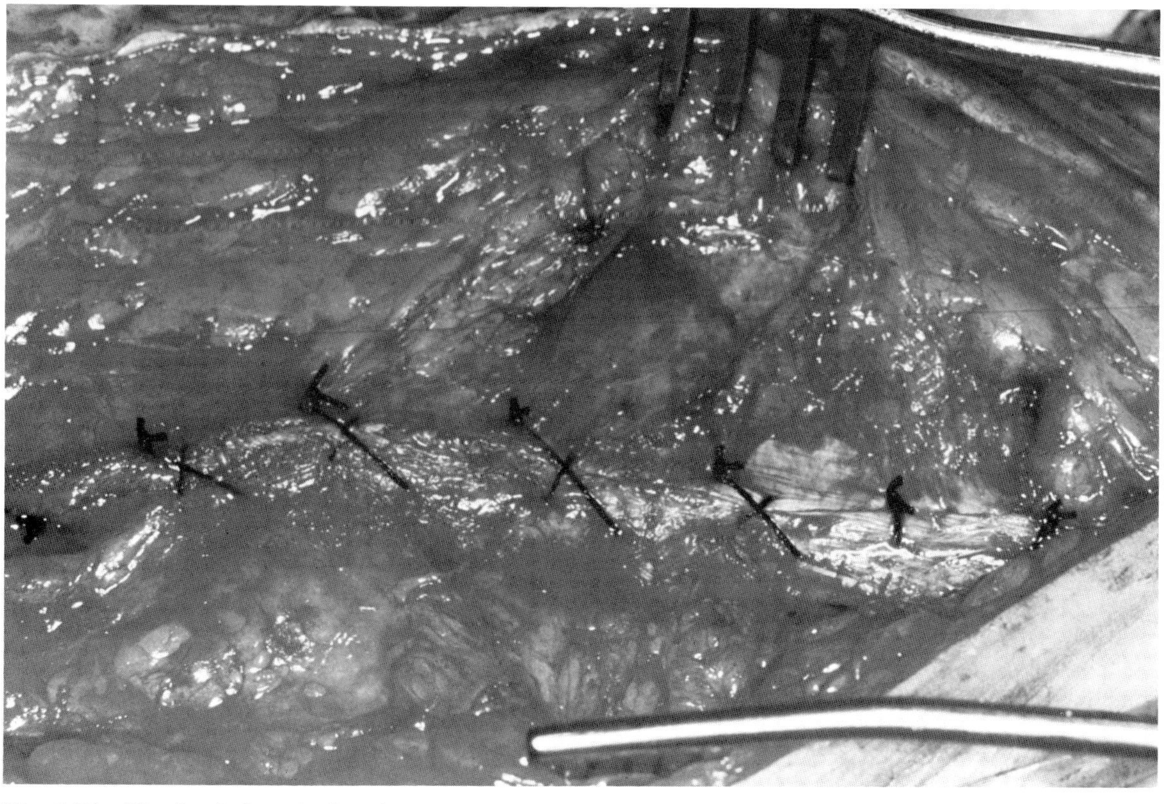

**Fig. 5-71** The fascia lata is closed.

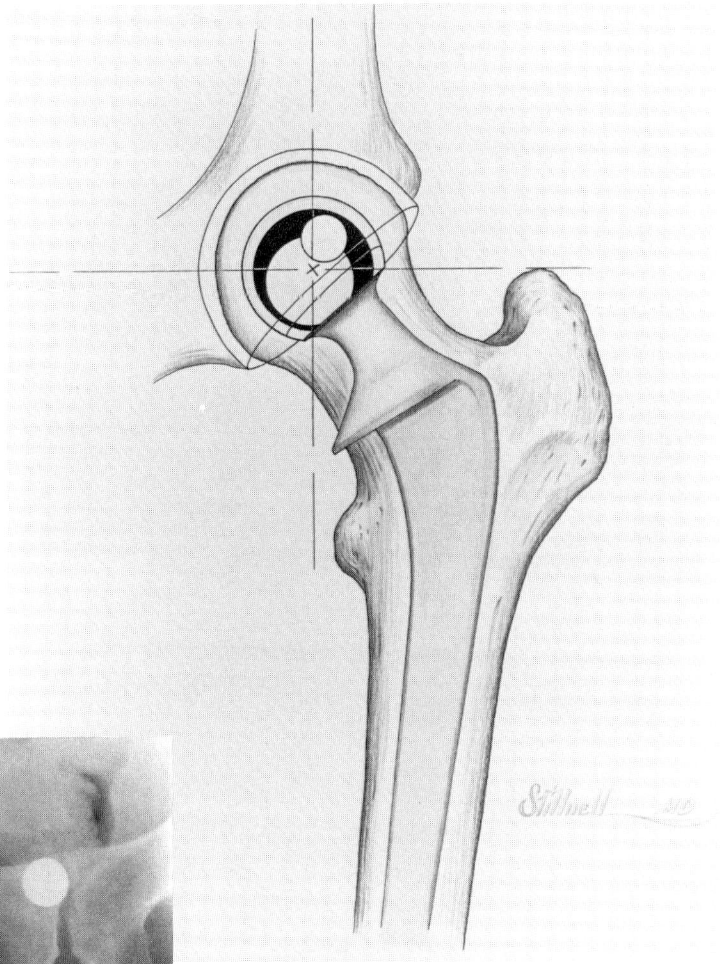

**Fig. 5-72** The orientation of the femoral prosthesis and the greater trochanter.

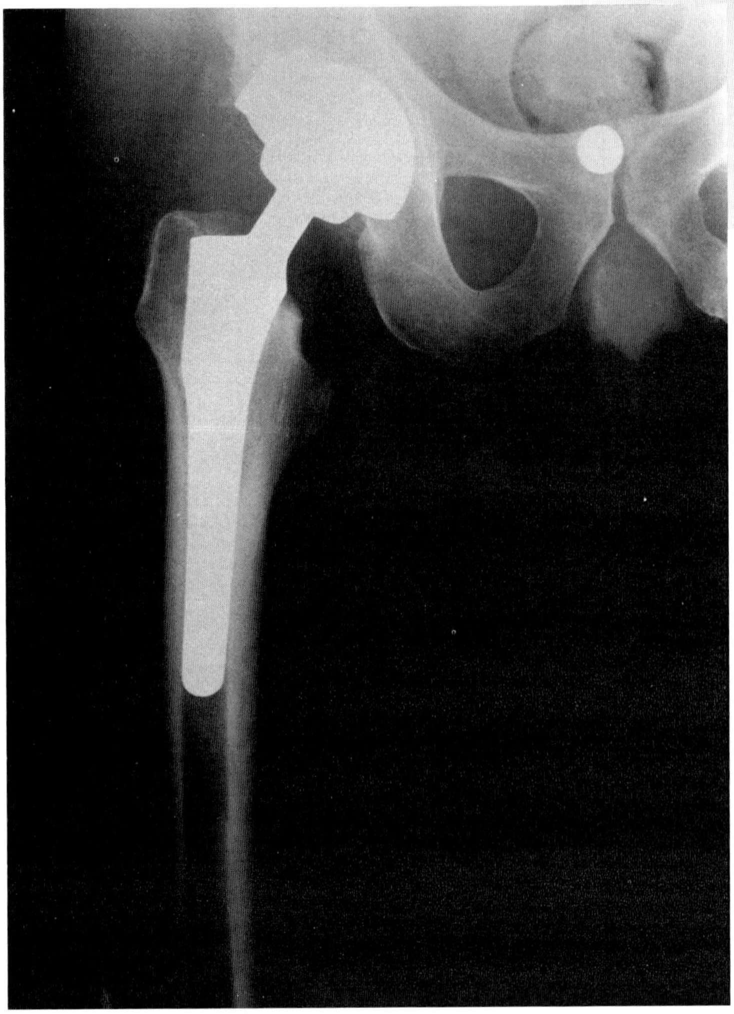

**Fig. 5-73** Anteroposterior view of a well-aligned cementless replacement.

# Knee Arthroplasty

# 6

W. Norman Scott
Richard D. Scott
William Thomas Stillwell

Although establishing a painless, mobile, and stable knee arthroplasty has been more difficult than developing a successful hip replacement, the present 10-year results are better than the comparable hip experience.[1] In the latter half of the nineteenth century, and most of the twentieth century, material interposition arthroplasty was not as successful as a knee arthrodesis. When molded femoral hemiarthroplasties were introduced in the first half of the twentieth century, application was limited.[2] Modest success was not universally achieved until the biaxial hinges were developed by Walldius[3] and d'Aubique.[4] However, these results were fraught with the anticipated mechanical problems, higher rates of infection, and patellofemoral problems. The concepts of a low friction arthroplasty stimulated the search for a successful surface replacement, a standard of the present era. As the quest for the ideal knee replacement continues, controversies surround prosthetic selection, surgical technique, indications, and the potential for future success.

## Prosthetic Selection

Selecting the appropriate knee replacement is more often based on philosophical rather than scientific criteria. Most prostheses today are available as a system, so the surgeon may select whichever type of replacement while using the same instrumentation and principles inherent in the design, e.g., Townley, P.C.A., or Kinematic systems.

There are two major categories of knee replacements: surface replacements and articulated designs, the latter of which is becoming somewhat extinct. The surface replacements are further divided into cruciate retaining and sacrificing models, with comparable short term success reported. The cruciate retaining prostheses range from uni- to tricompartment. Unicompartment designs have had a resurgence in interest and successful results.[5] Widening the surface area of both the femoral and tibial runners while improving the surgical technique and narrowing the indications for use has accounted for the improved early results. Anterior cruciate retaining prostheses, e.g., Oxford and New Jersey designs, are infrequently used due to the often-encountered pathological state of the ligament. All bicompartment prostheses resurface the anterior aspect of the femur, leaving the patella replacement as optional. It is estimated that approximately 55% of all replacements performed in the United States are cruciate retaining, the most popular ones being the P.C.A., Townley, Duopatella, Brigham, and Miller-Galante knees. The essential features include an anatomic femoral resurfacing using either a chrome cobalt alloy, stainless steel, or a titanium composite. The intercondylar area allows room for the excursion of the posterior cruciate ligaments, with small anchoring pegs for immediate positioning. Likewise, the tibial components have a reciprocal cutout area on the midportion with a relatively flat surface in both a coronal and sagittal plane. Stability is thus imparted by the integrity of the ligaments and not just by prosthetic conformity. Both cemented and noncemented methods of fixation are now available. The early results with the porous designs are encouraging; yet, equaling the mechanical success rates of the cemented replacements presents a formidable obstacle in itself.[6]

The cruciate sacrificing replacements have the longest follow-up, 12 years, and represent approximately 45% of the currently used designs. Owing to the resection of the posterior cruciate ligament, the tibial plateau covers the entire subchondral surface. Although neither component allows room for the cruciate ligaments, loss of stability is compensated for by prosthetic conformity throughout the range of motion. Dishing of the plateau in both a coronal and sagittal direction, allowing contact throughout the rollback and sliding stages of motion, is an essential design feature for all cruciate sacrificing designs. The initial Total Condylar replacement, while still in existence, has had two subsequent design modifications: sloping the tibial plateau (Insall-Burstein Total Condylar) and enhancement of the intercondylar notch (Insall-Burstein Posterior Stabilized) to improve motion and anterior-posterior stability. In addition to the above, the most commonly used prosthesis in this category includes the Freeman-Samuelson, ICLH, Townley, and R.M.C. designs.

It is generally conceded that the "hinge is dead"; yet there are some instances for using triaxial hinges such as the Spherocentric and Kinematic rotating hinge. This last group of knee designs has narrow indications as evidenced by the relatively infrequent use (less than 5%). The specific indications relate to "grossly unstable" knees and those revisions with excessive bone loss. It is somewhat debatable whether all "grossly unstable" knees can be treated by a ligament balancing and surface replacements, although most experienced surgeons feel that such is the case. Based on clinical experience, rotating hinges or articulated designs used for stability purposes usually represent individual preference. Excessive bone loss problems can usually be treated with articulated designs, but more recently have been addressed by customizing surface replacements, for specific areas of bone loss.

Although it is often stated that knee arthroplasty is technically more demanding than hip arthroplasty, there is no universally accepted surgical technique. In this chapter we try to delineate the different approaches by highlighting the principles of insertion. Regardless of the specific knee system, there are three basic "cuts" that ensure prosthetic stability and alignment. Stability can be thought of in terms of flexion and extension spaces. The former encompasses the combination of proximal tibia and posterior femur, whereas the proximal tibia and distal femur comprise the extension space. Theoretically, these spaces should be equal, thus ensuring stability throughout the range of motion. Similarly, it is the extension space, proximal tibia and distal femur, that determines the overall limb alignment. All methods of instrumentation achieve this balance by resecting either of the three major cuts, proximal tibia and posterior and distal femur, in a different sequence. It is not our objective to champion any specific approach, but rather to depict the differences. Shaping the bone to accept the individual components is design dependent, and several systems are illustrated.

The success of knee arthroplasty has continually broadened its horizon while narrowing the indications for debridement, osteotomy, and arthrodesis. A pathological diagnosis involving the knee of any inflammatory arthritis, osteoarthritis, or posttraumatic arthritis represents the most usual indications for primary total knee replacement. Failed arthroplasties, septic or mechanical, fractures about the knee, and rare neuropathic situations comprise the remainder of pathological instances in which a total knee replacement is potentially indicated. The clinical setting, disability, age, and lifestyle expectations become the determining factors in helping the patient select the best treatment. In general, osteotomies have a statistically predictable success rate of approximately 75% for 5 years, with decreasing effectiveness after that interval. Knee arthroplasties, on the other hand, have, at 10 years, a level of success in over 90% of patients. The population, however, has been an older, less active group than a typical osteotomy patient. The mechanical effectiveness of the knee replacement in a young active individual must still be ascertained. The osteotomy patient with isolated unicompartment disease is likewise a candidate for a unicompartment replacement. For this group of designs, the best results seem to be confined to those patients whose disease is strictly limited to either the medial or lateral tibial femoral compartment. Arthroscopic debridements are, at best, temporizing procedures that interestingly satisfy the expectations of many patients who otherwise would be considered for a replacement. In general, patients with minimal deformities and a good range of motion are the best candidates for this procedure.

In summary, the choice of a specific prosthesis is based more on the individual surgeon's preference than on scientific data. Similarly, the indications for knee arthroplasty are only limited by the continual clinical evaluation as to survival in both the older population and younger athletic generation. Surgical technique, however, seems to be the single most important factor in realizing the excellent success rates already achieved. It is with this understanding that the following pictorial on the principles of knee arthroplasty is presented.

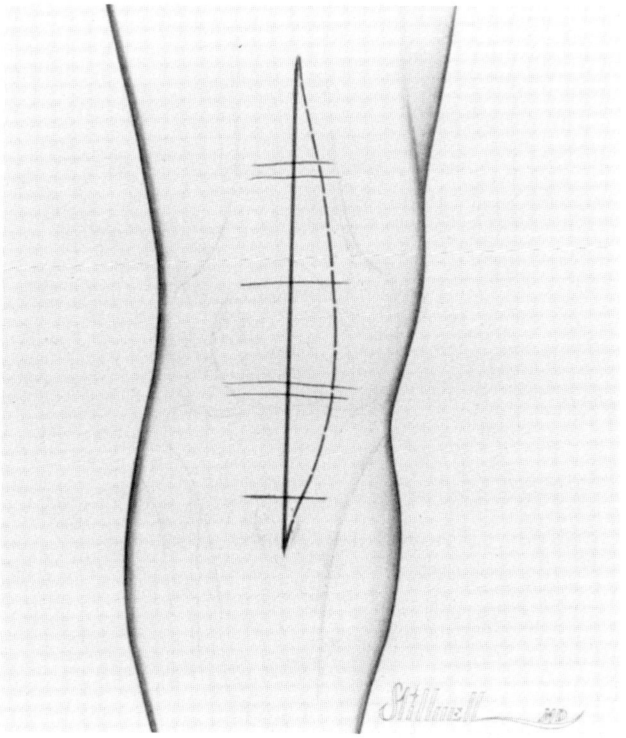

**Fig. 6-1A** Straight midline incision with limited medial flap.

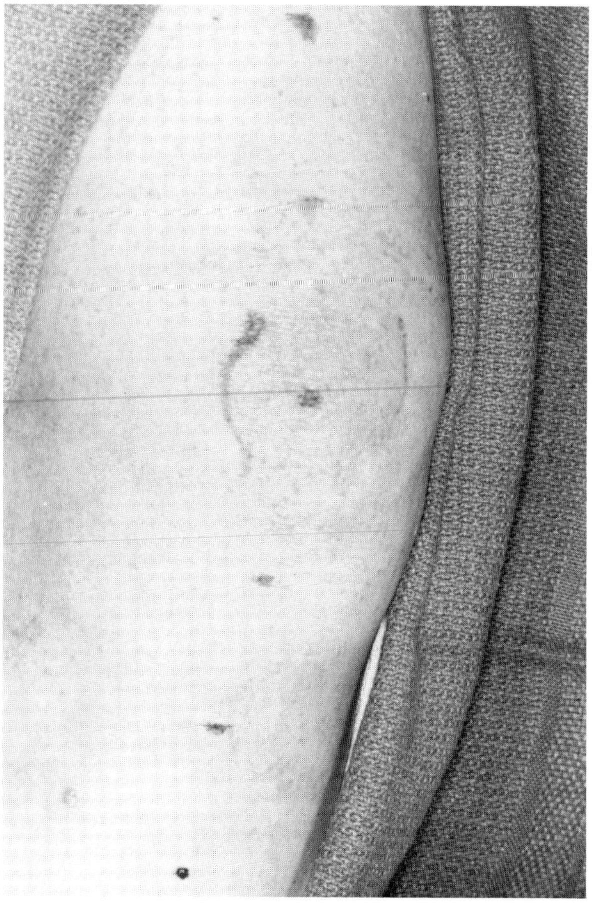

**Fig. 6-1B** Midline incision centered over patella.

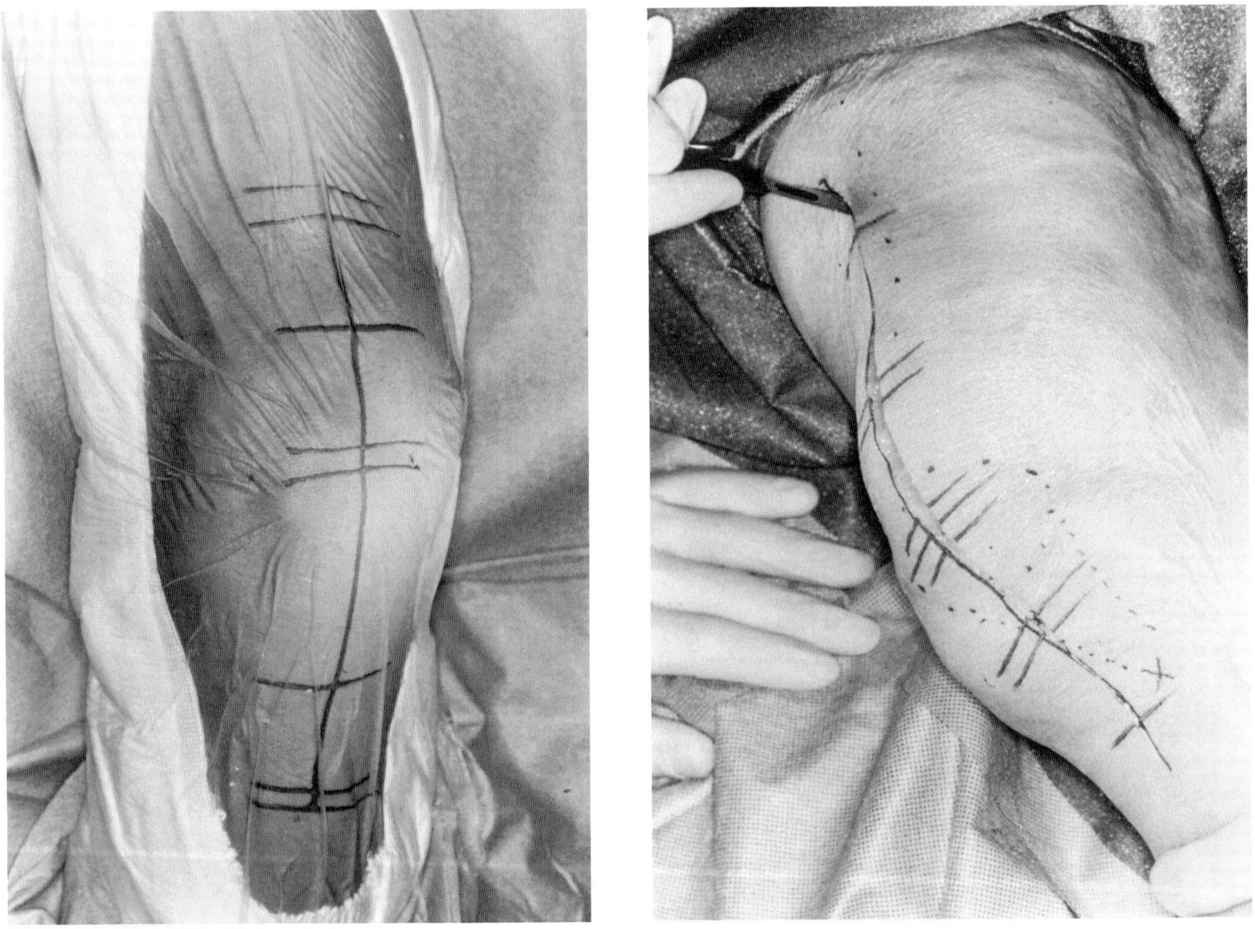

**Figs. 6-1C and D** Cross hatching to facilitate skin approximation.

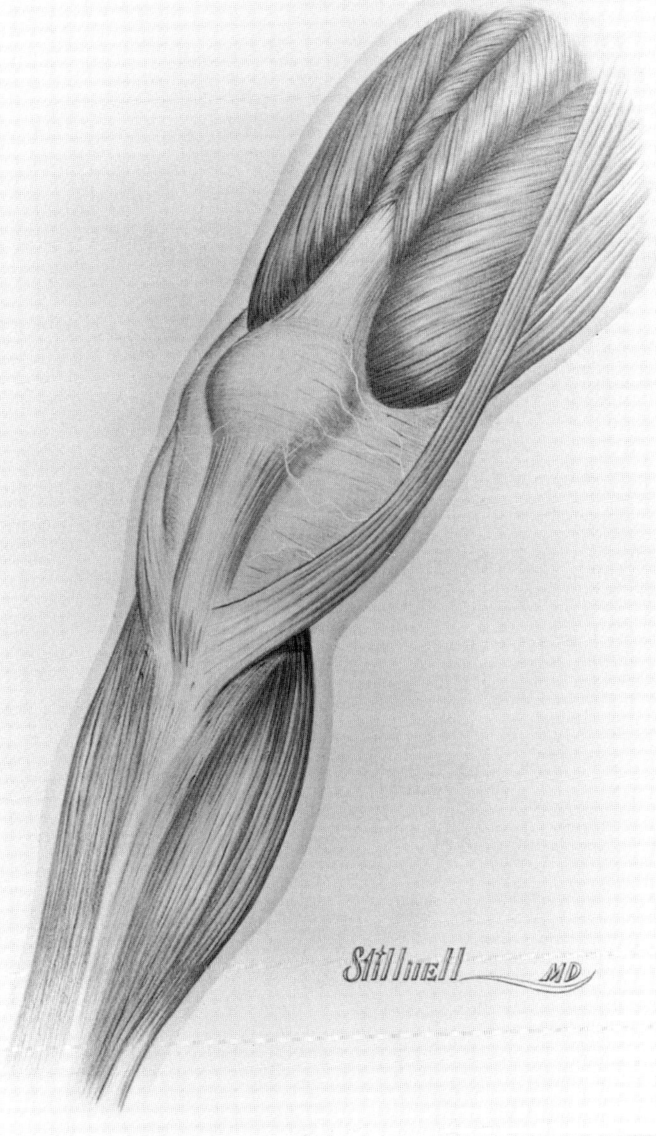


**Fig. 6-2A** Normal muscle, capsule, tendon, and patella relationship.

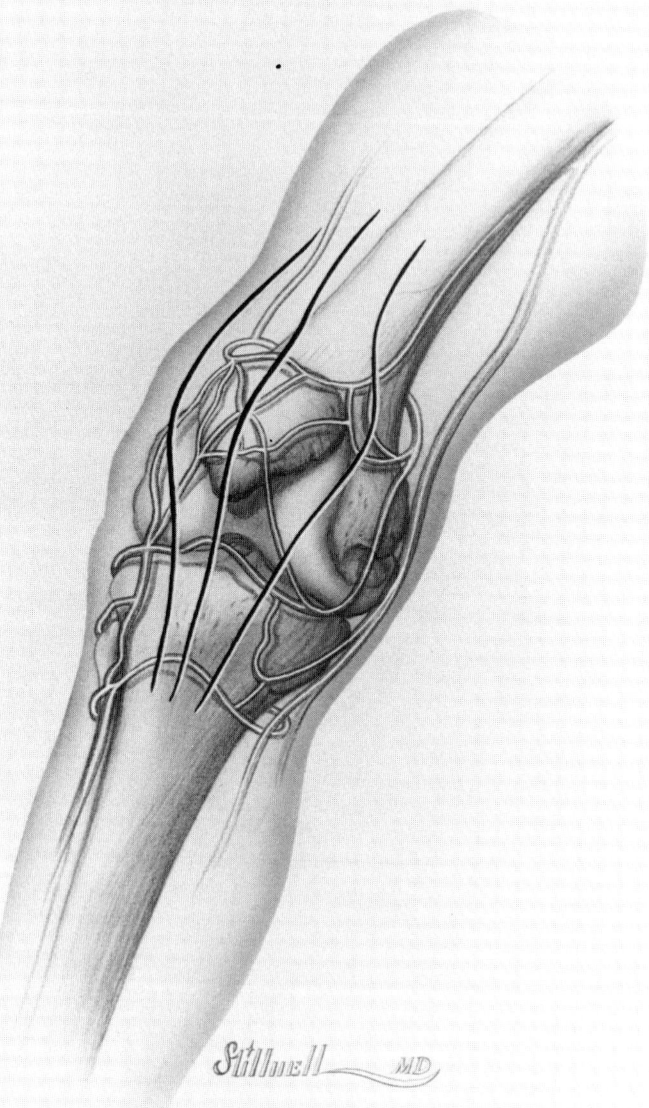

**Fig. 6-2B** Relationship of capsular incisions to geniculate blood supply.

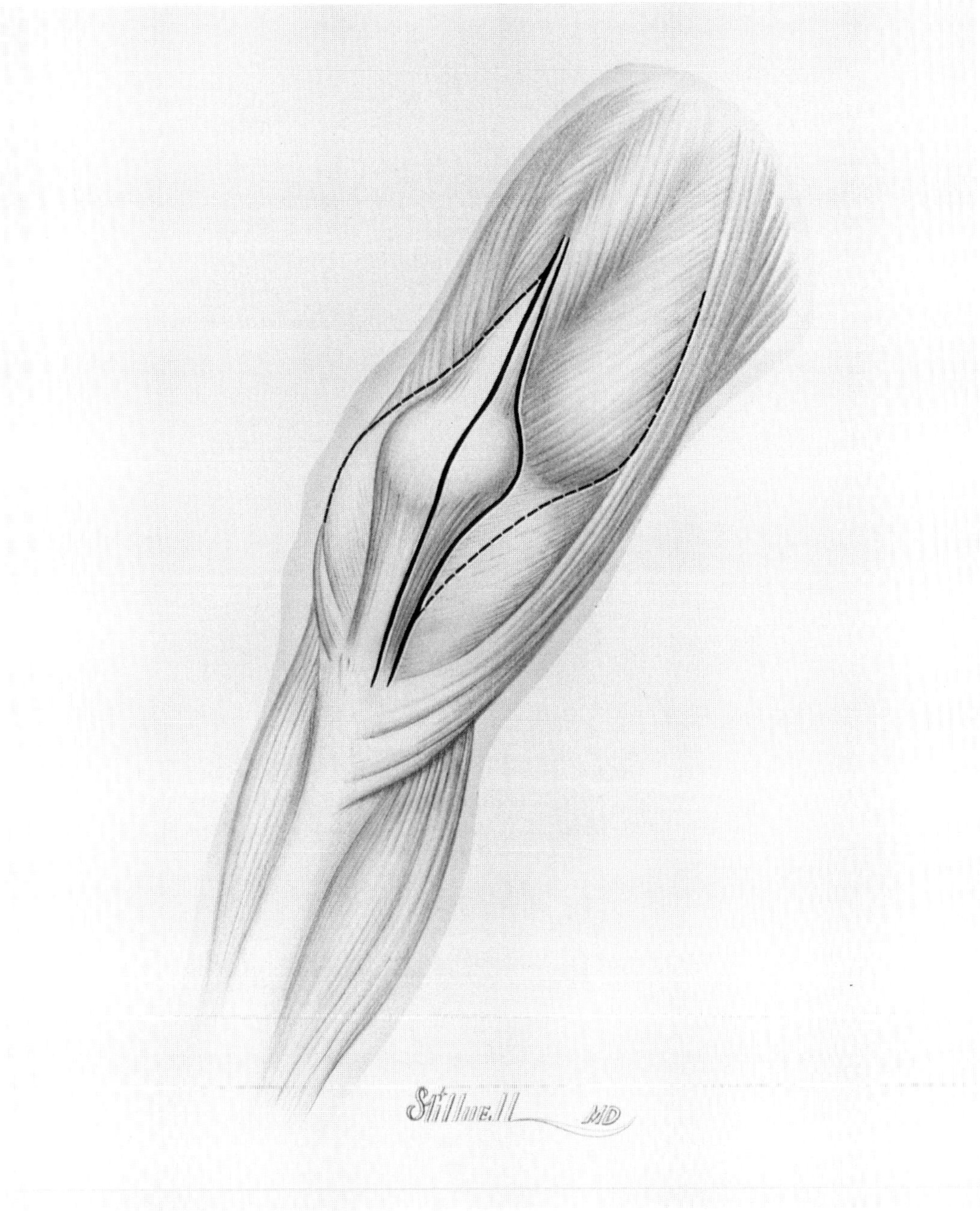

**Fig. 6-2C** Various capsular approaches.

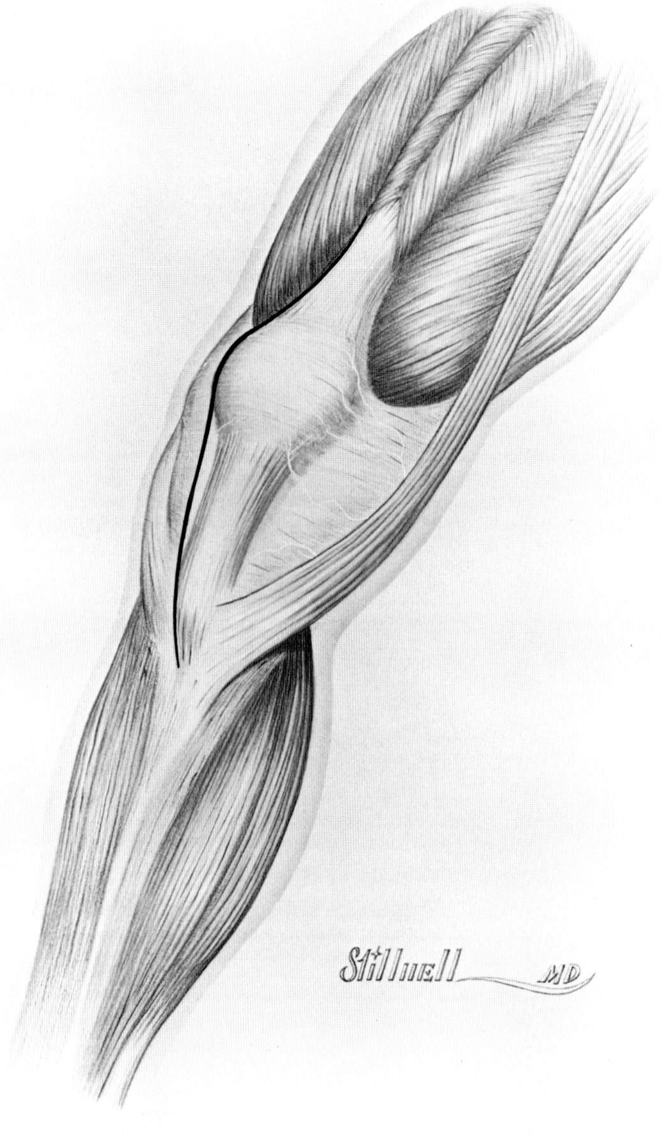

**Fig. 6-3A** Lateral capsular incision.

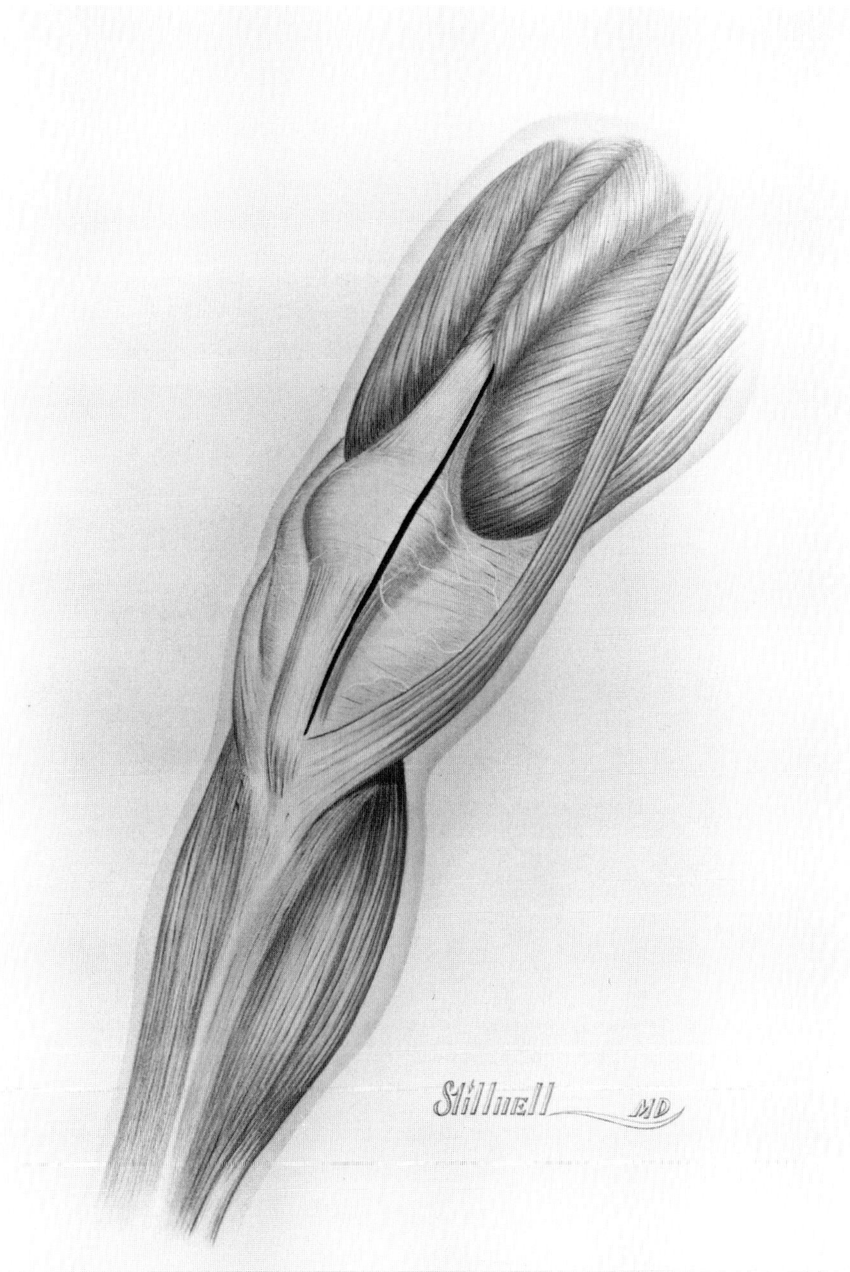

**Fig. 6-3B** Medial patella incision elevating periosteal patella flap.

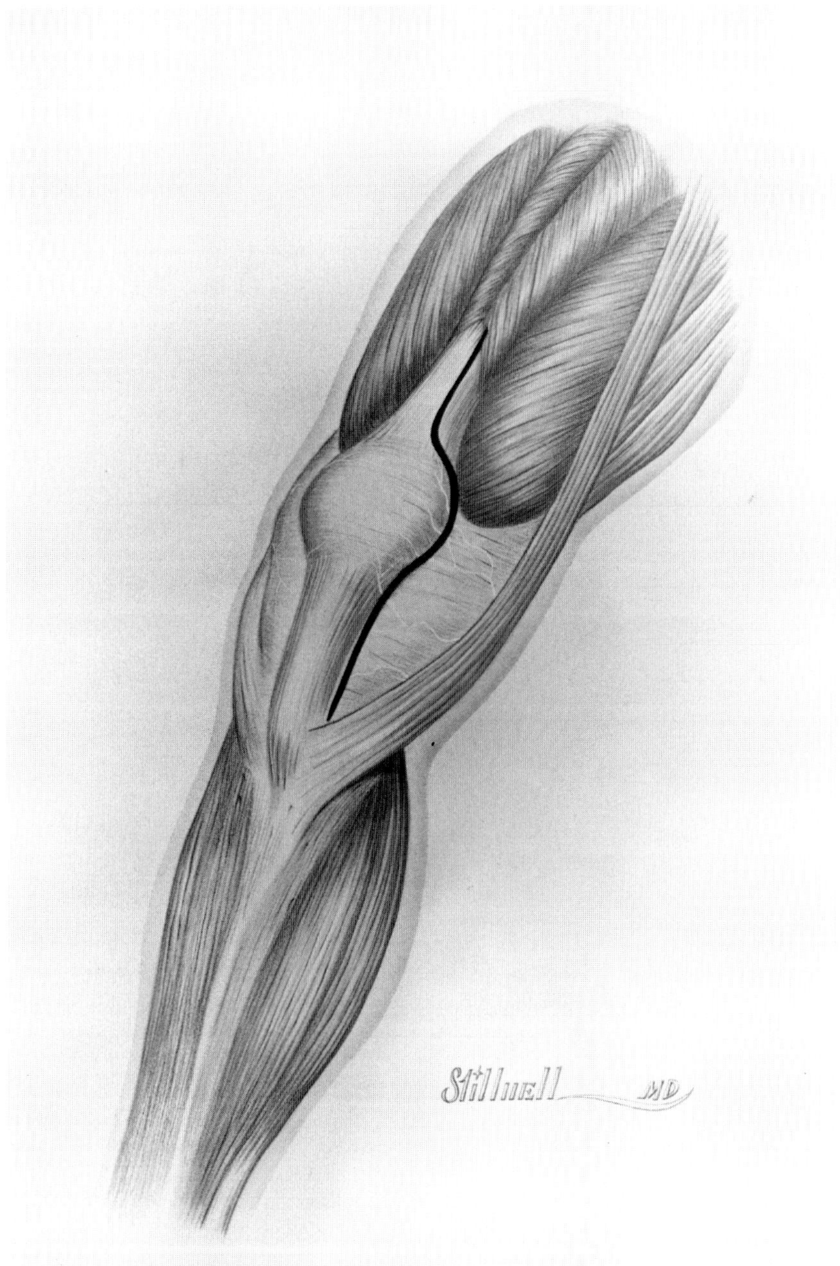

**Fig. 6-3C** Medial parapatella quadriceps and capsular incision.

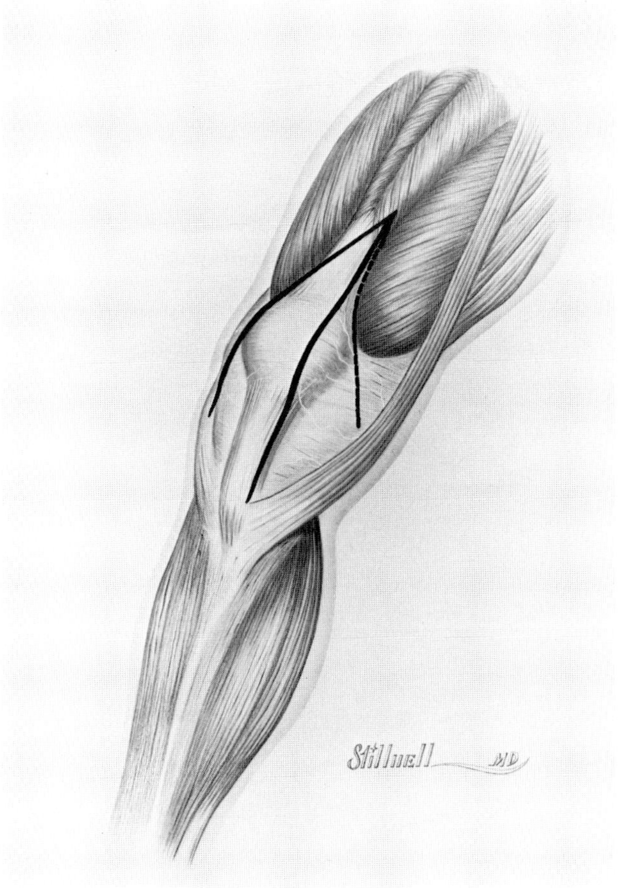

**Fig. 6-4A** Coonse-Adams (Y-V) approach and modification (dotted line).

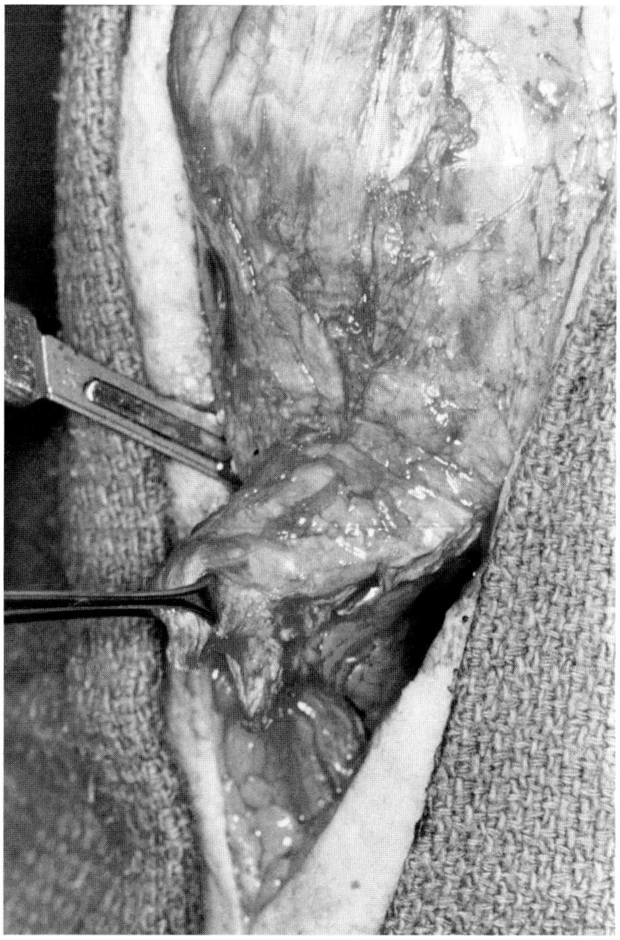

**Fig. 6-4B** Elevating quadriceps in Coonse-Adams approach.

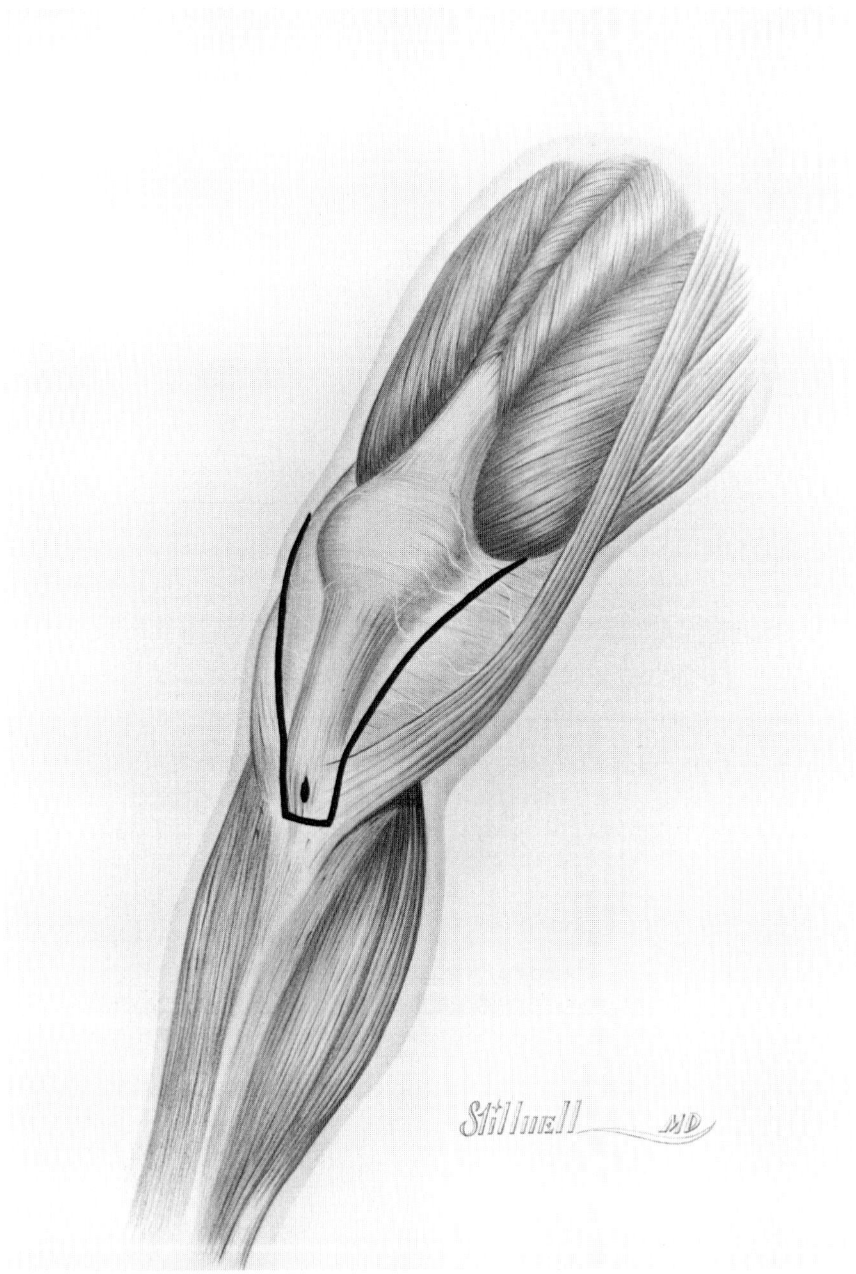


**Fig. 6-5A** Tibial tubercle elevation.

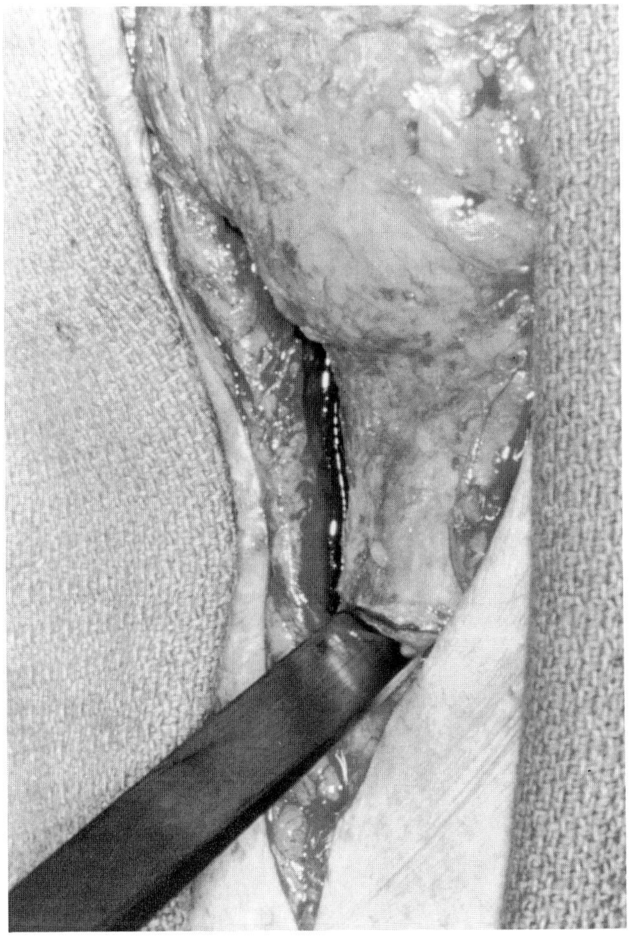

**Fig. 6-5B** Osteotome elevation of tubercle.

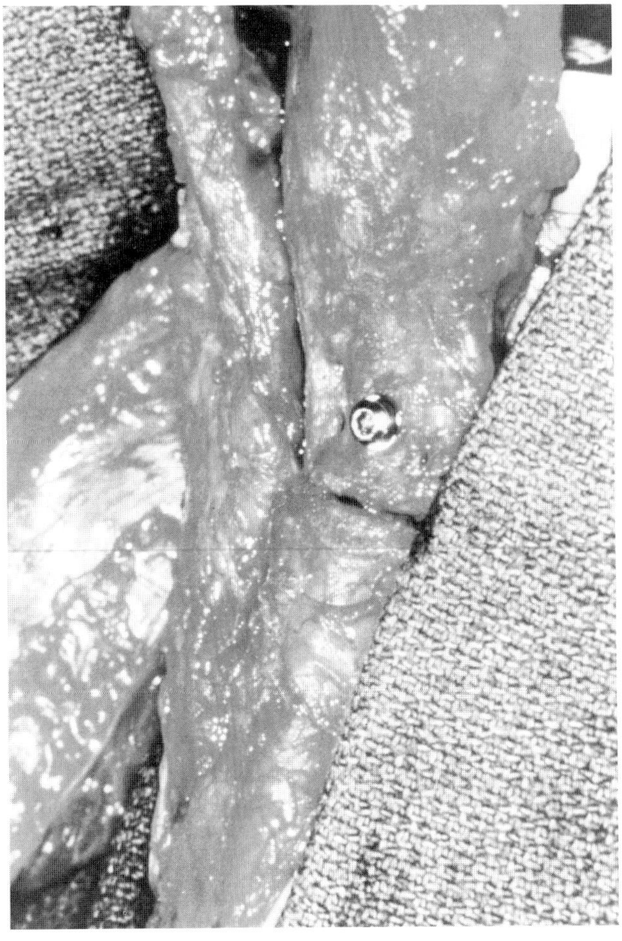

**Fig. 6-5C** Screw fixation of the tibial tubercle is preferred.

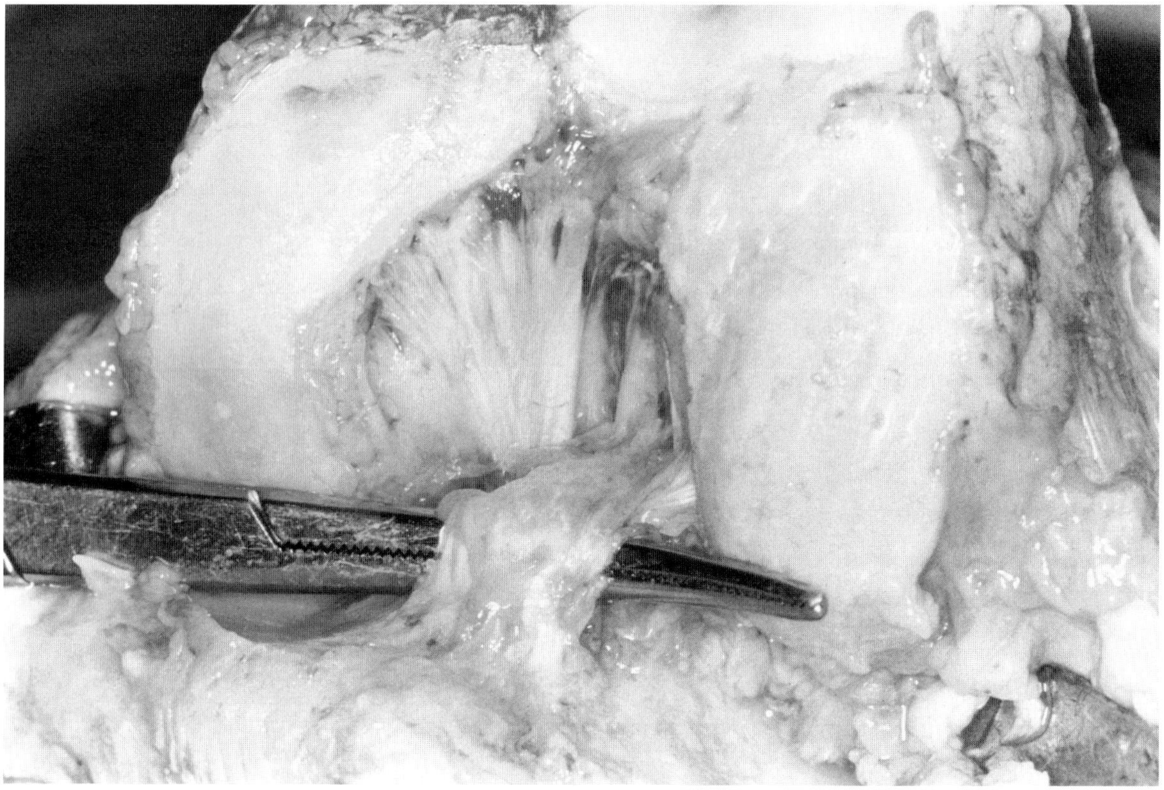

**Fig. 6-6A** The anterior cruciate ligament is infrequently present and often nonfunctional in the arthritic knee.

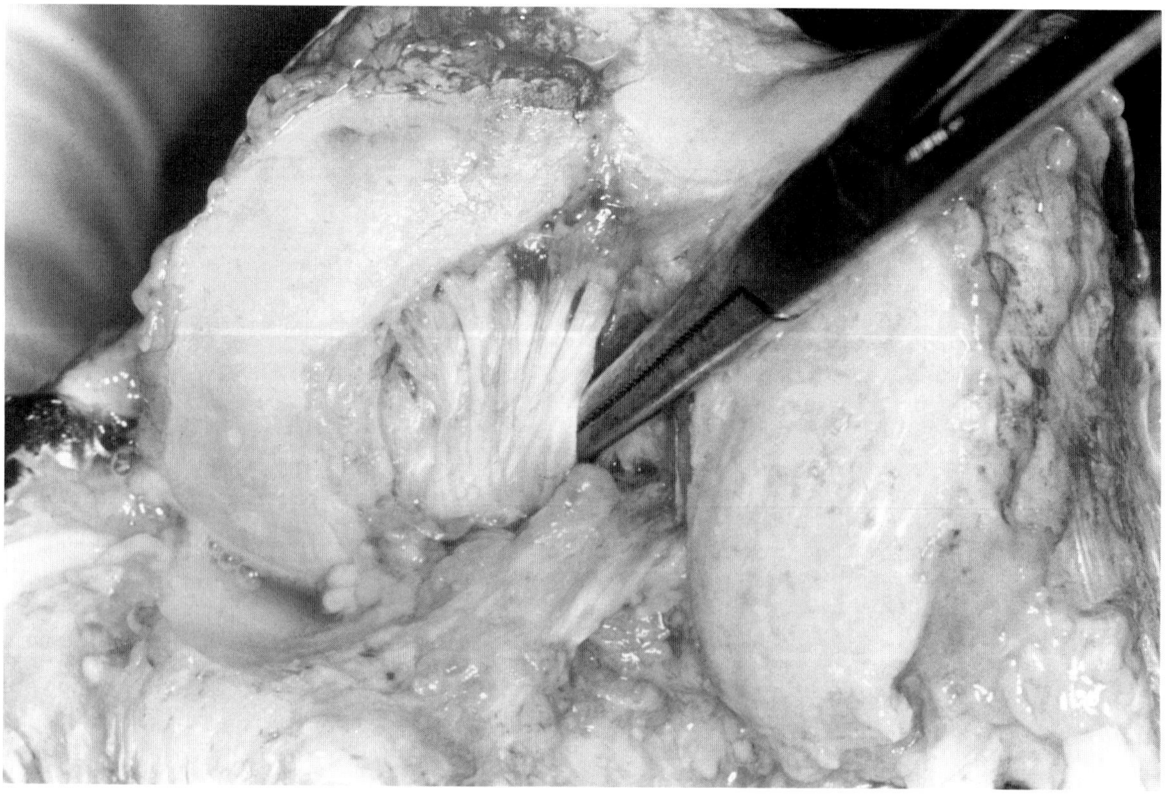

**Fig. 6-6B** Excision or retention of the posterior cruciate ligament remains a major point of controversy.

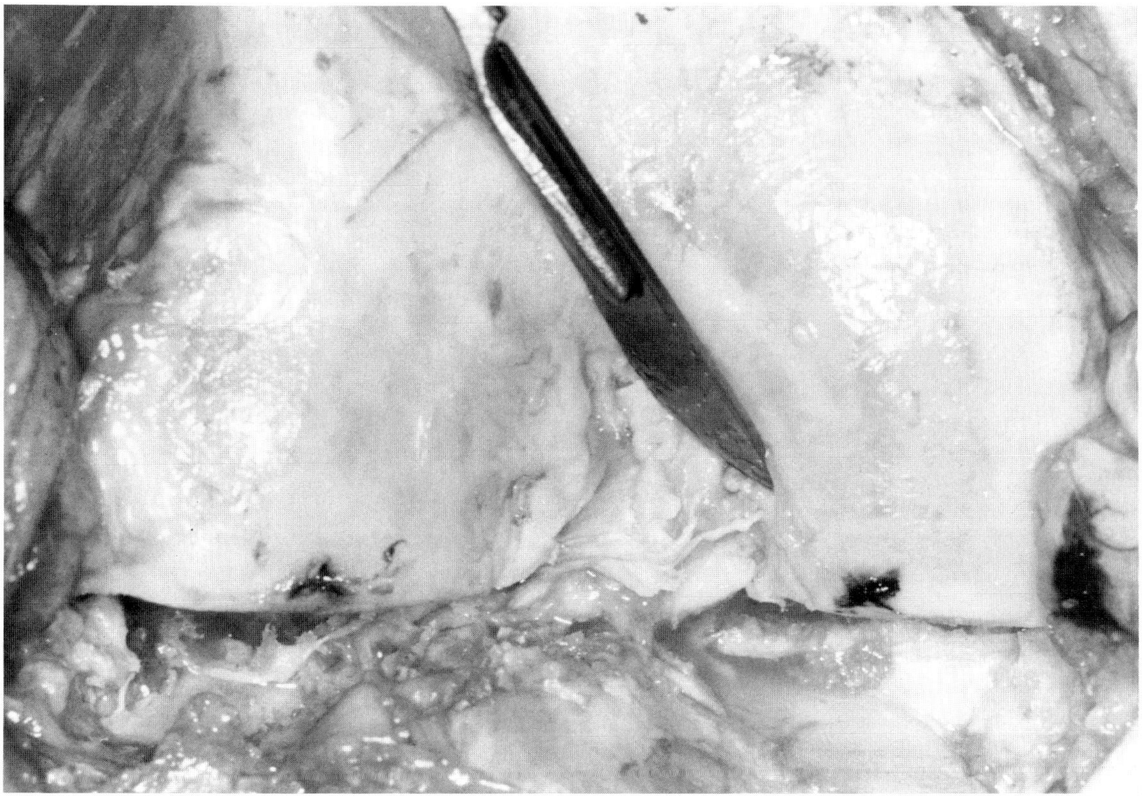

**Fig. 6-6C** Excision of the posterior cruciate ligament is most easily done from its origin at the lateral aspect of the medial femoral condyle.

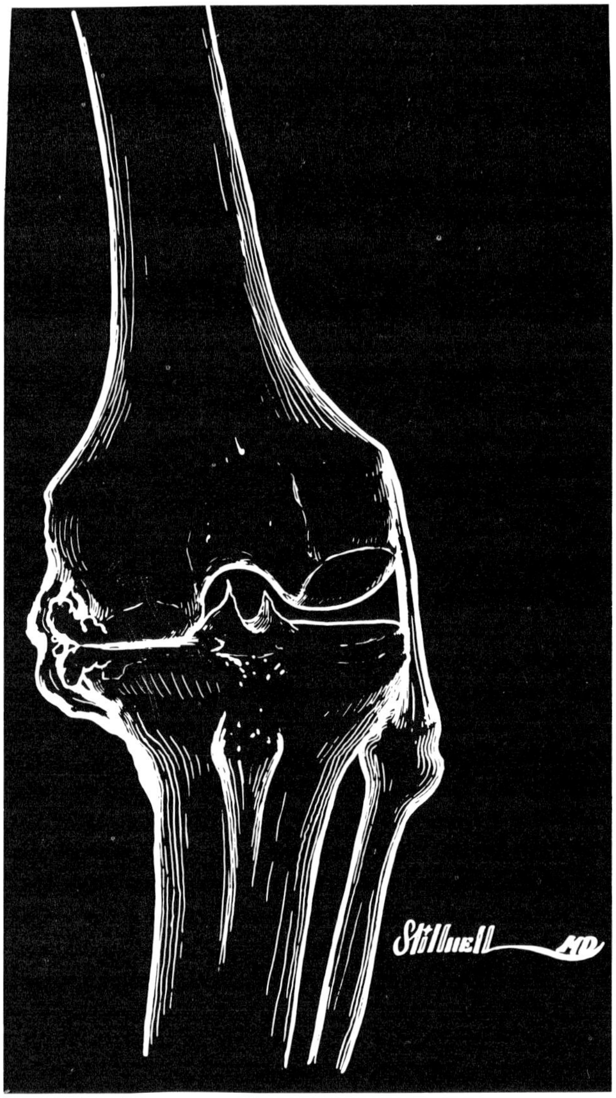

**Fig. 6-7A** The varus knee.

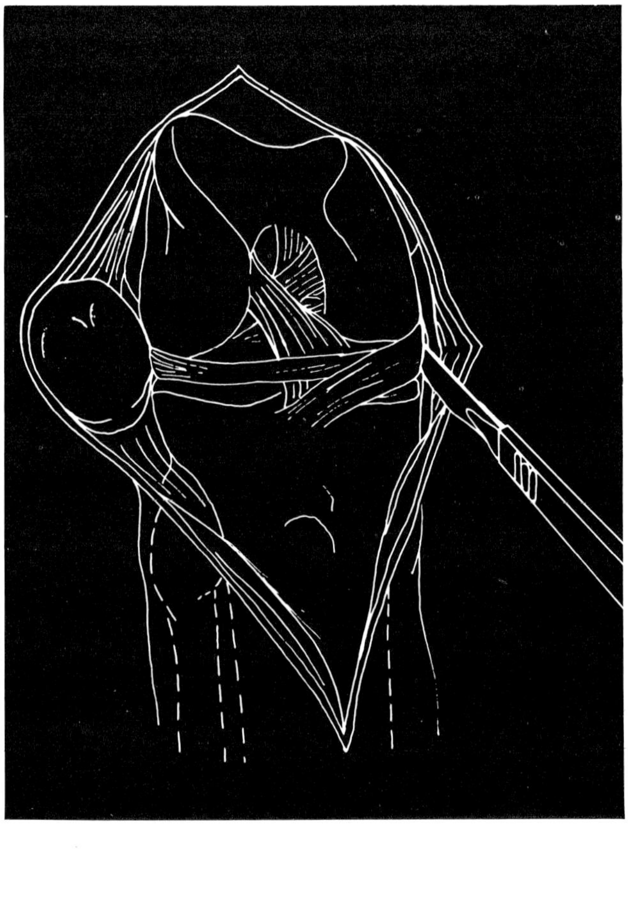

**Fig. 6-7B** In all knees medial exposure may be developed to the semimembranosus to ensure adequate visualization.

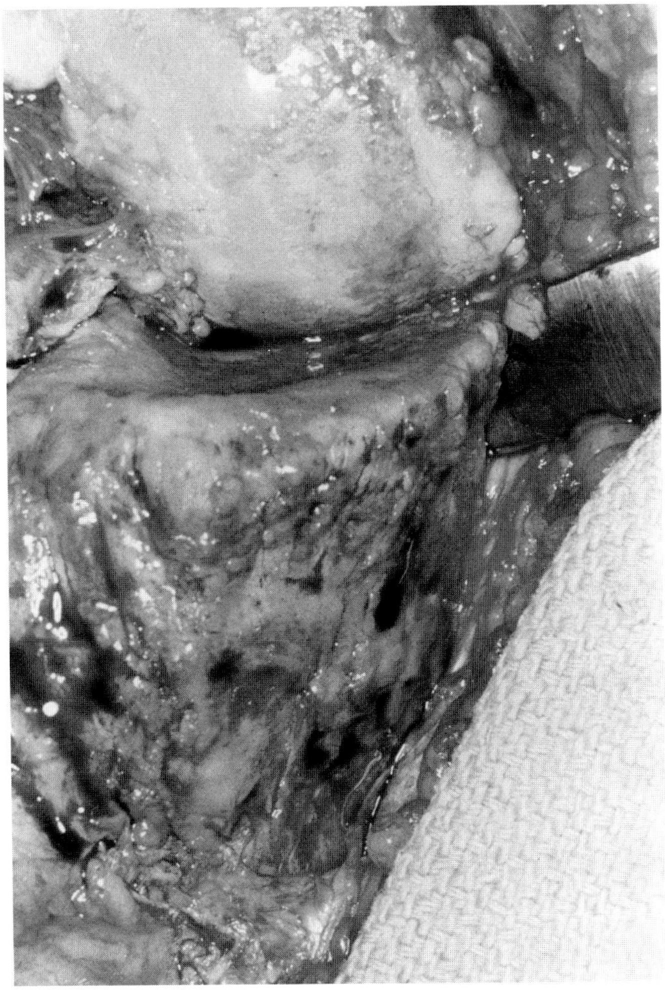

**Fig. 6-7C** The retractor indicates the area of insertion of the semimembranosus.

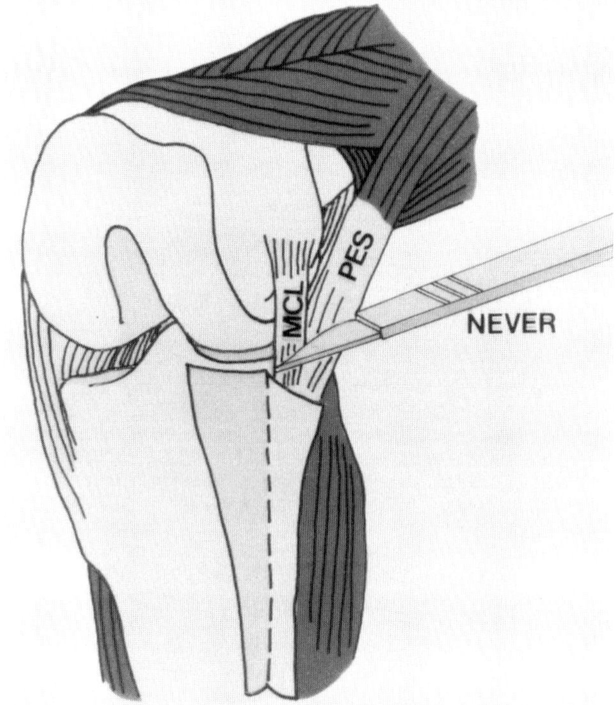


**Fig. 6-8A** The medial release for a varus knee should never be accomplished by transecting the medial collateral ligament and pes anserinus.

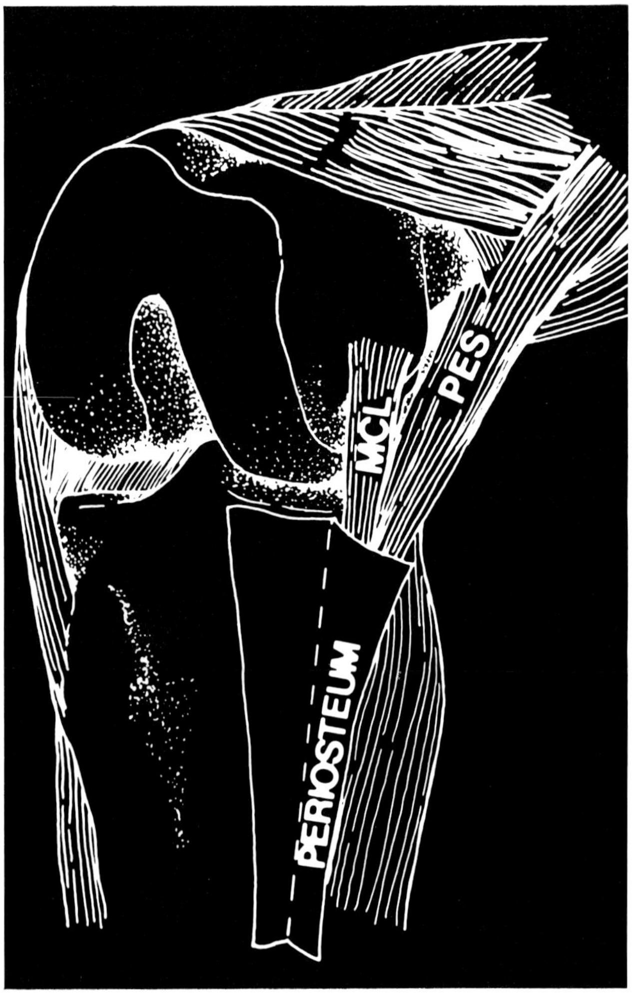


**Fig. 6-8B** The constituents of the medial release include a subperiosteal elevation of the medial collateral ligament and pes anserinus.

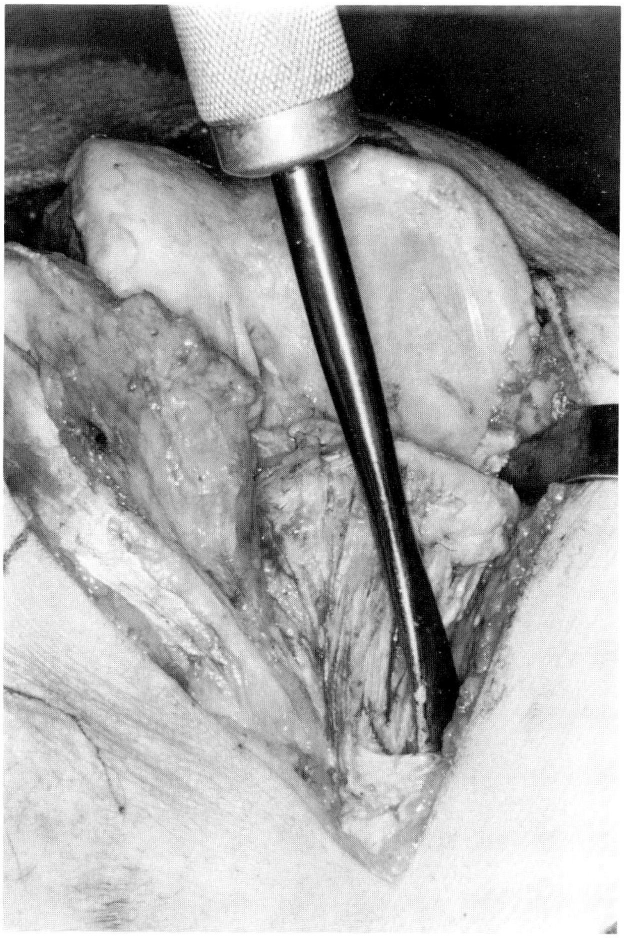

**Fig. 6-8C** Identification of the most anterior border of the pes anserinus tendon.

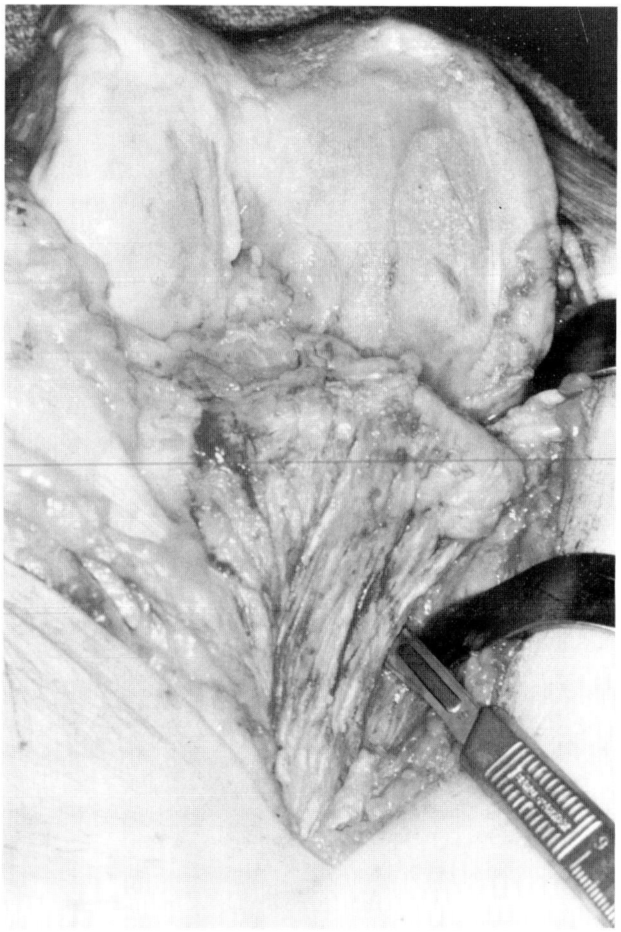

**Fig. 6-8D** Sharp elevation of the superficial medial collateral ligament.

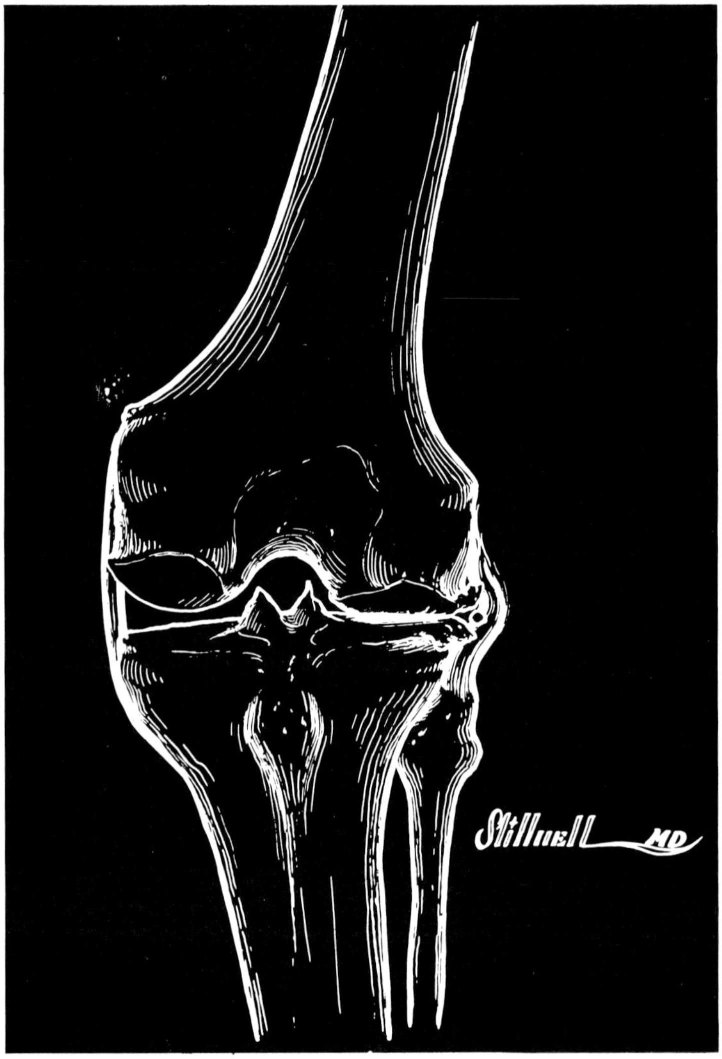


**Fig. 6-9A** The valgus knee.

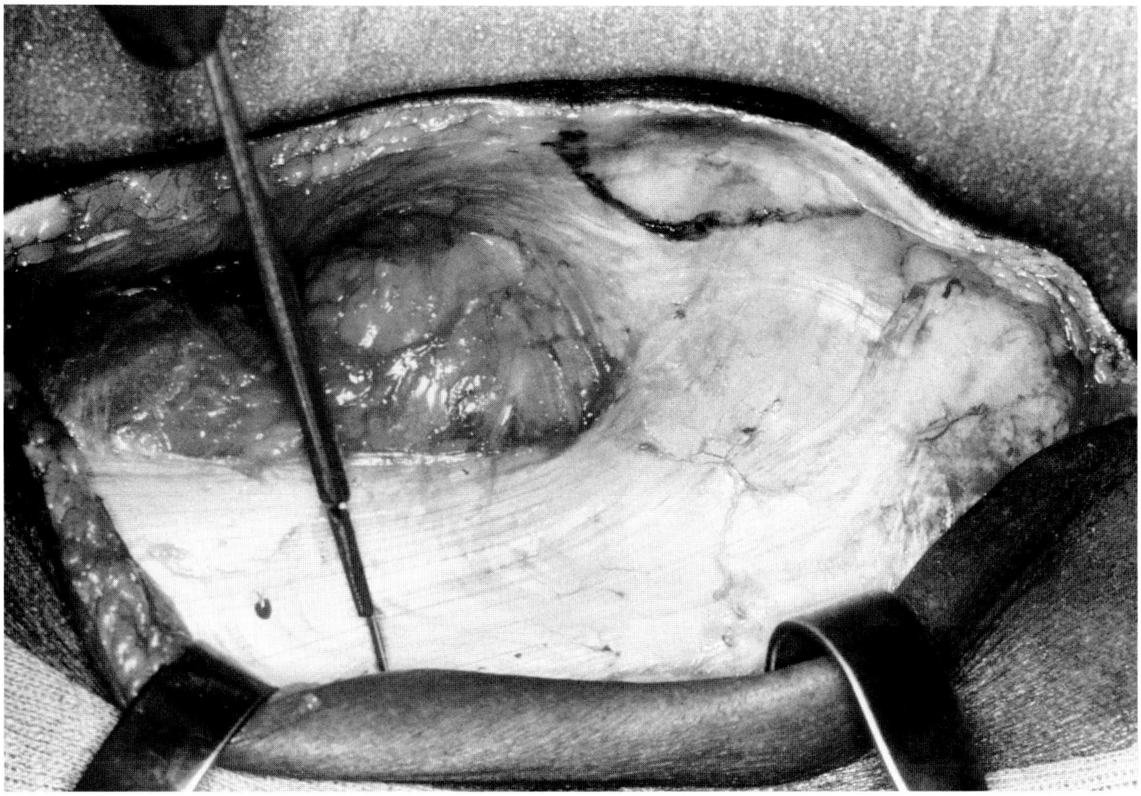

**Fig. 6-9B** The extraarticular component of the valgus knee; the iliotibial band may be transected anywhere along its course.

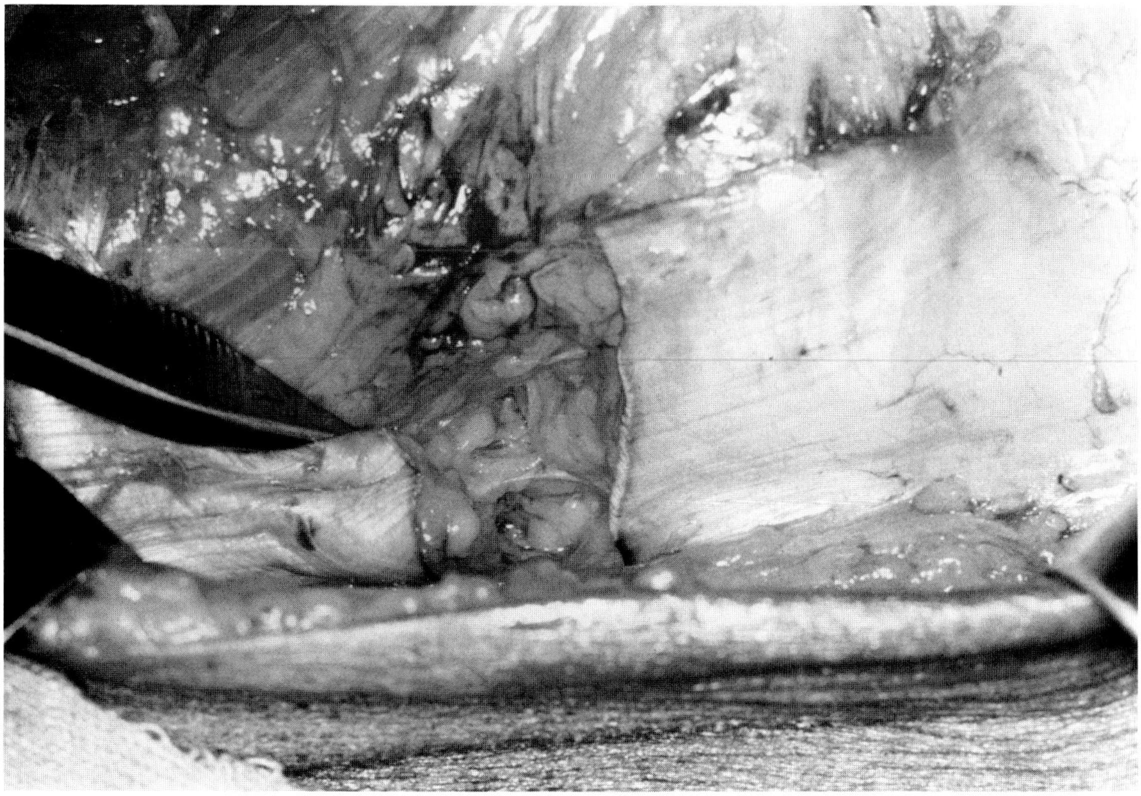

**Fig. 6-9C** Transection of the iliotibial band must be complete to eliminate the deforming force.

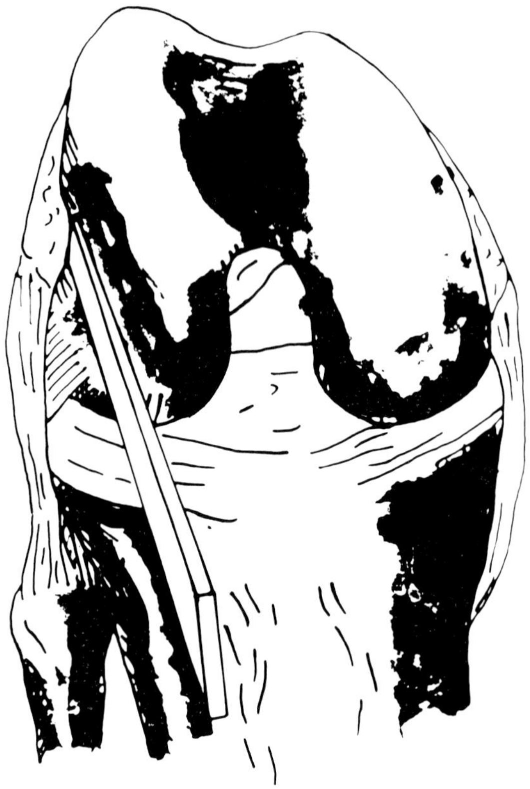

**Fig. 6-10A** The intraarticular valgus correction requires releasing the popliteus and lateral collateral ligament.

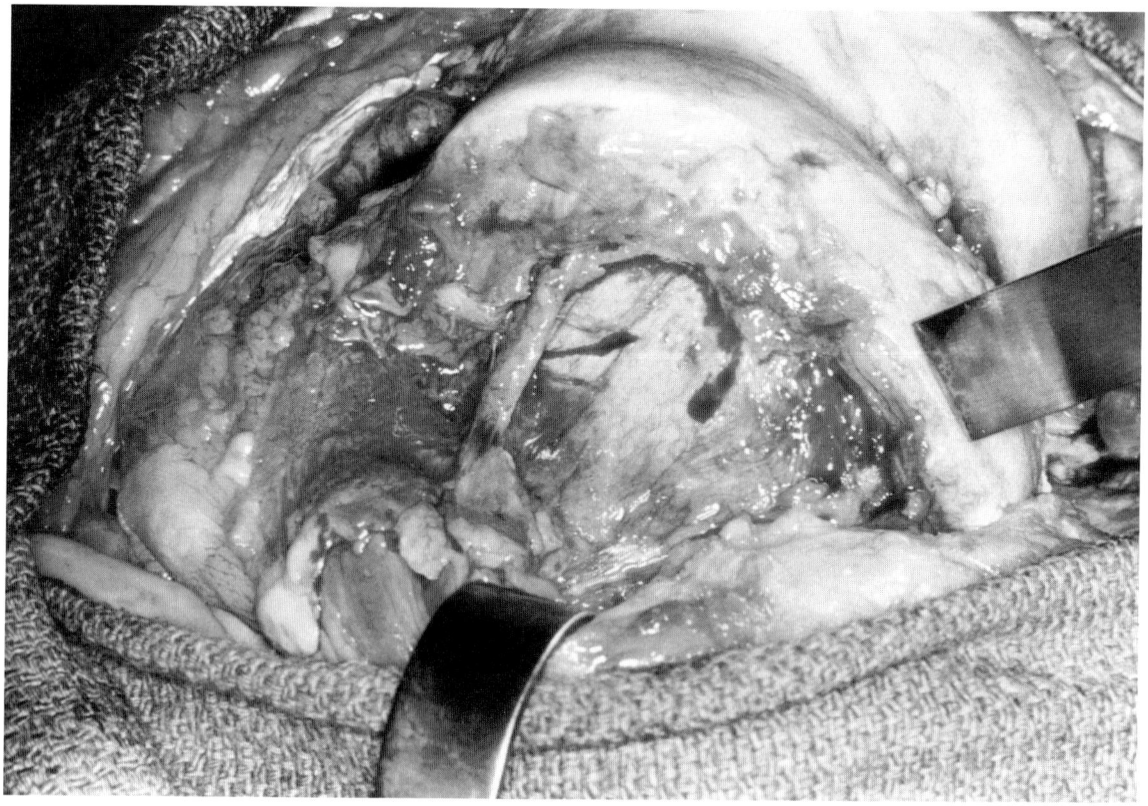

**Fig. 6-10B** The popliteus and lateral collateral may be elevated either sharply or with their bone attachment to the lateral femoral condyle.

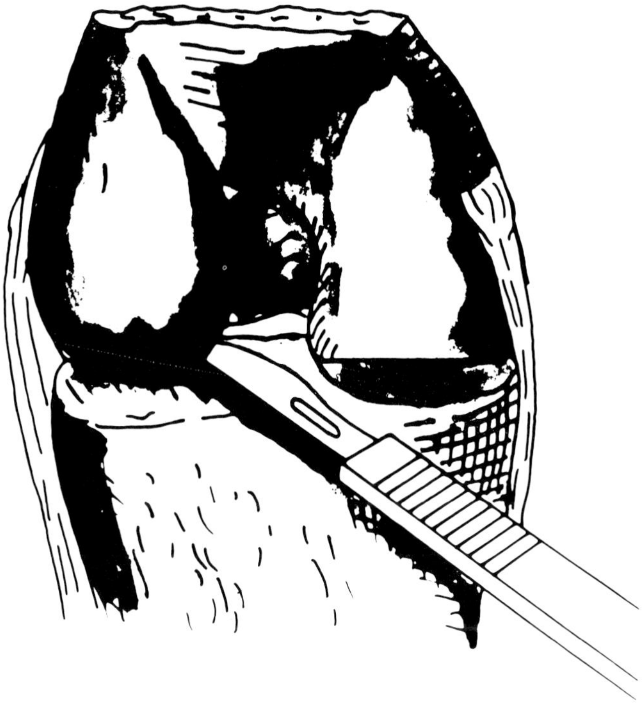

**Fig. 6-11A** A flexion contracture can be corrected by bone (distal femur-proximal tibia) resection and posterior capsule release.

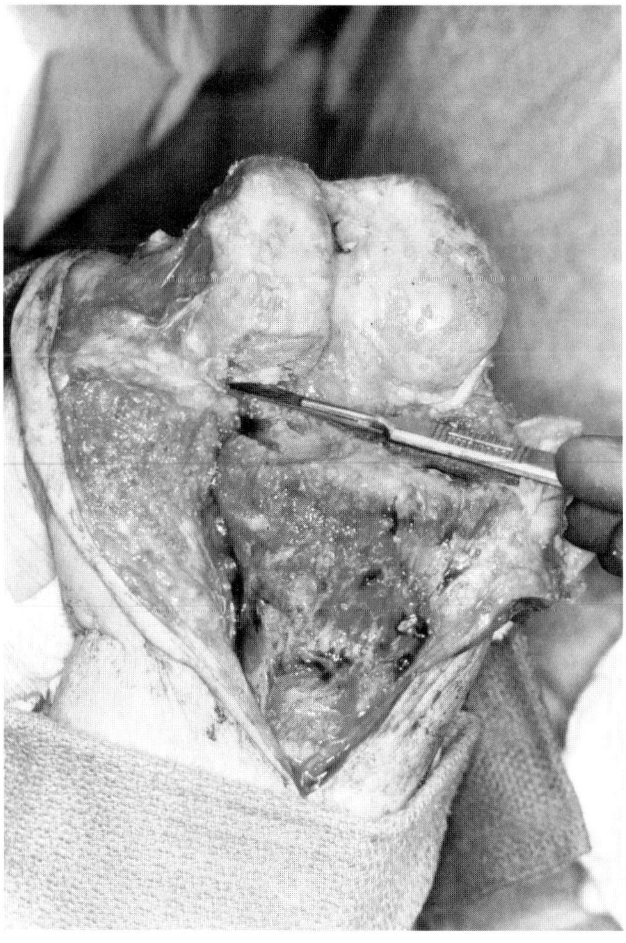

**Fig. 6-11B** Having removed the posterior condyles, the capsule can be directly identified.

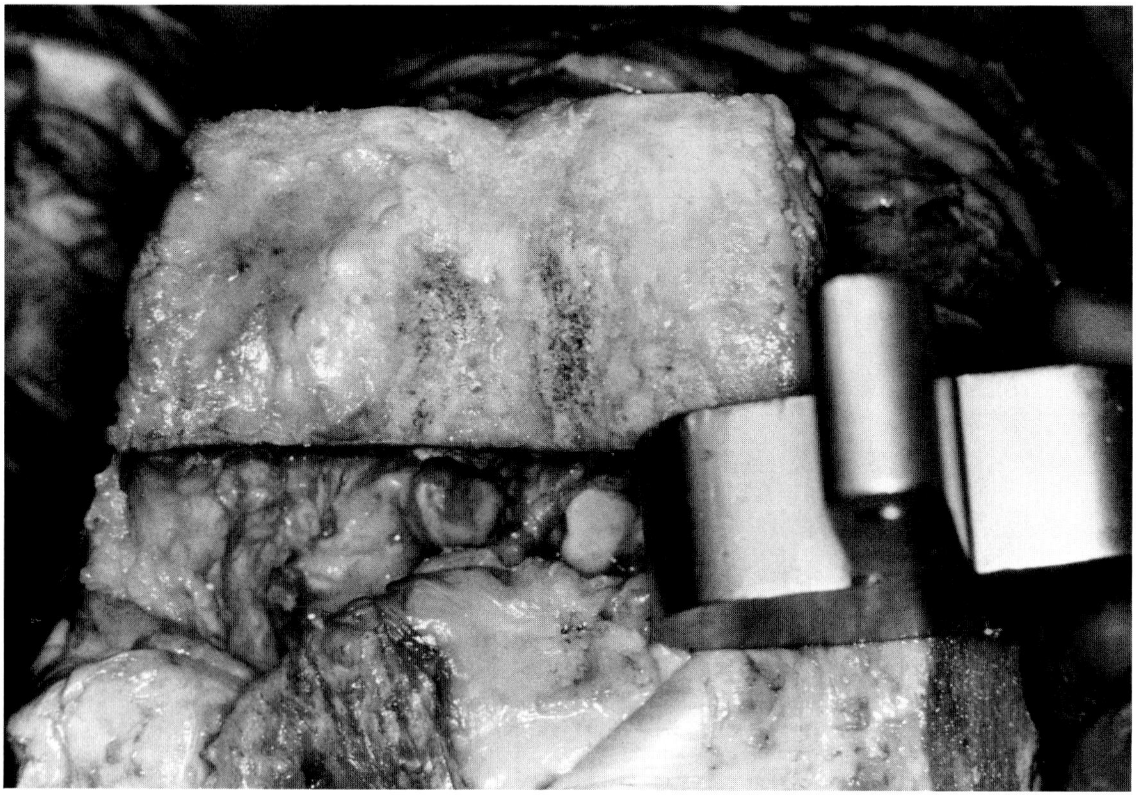

**Fig. 6-11C** Release of the bone and soft tissue component of the flexion contracture allows adequate spacing.

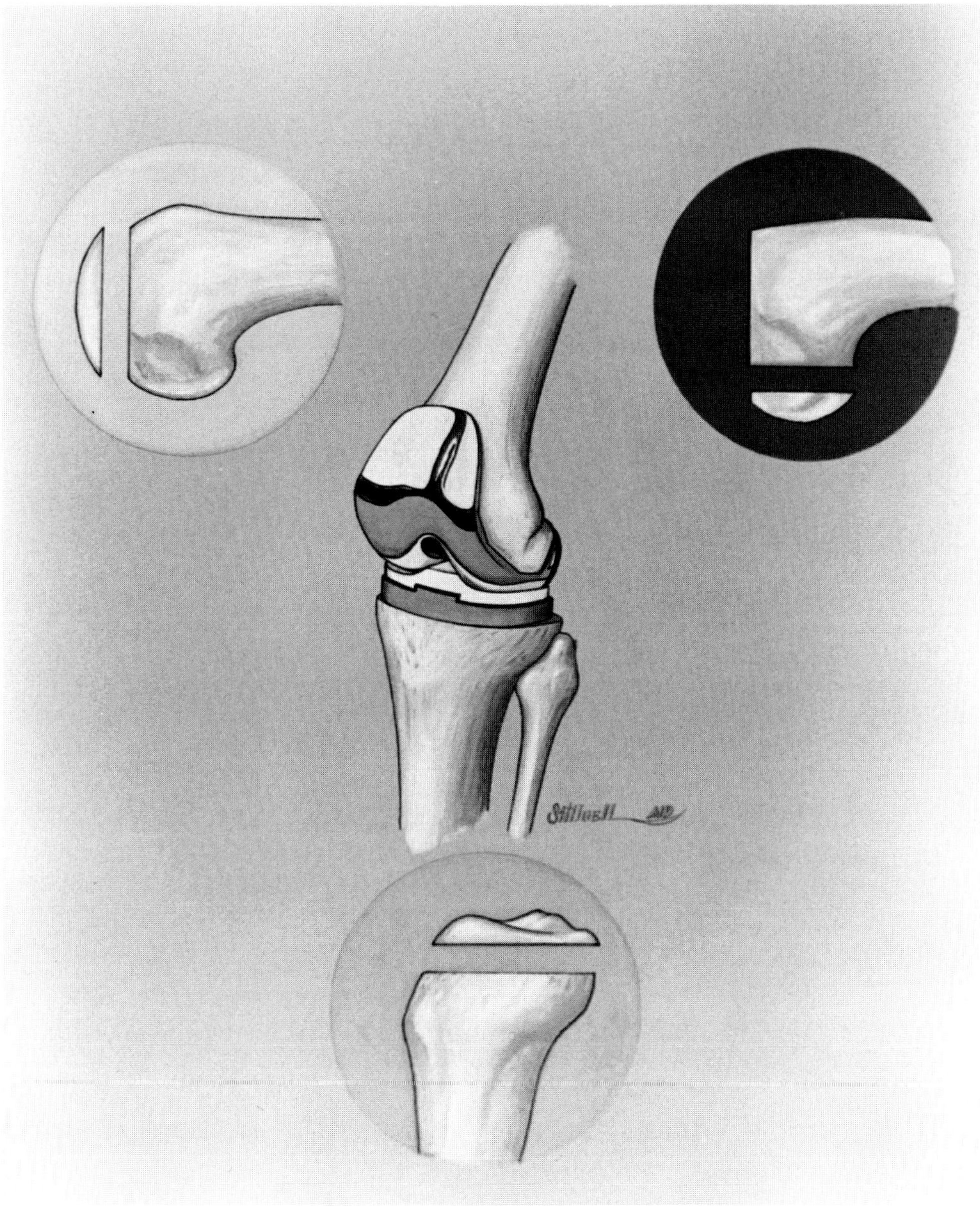

**Fig. 6-12** The basic bone cuts for alignment and stability in all types of knee arthroplasty.

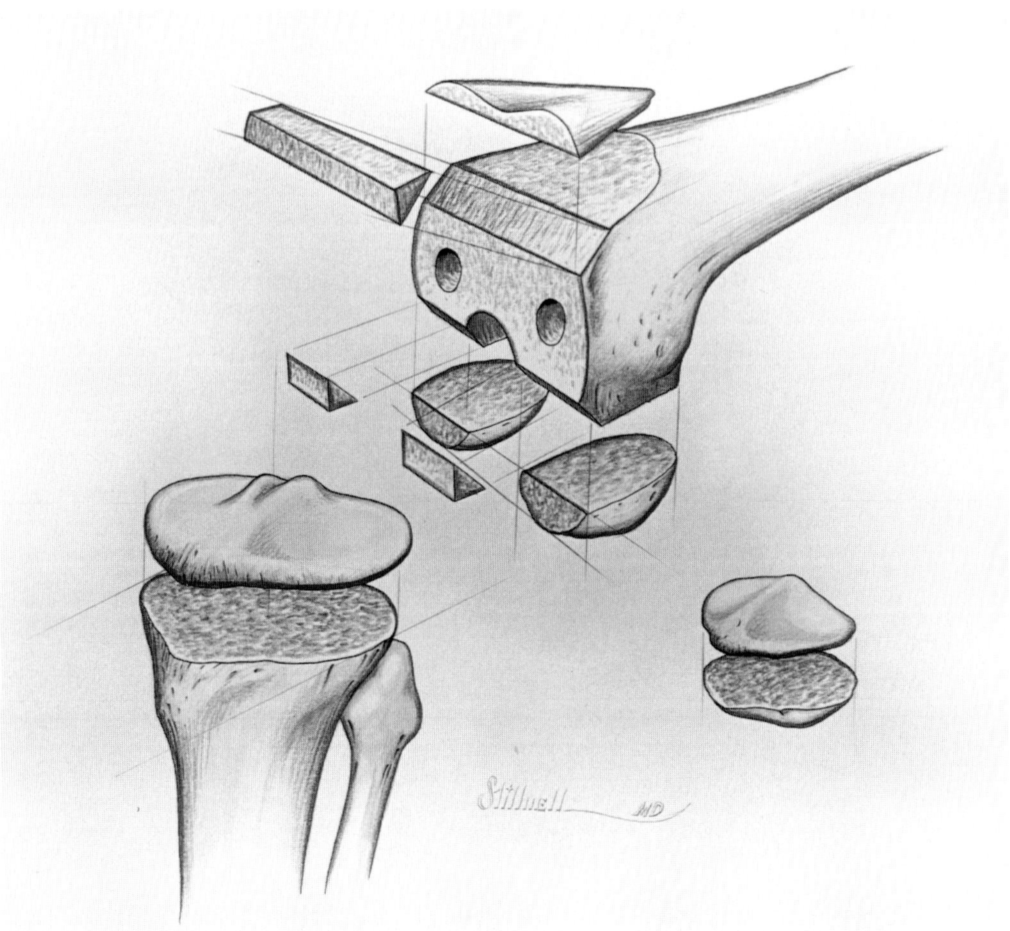


**Fig. 6-13** Bone resection for basic and chamfering cuts.

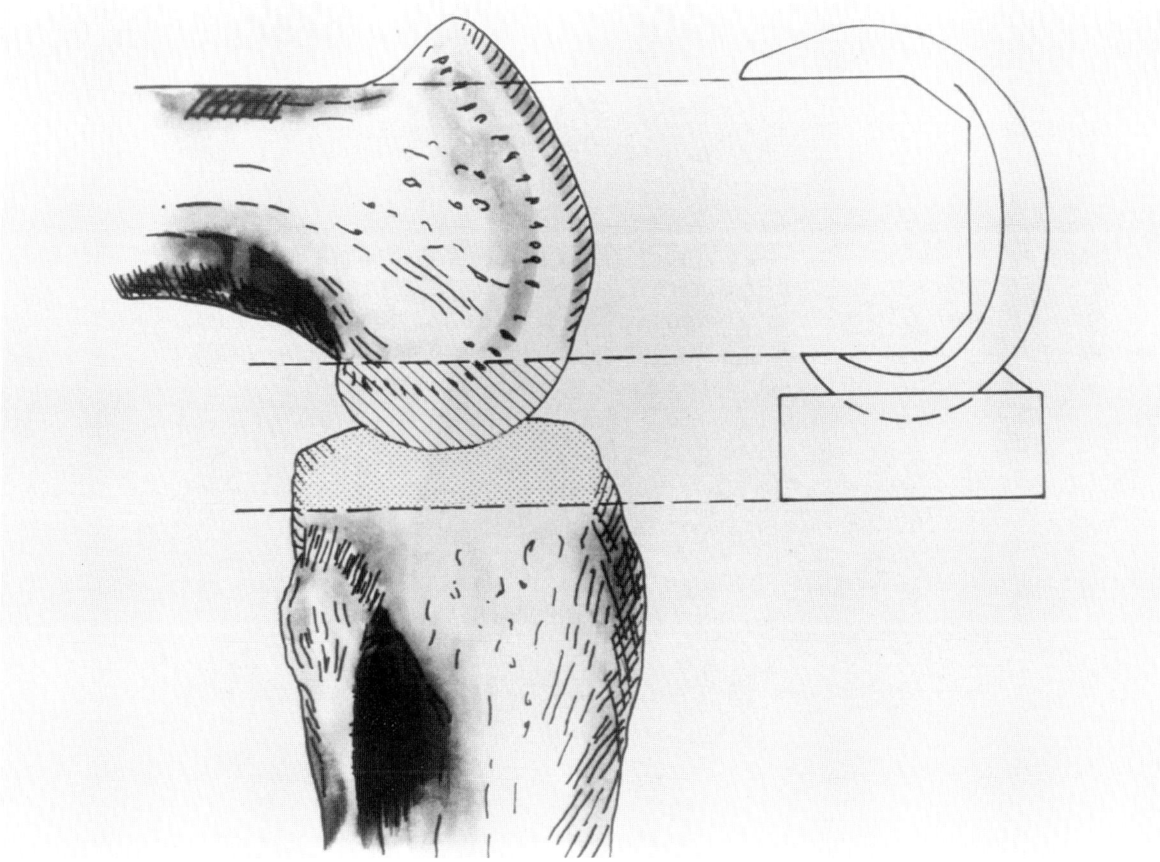

**Fig. 6-14A** Flexion space as identified by bone resection and prosthetic components. The anterior femoral cut is for leveling the bone to accommodate the femoral component.

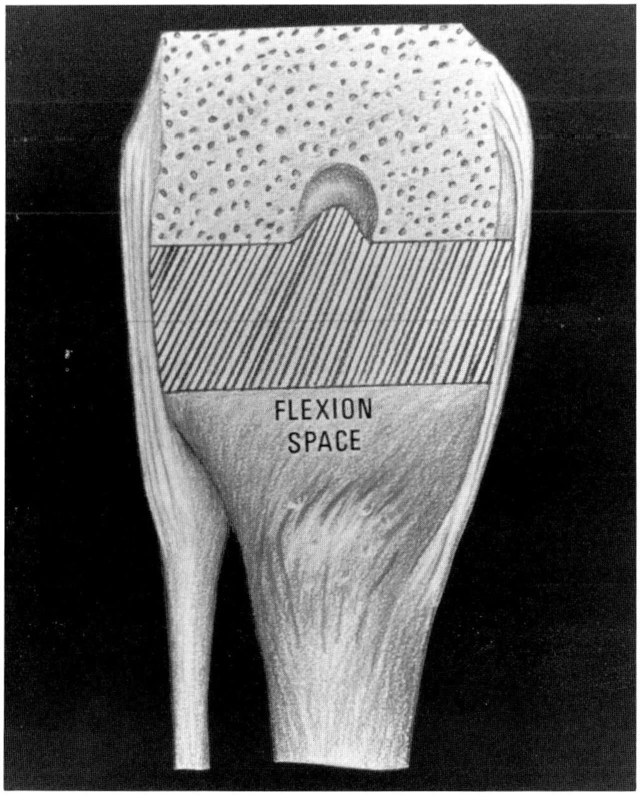


**Fig. 6-14B** Diagrammatic representation of flexion space as viewed in a frontal plane.

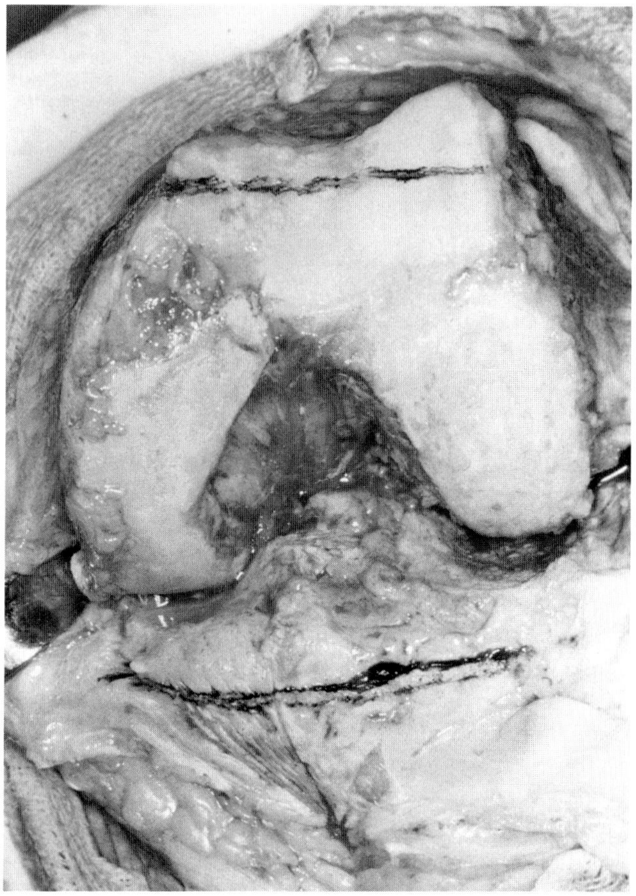

**Fig. 6-15A** Operative photograph indicating the level of resection of anterior and posterior femur and proximal tibia.

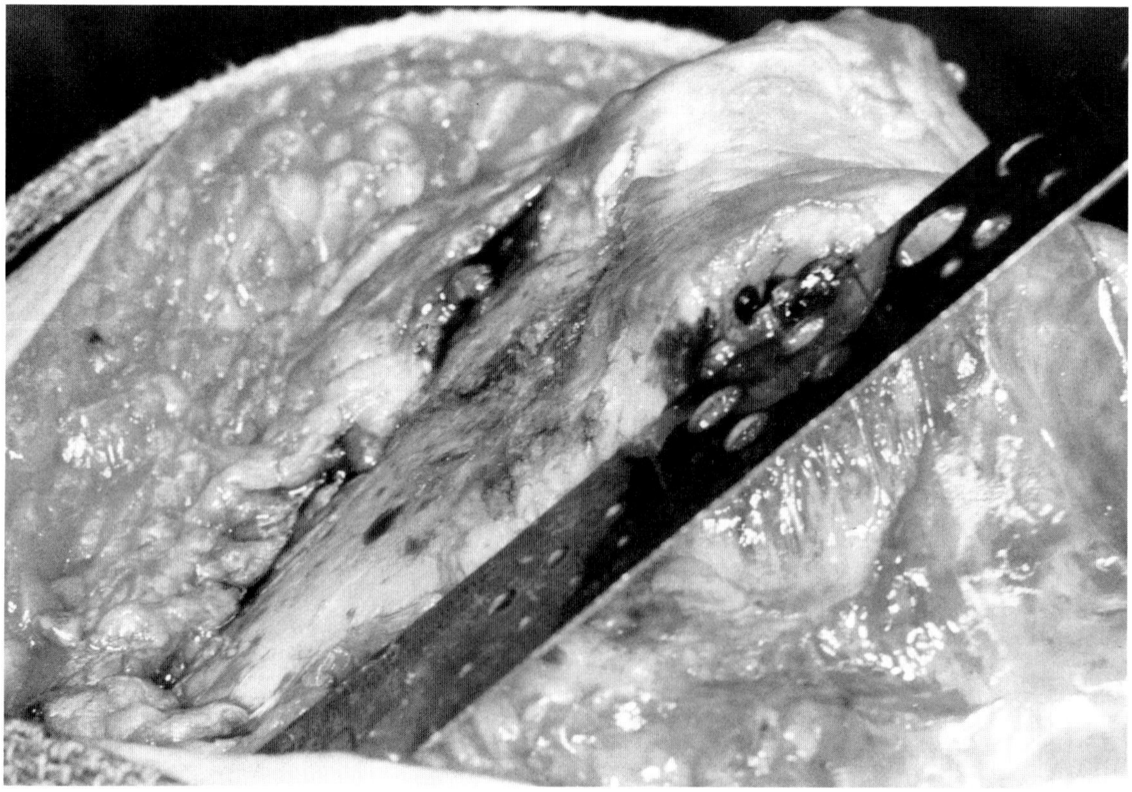

**Fig. 6-15B** A ruler used as a reference point to delineate the anterior femoral shaft.

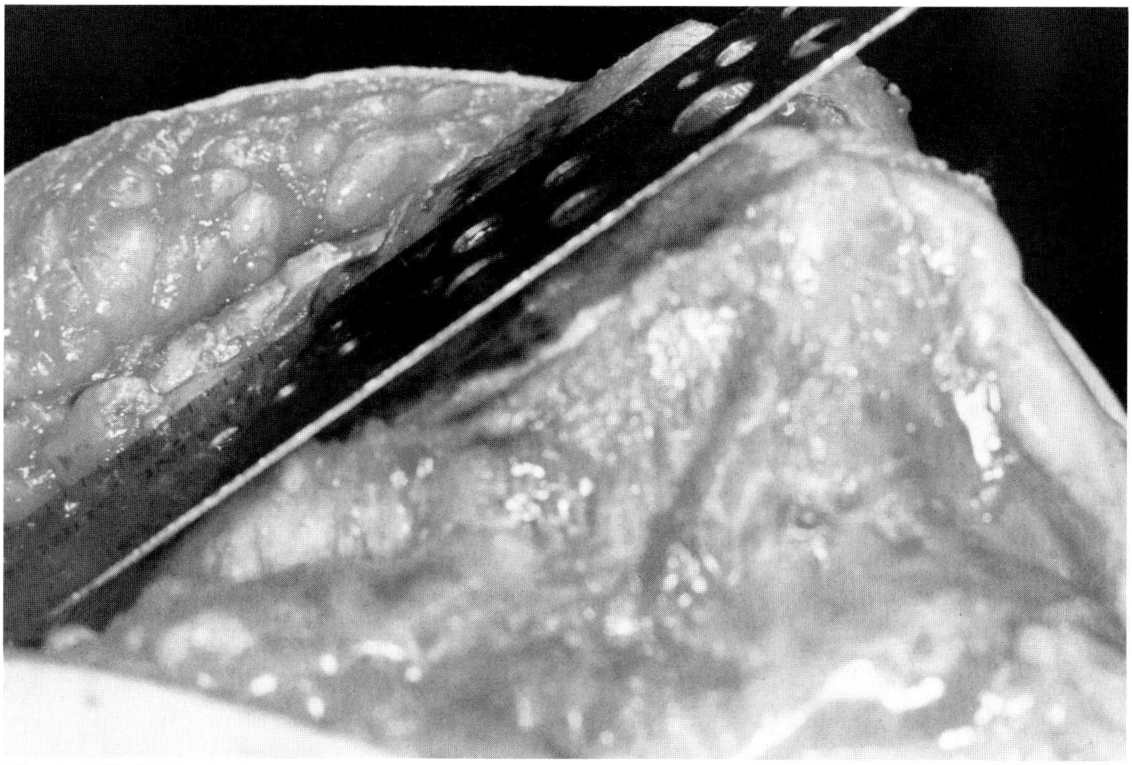

**Fig. 6-15C** With the bone resected, the ruler rests evenly on the anterior aspect of the femur.

**Fig. 6-15D** The resected anterior femoral bone is removed with an osteotome.

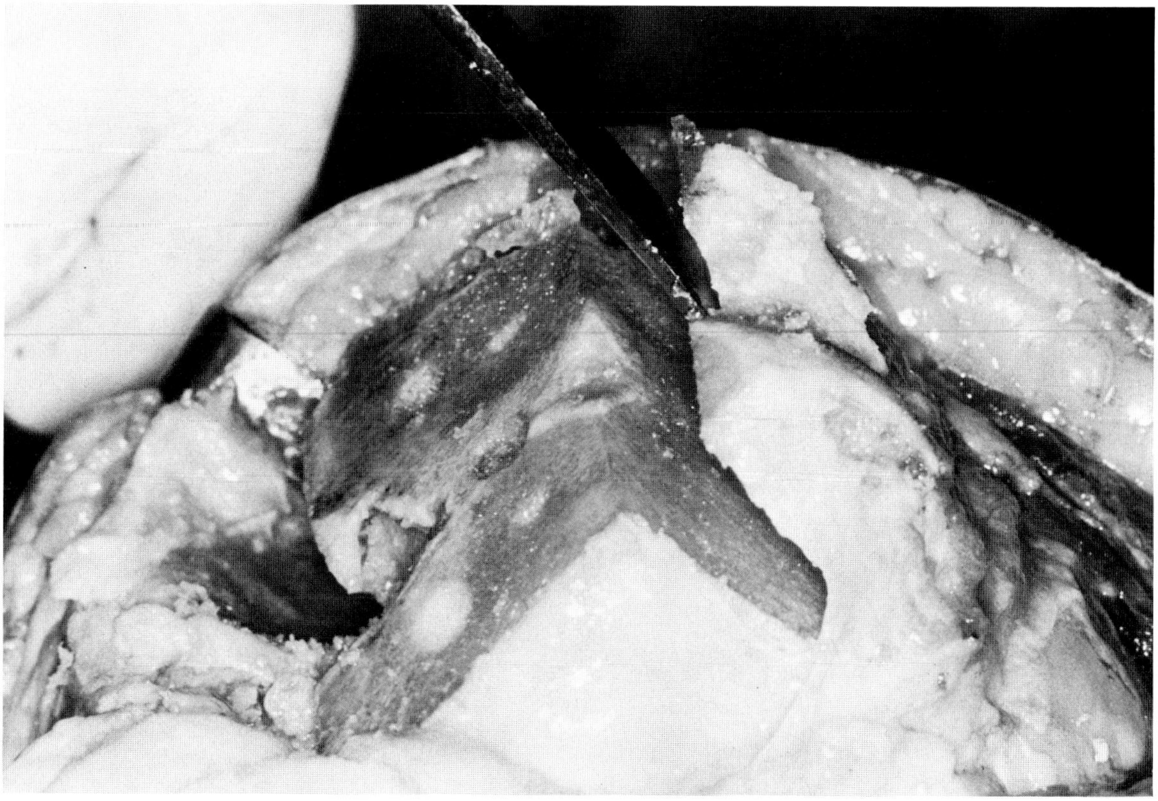

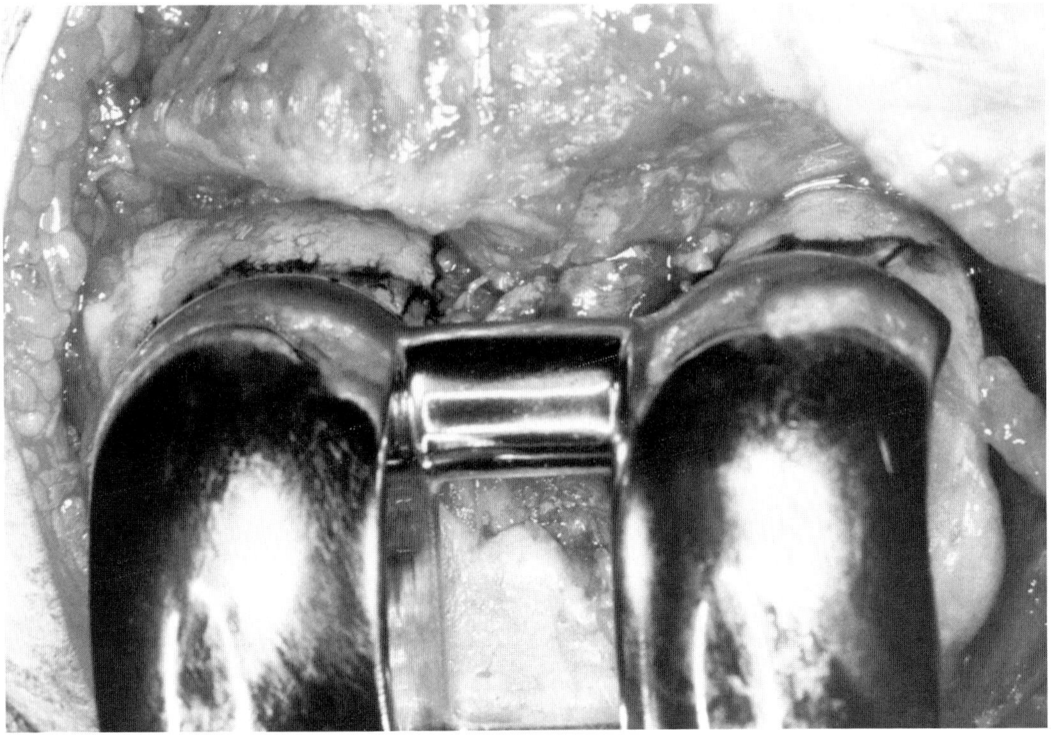

**Fig. 6-16A** "Dummy" prosthesis in situ to confirm the level of posterior femoral resection.

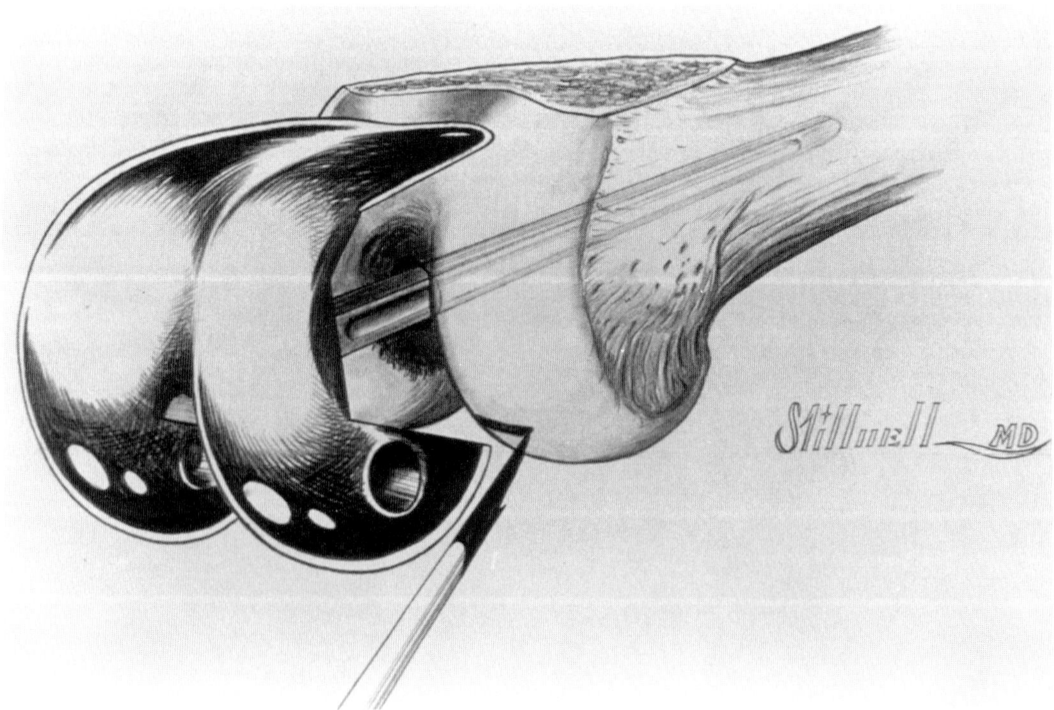

**Fig. 6-16B** Different systems use spacing blocks or trial prosthesis to identify the level of bone resection.

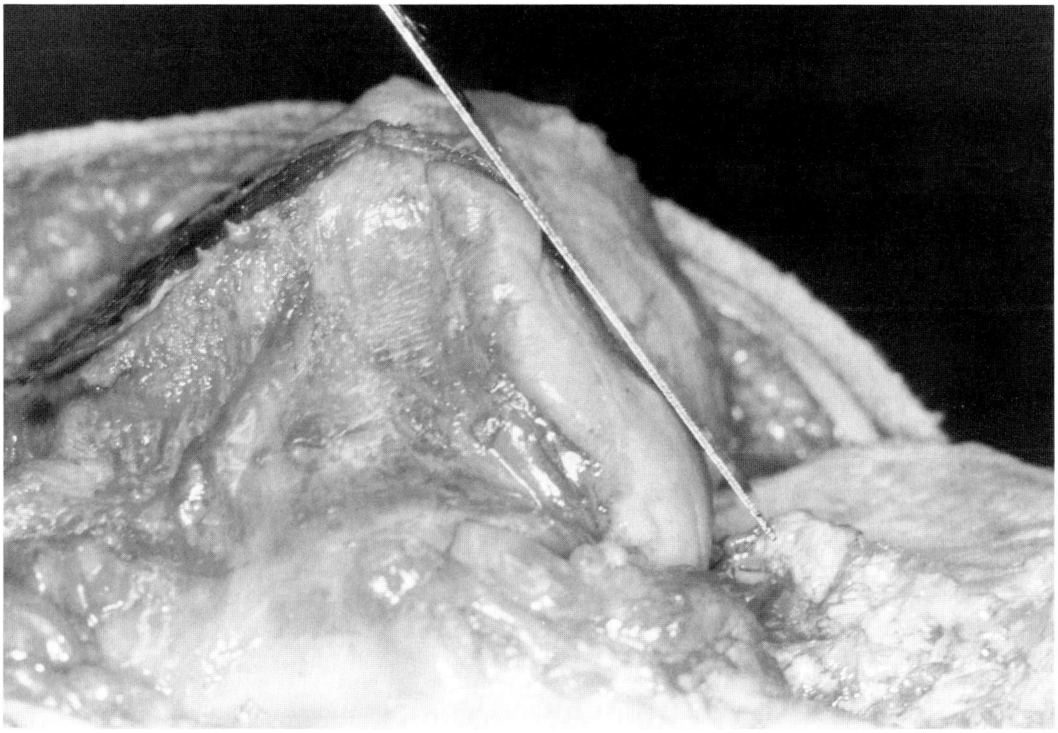

**Fig. 6-16C** A ruler marks the anterior/posterior dimension of the distal femur.

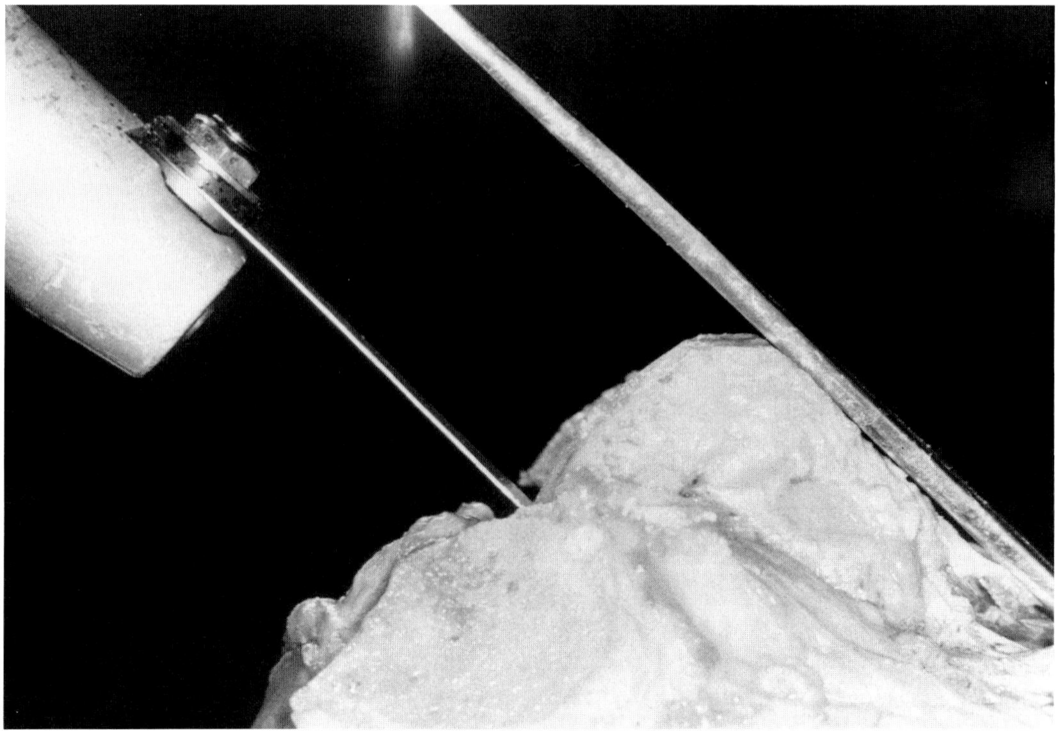

**Fig. 6-17A** The posterior femur is resected parallel to the anterior cortex.

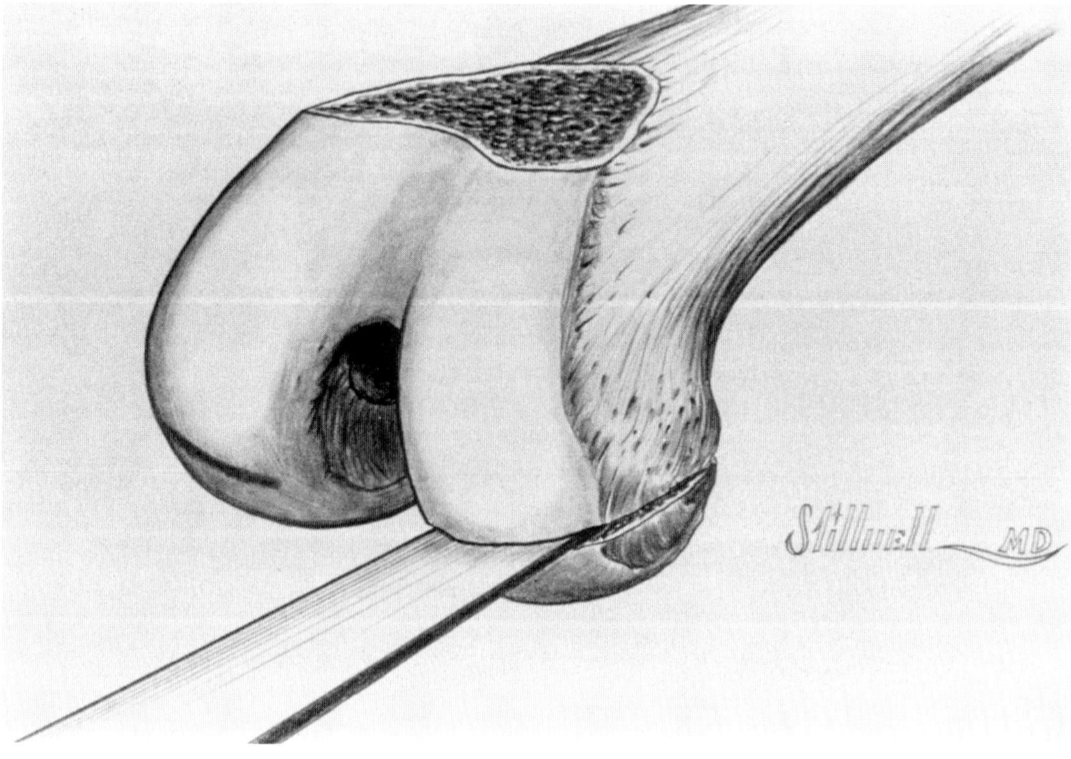

**Fig. 6-17B** The posterior femoral bone is removed with an osteotome.

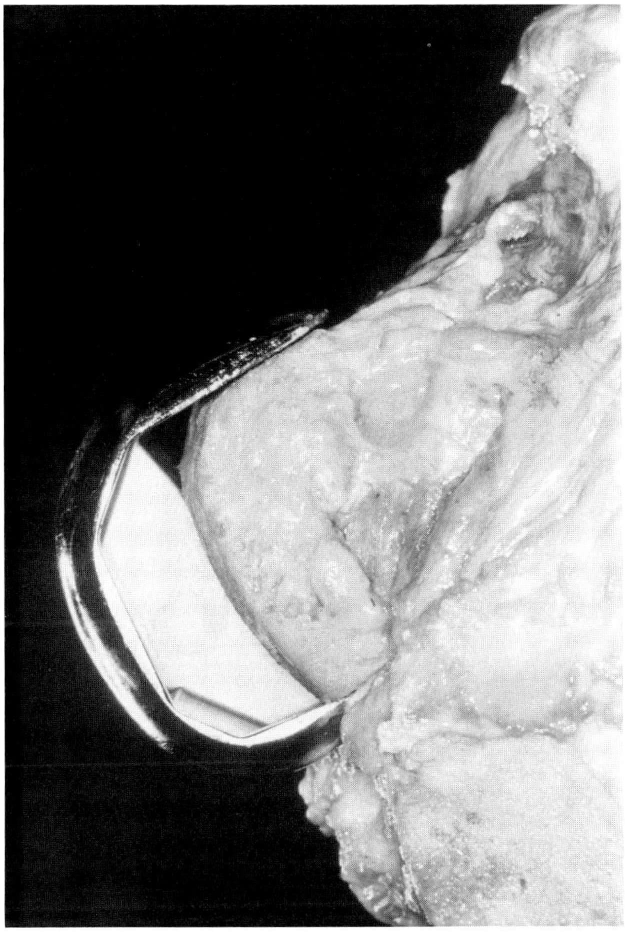

**Fig. 6-17C** A trial prosthesis confirms the area of anterior and posterior femoral bone resection.

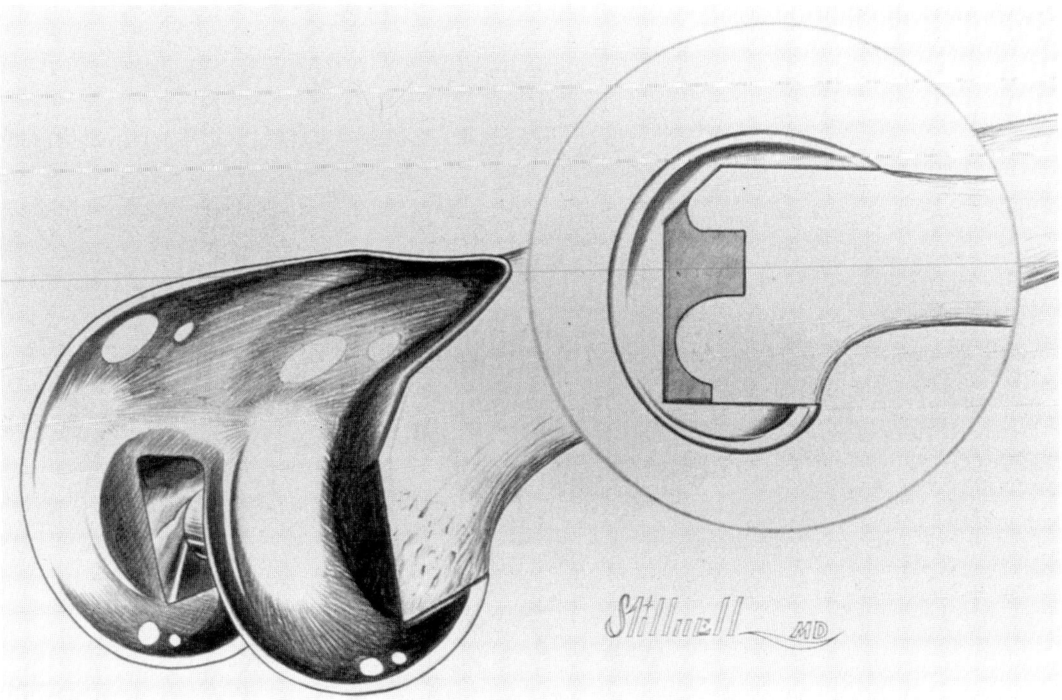

**Fig. 6-17D** A composite of a shaped femur and its trial component.

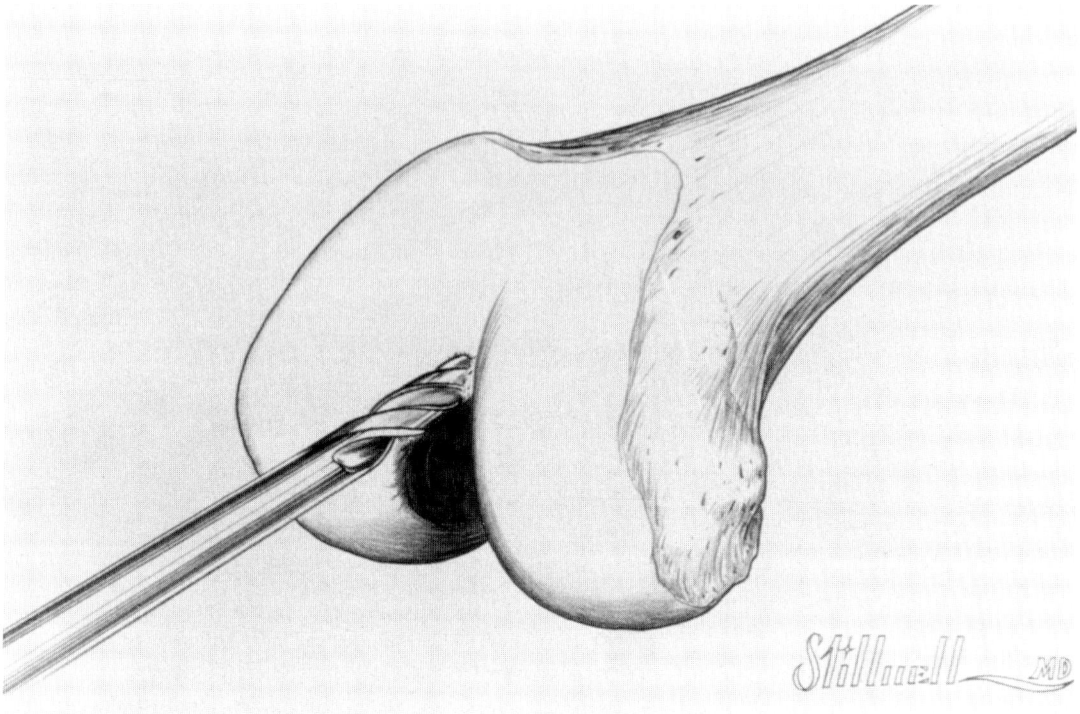

**Fig. 6-18A** For a "stemmed" femoral component, a centering hole is made in the distal femur.

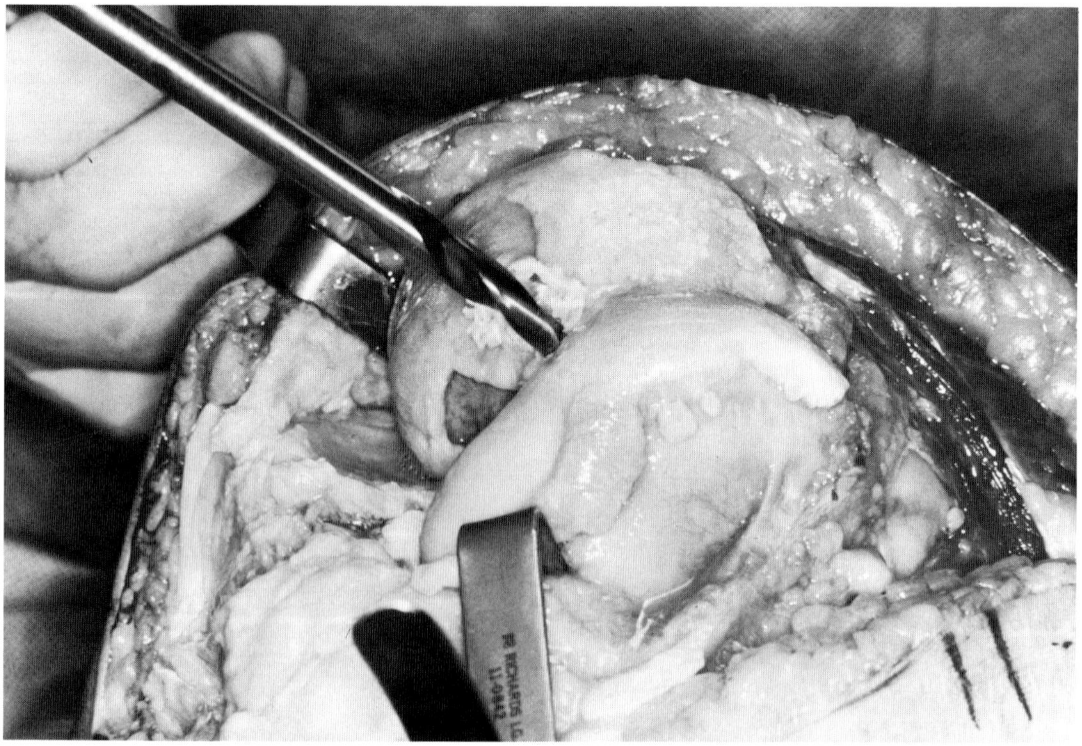

**Fig. 6-18B** The hole is usually centered at the level of the posterior cruciate ligament.

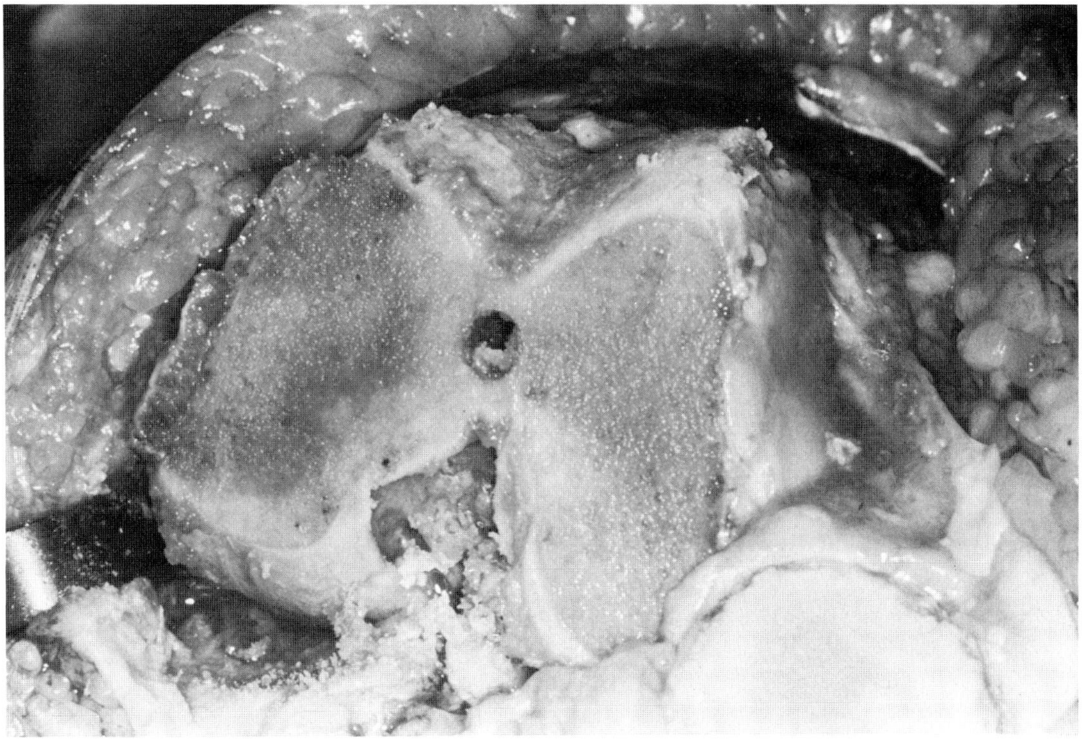

**Fig. 6-18C** Resecting the distal femur constitutes completion of one-half of the extension space.

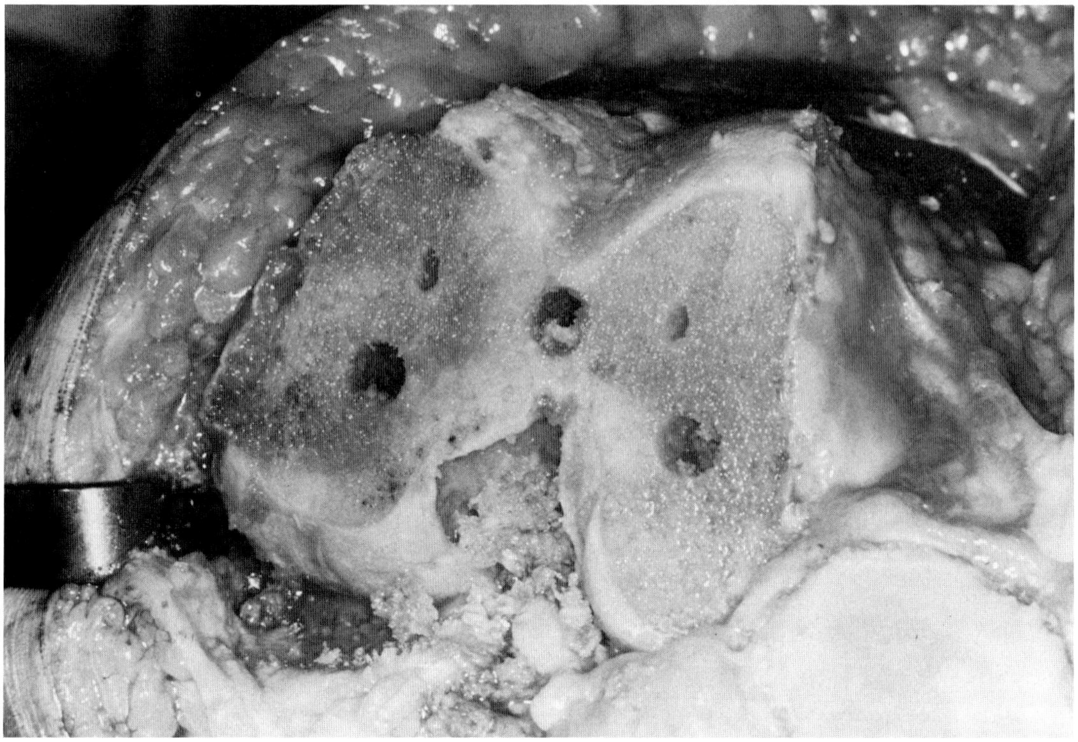

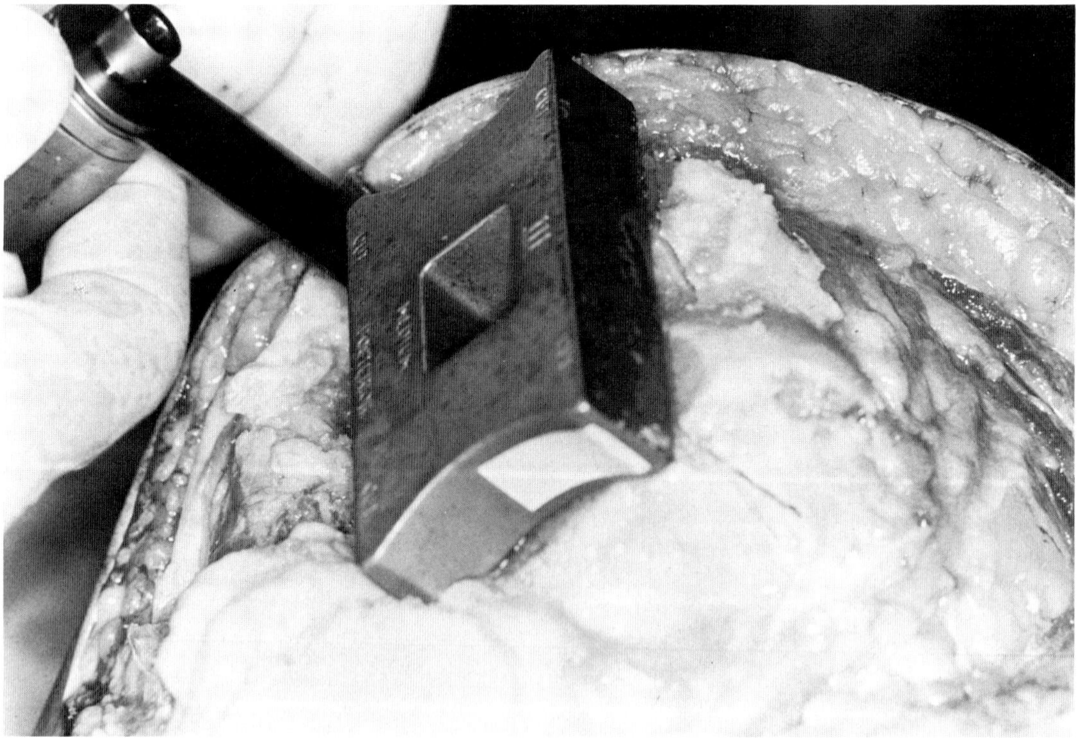

**Figs. 6-19A and B** Cutting block for anterior and posterior femur.

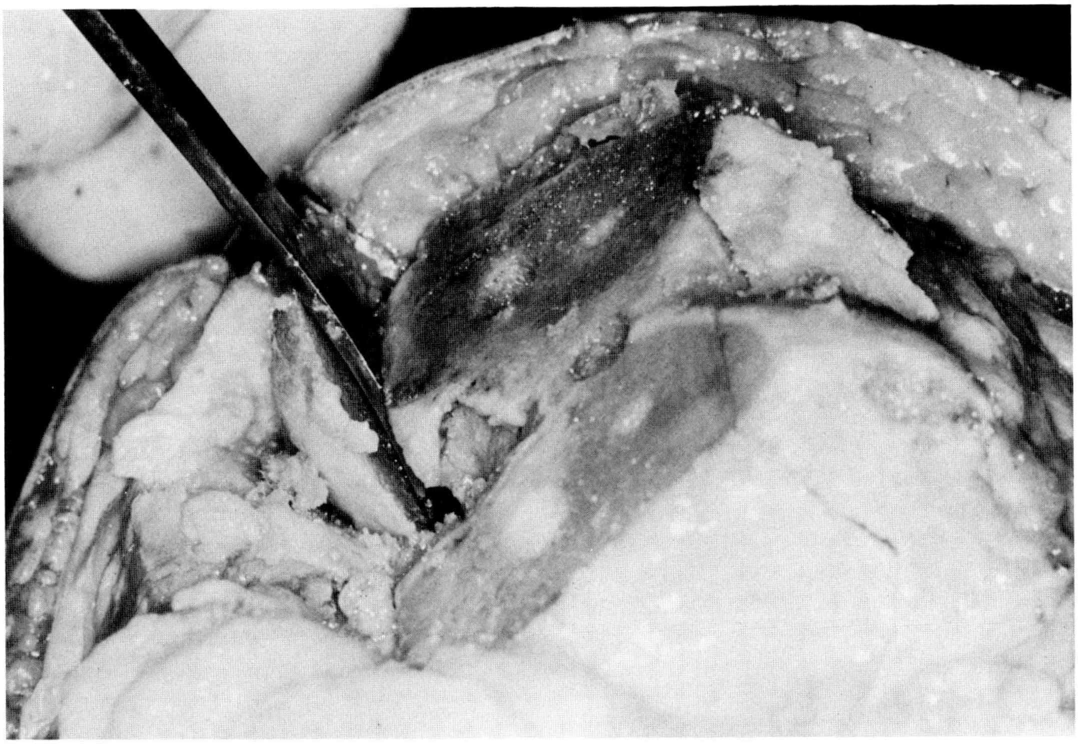

**Fig. 6-19C** In some procedures the posterior femoral resection is after the distal femur.

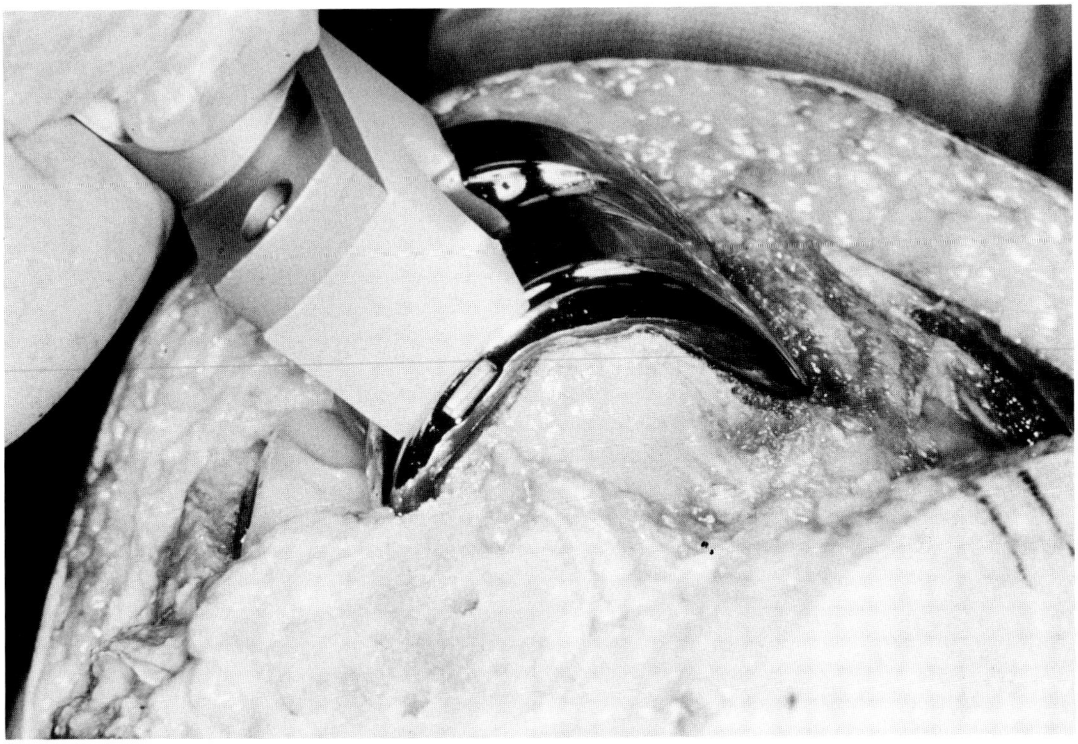

**Fig. 6-19D** Press fit of the femoral component.

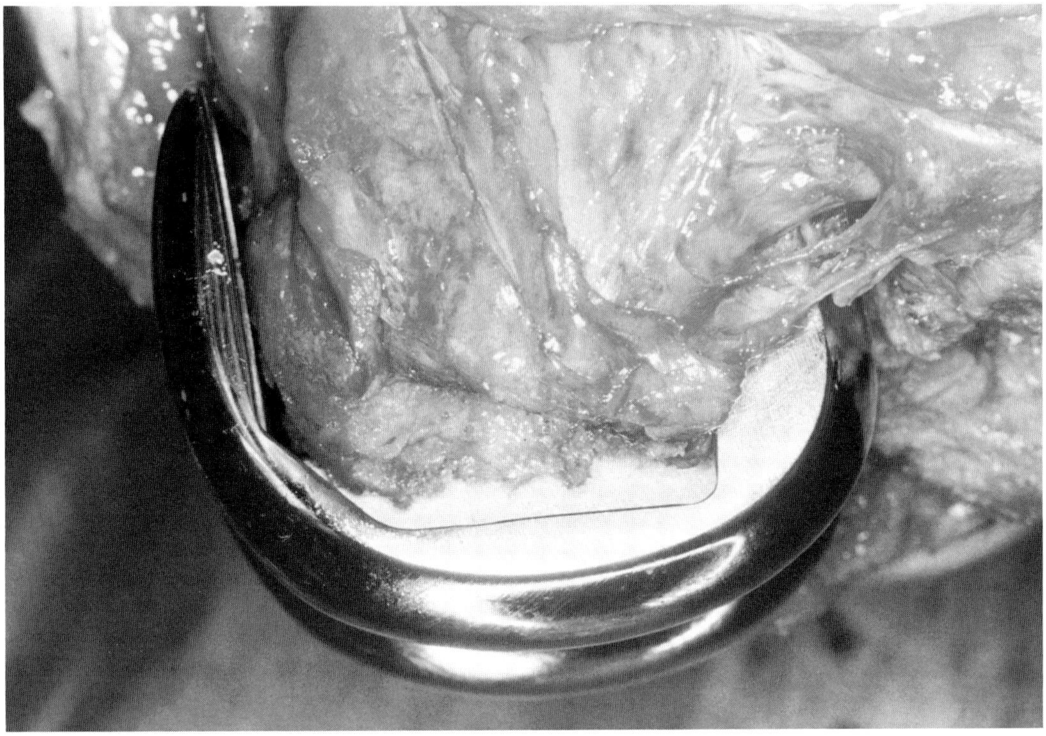

**Fig. 6-20A** A built-up femoral component can compensate for specific bone loss, e.g., posterior femur.

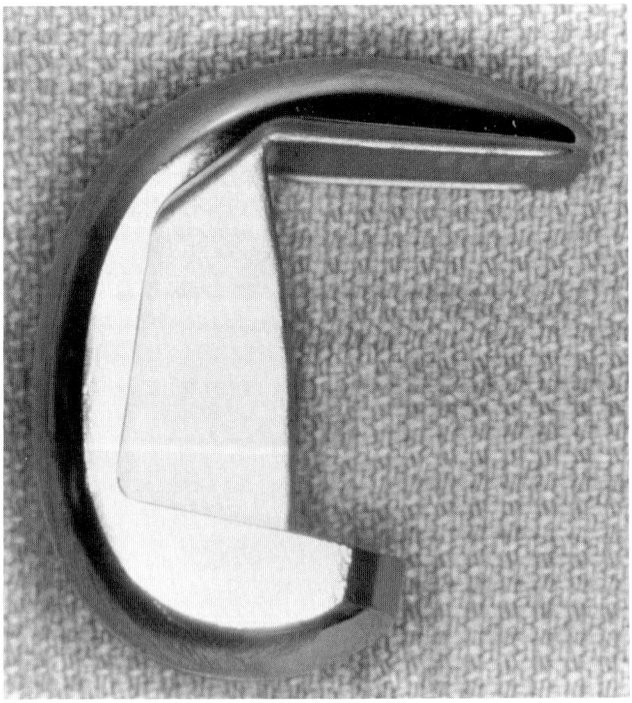

**Fig. 6-20B** A typical femoral component is available in several different anterior-posterior dimensions and can even be further augmented to compensate for bone loss.

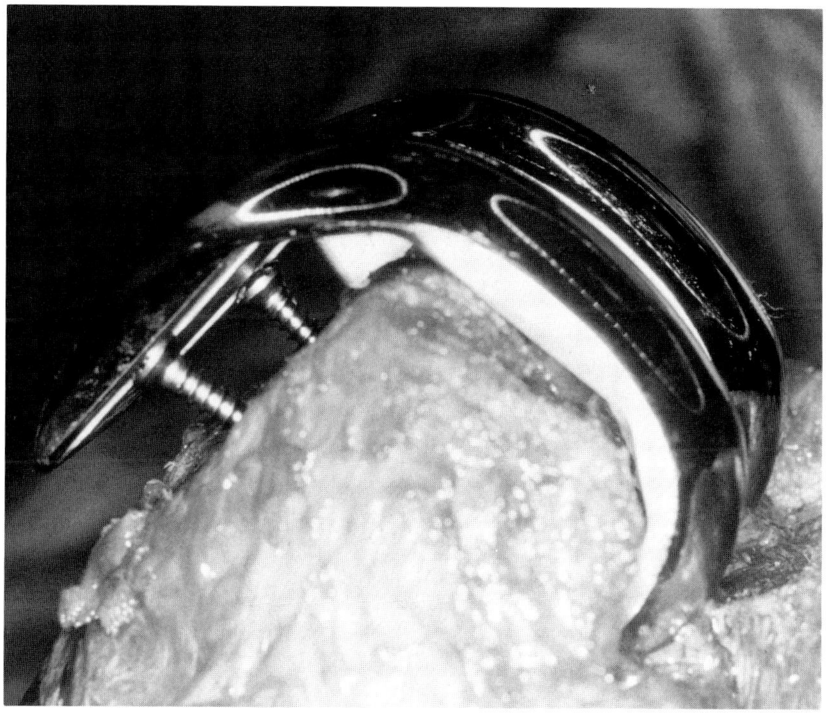

**Fig. 6-20C** Bone loss can also be accommodated for with screws and cement build-up.

Fig. 6-21A The extension space is composed of the distal femur and proximal tibia.

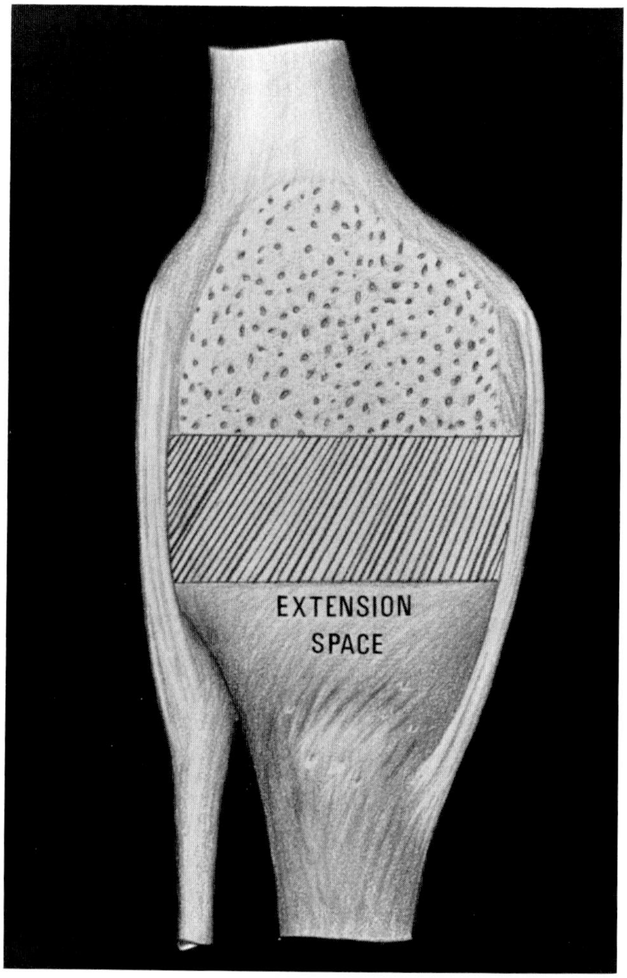


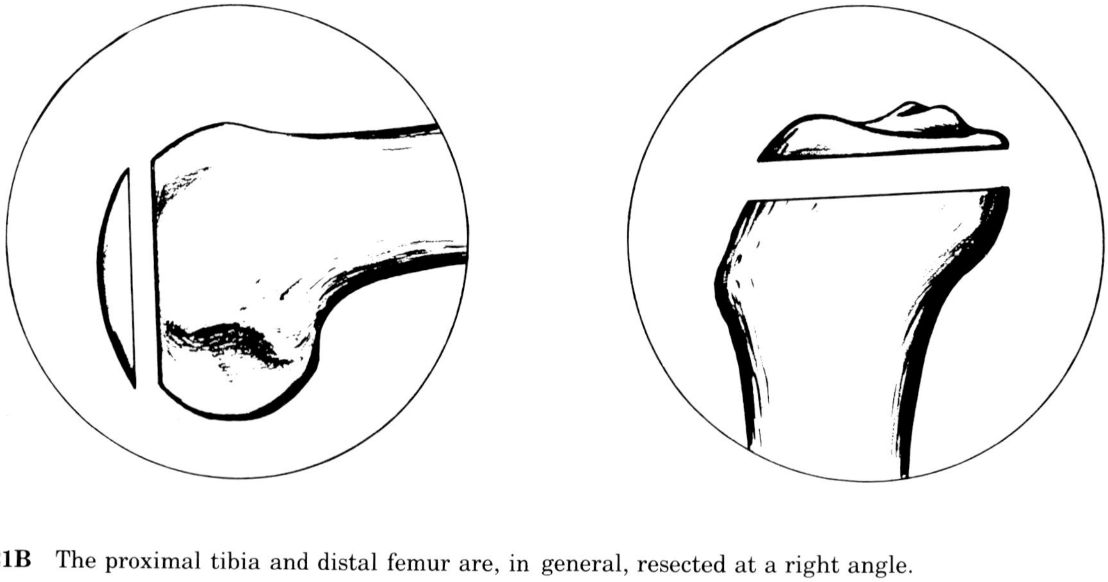

Fig. 6-21B The proximal tibia and distal femur are, in general, resected at a right angle.

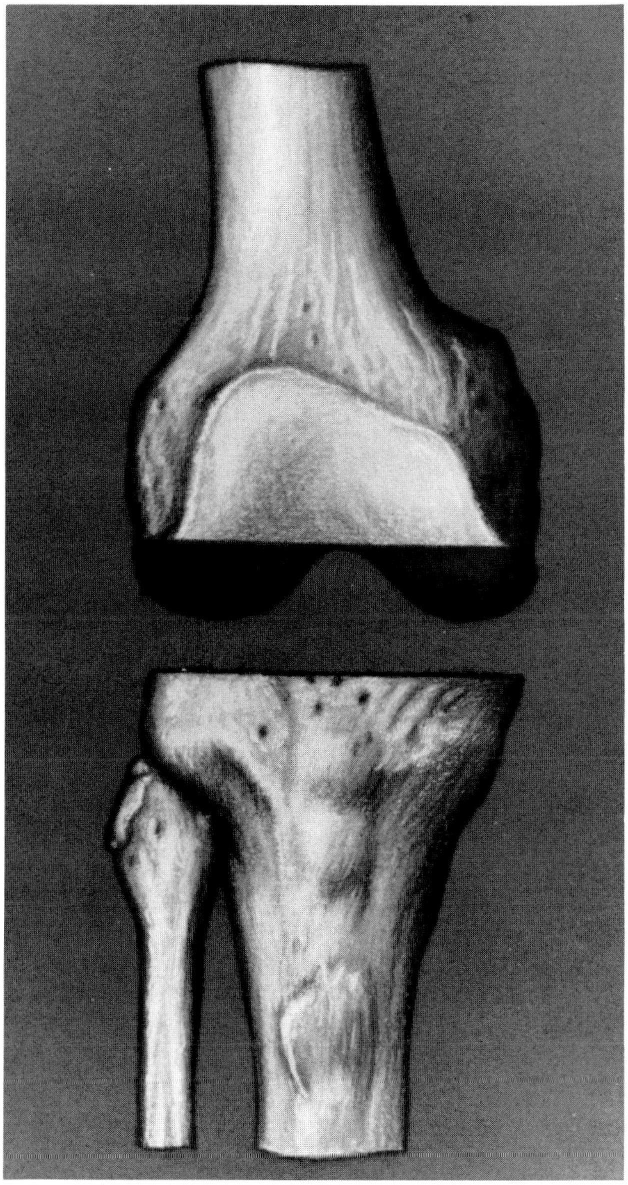

**Fig. 6-22A** If the procedure entails resection of the proximal tibia first, the remainder of the extension space, distal femur, must be cut parallel to the resected tibia.

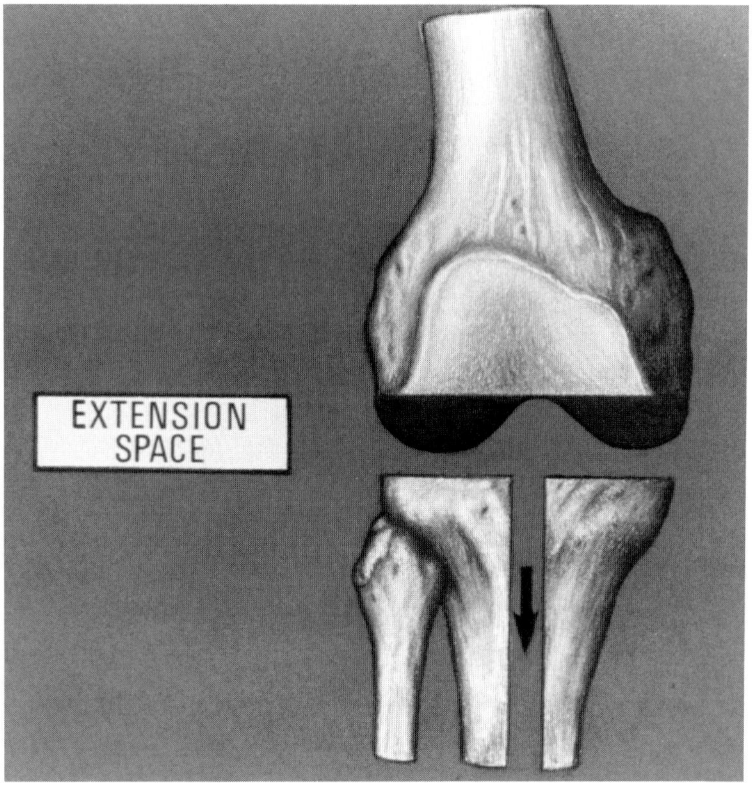


**Fig. 6-22B** The distal femur is resected after distraction to ensure minimal bone removal.

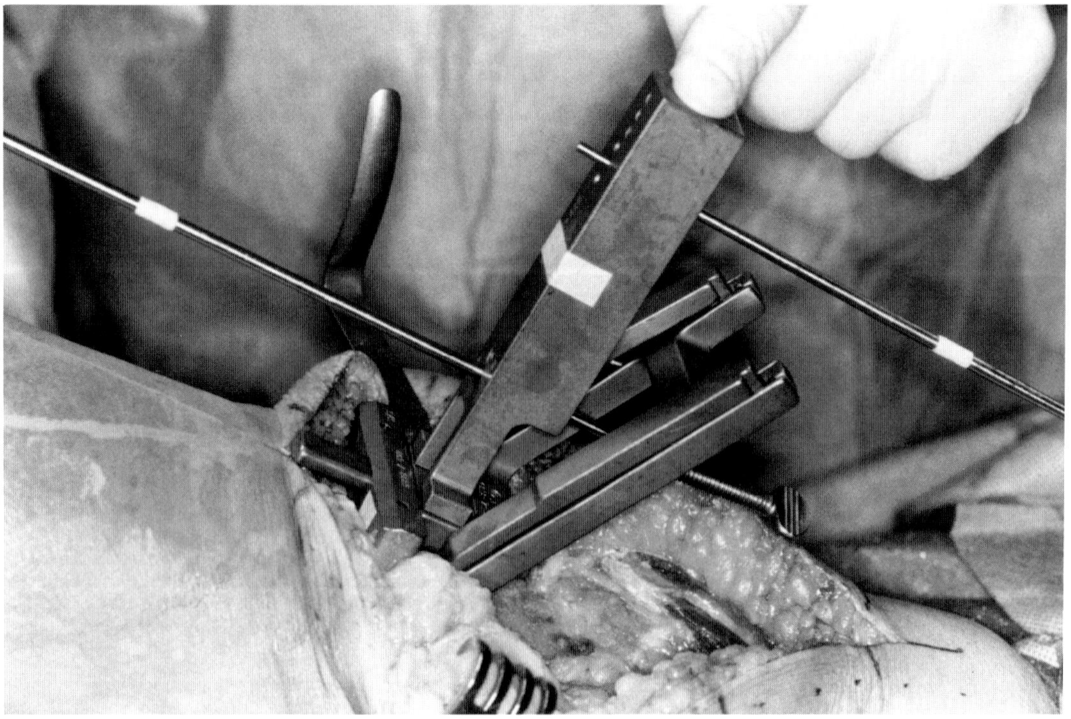

**Fig. 6-22C** In some systems the distal femur is resected first using aligning rods to delineate the mechanical or anatomical axis.

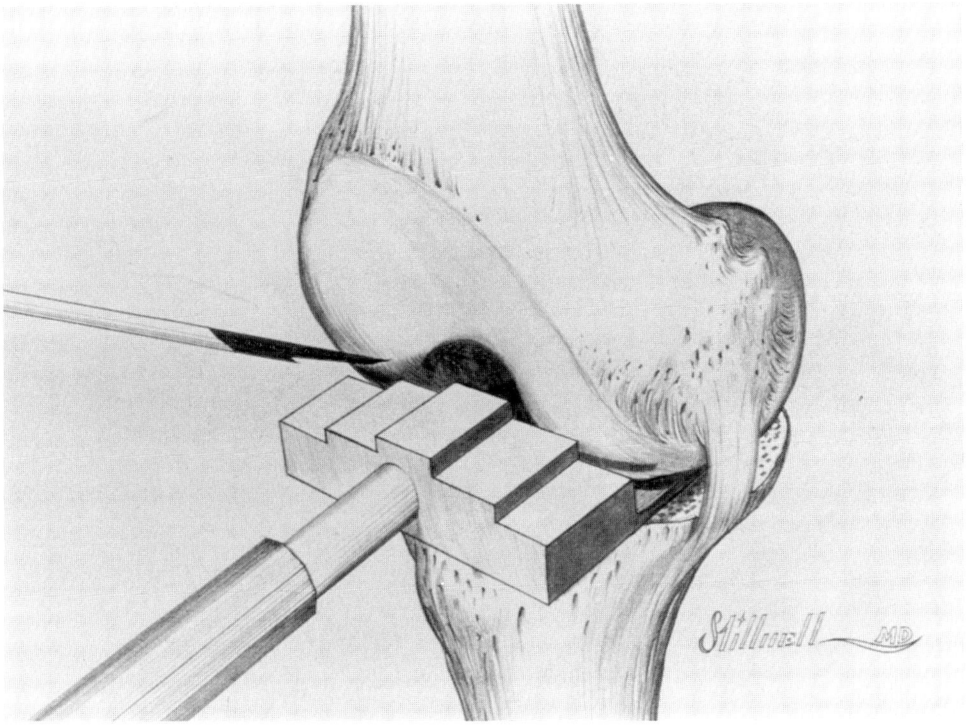

**Fig. 6-23A** In some techniques, the distal femur is resected without distraction.

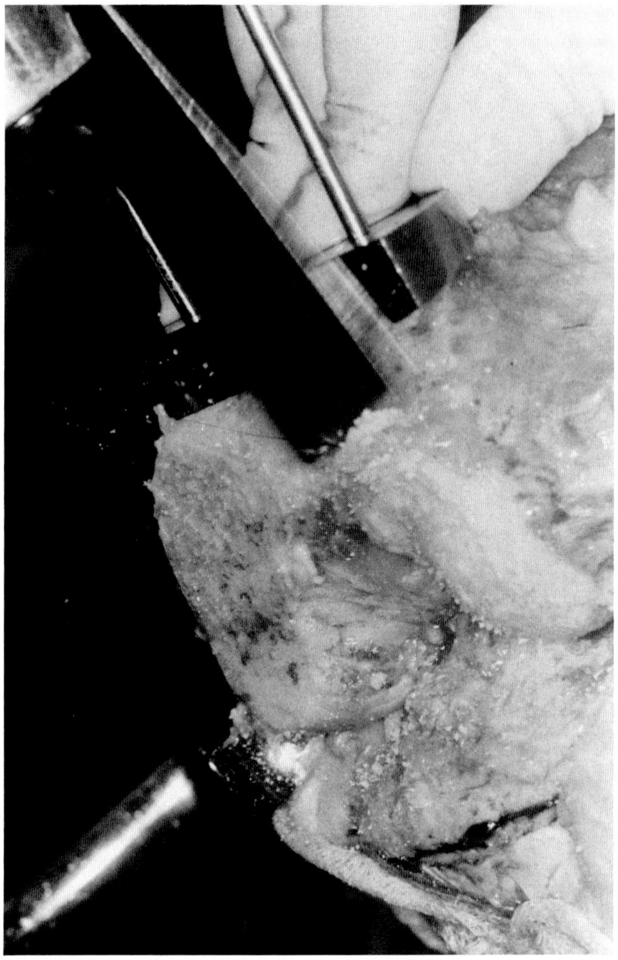

Fig. 6-23B The distal femur is cut with an oscillating saw.

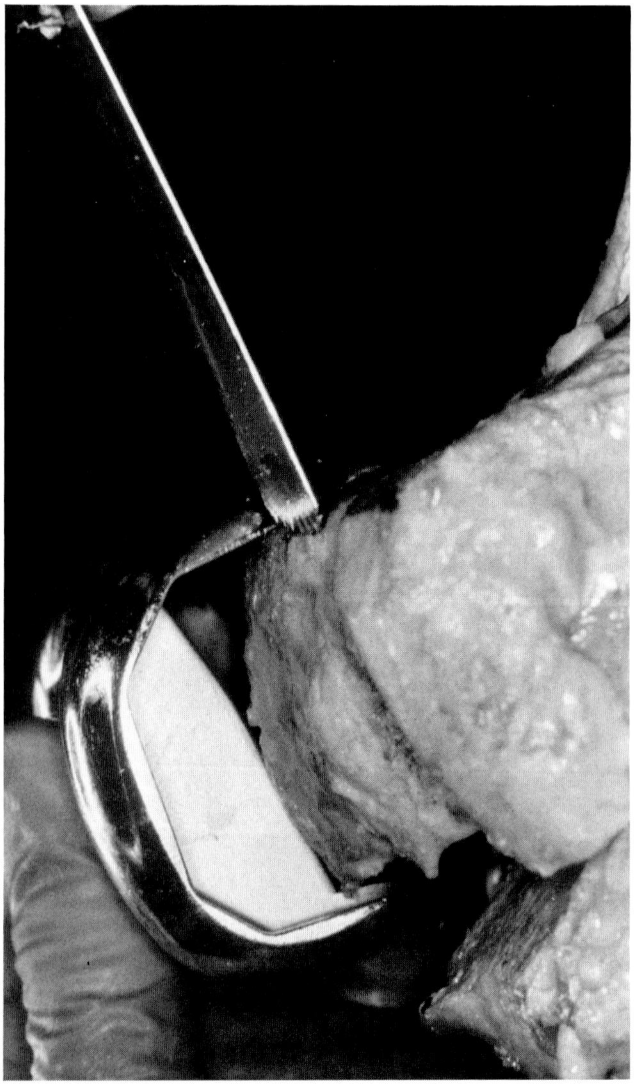

Fig. 6-23C The distal femoral cut is parallel to the femoral component while in position.

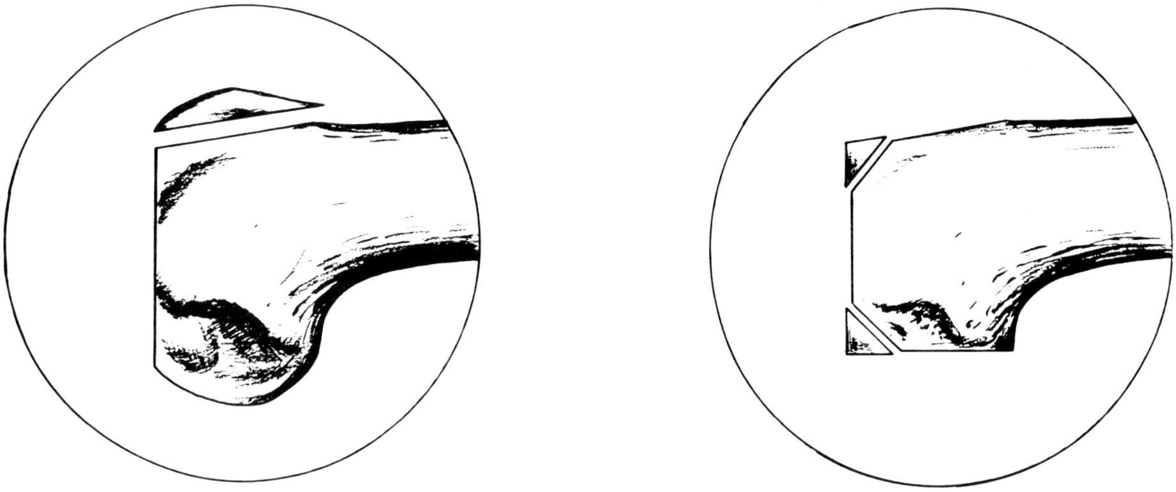

**Fig. 6-24A** These cuts do not effect overall alignment or stability, but rather allow the fit of the component to the femur.

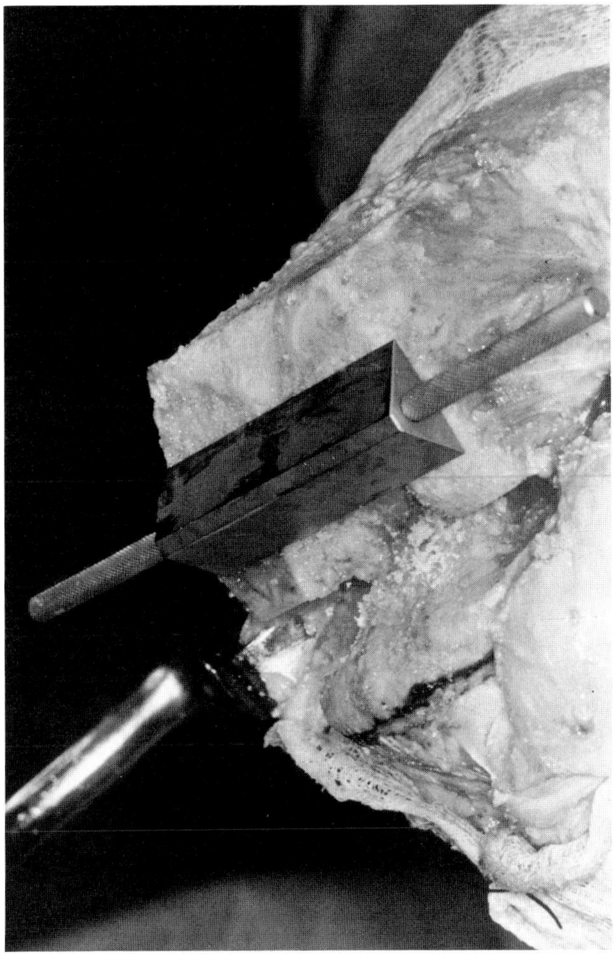

**Fig. 6-24B** A typical chamfering guide for the distal femur.

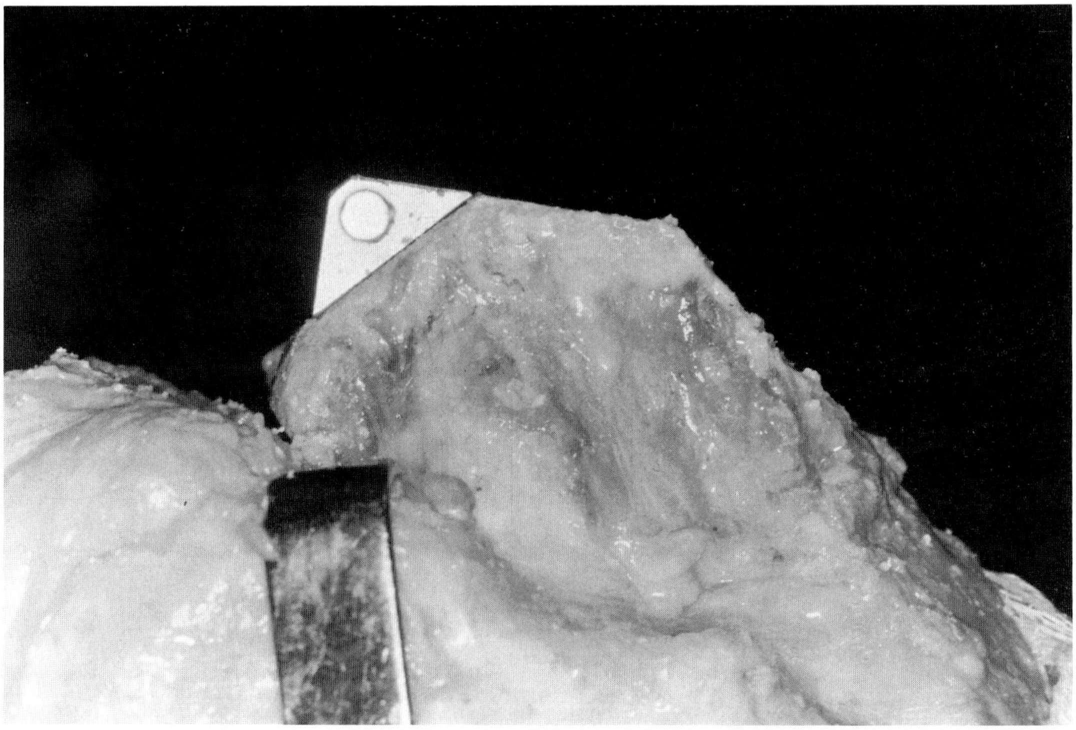

**Fig. 6-24C** A side view of the chamfering guide.

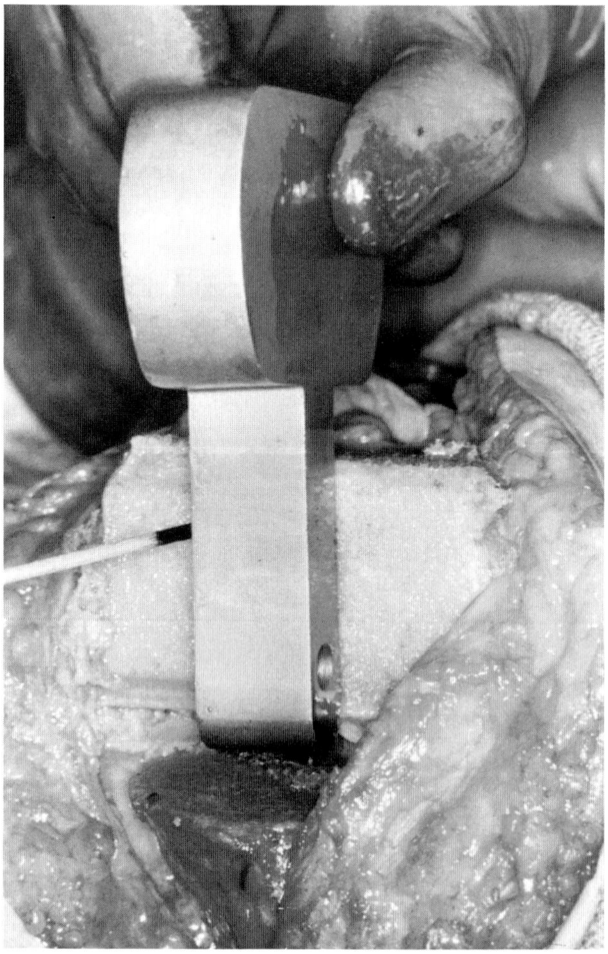

**Fig. 6-25A** For the posterior-stabilized design, the central portion must be resected to accommodate the housing of the femoral component.

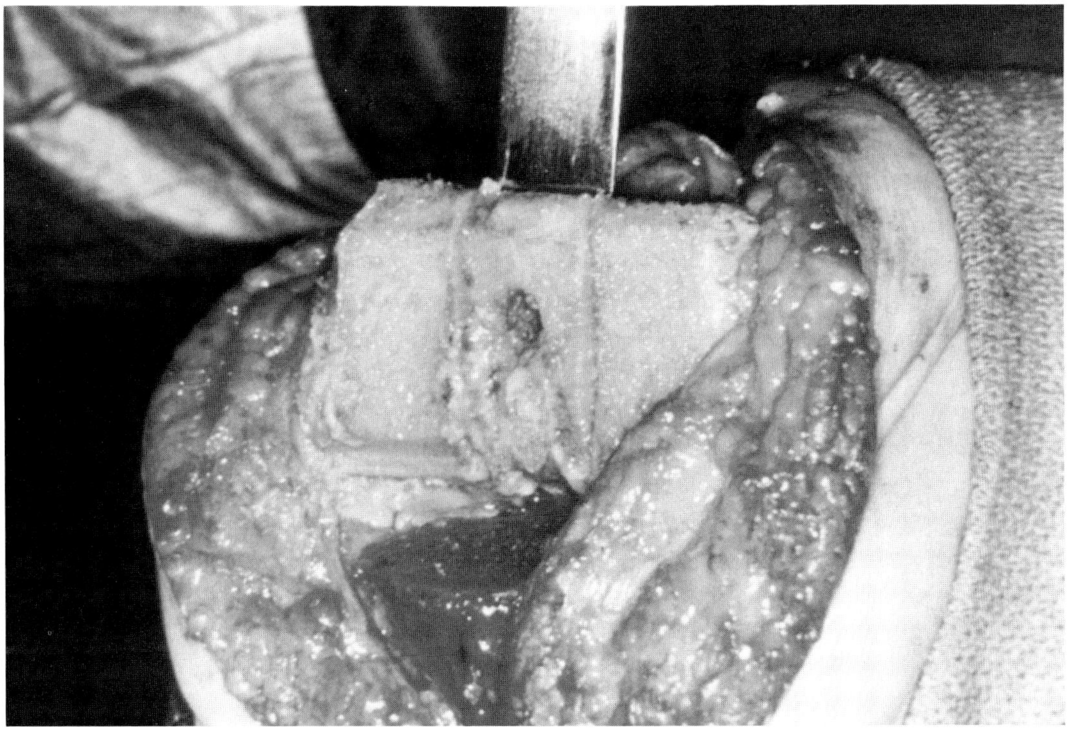

**Fig. 6-25B** It is best to remove bone in this area with an osteotome, not a saw.

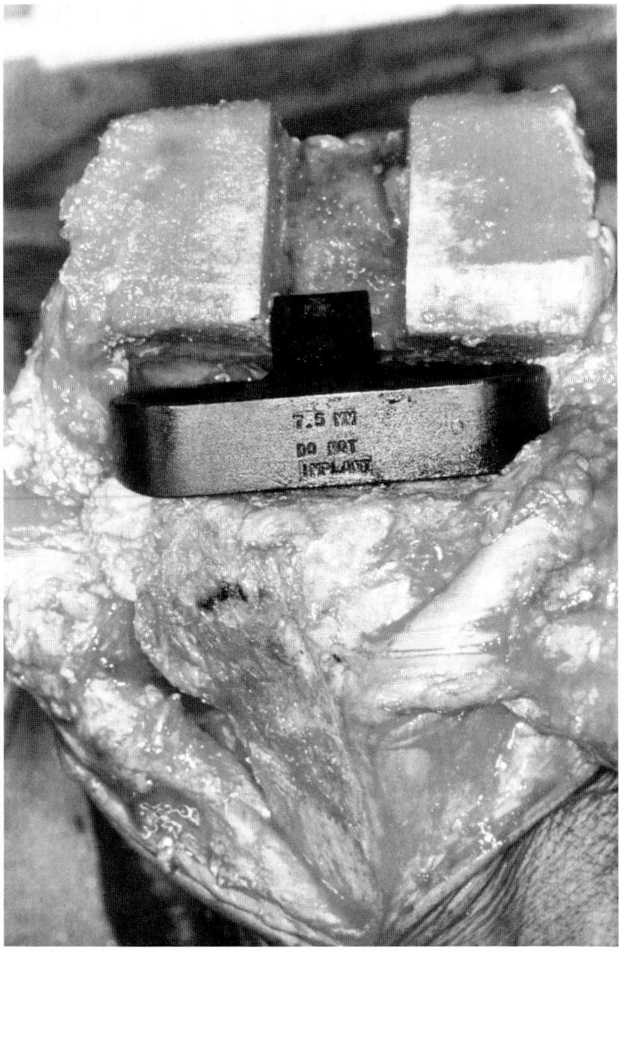

**Fig. 6-25C** With some designs, such as the posterior-stabilized, the alignment in flexion can be checked by assessing the intercondylar eminence with the femoral housing.

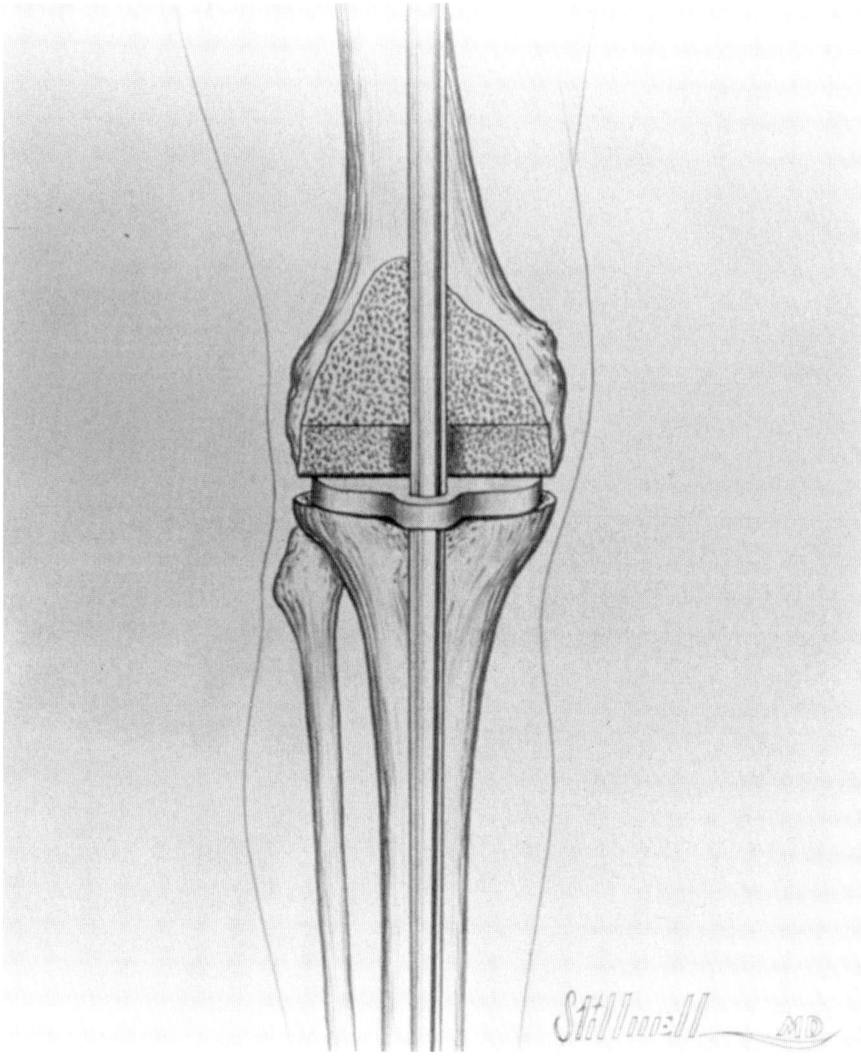


**Fig. 6-26A** Spacing and alignment is checked with a rod approaching the anterior superior inferior iliac crest with the midmalleolar axis.

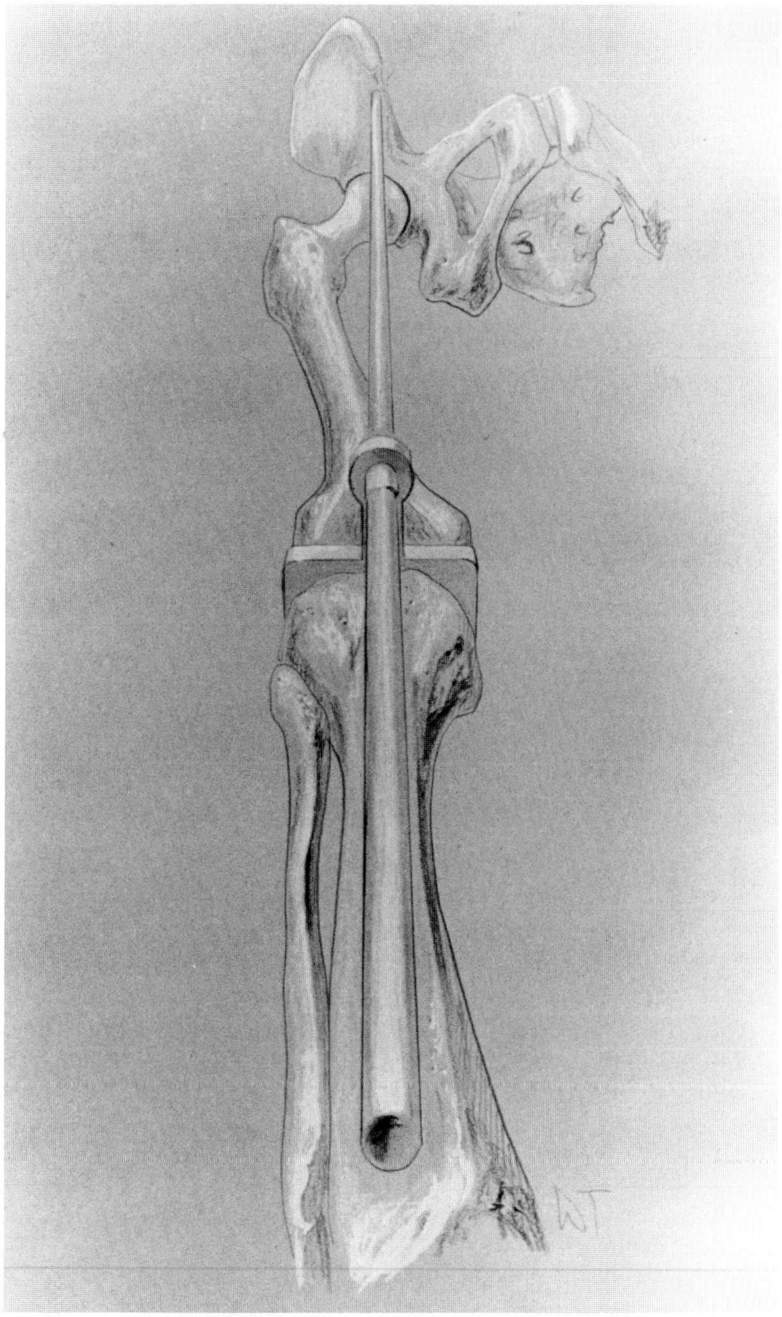

**Fig. 6-26B** An overall view of the aligning rod and its anatomical relationships.

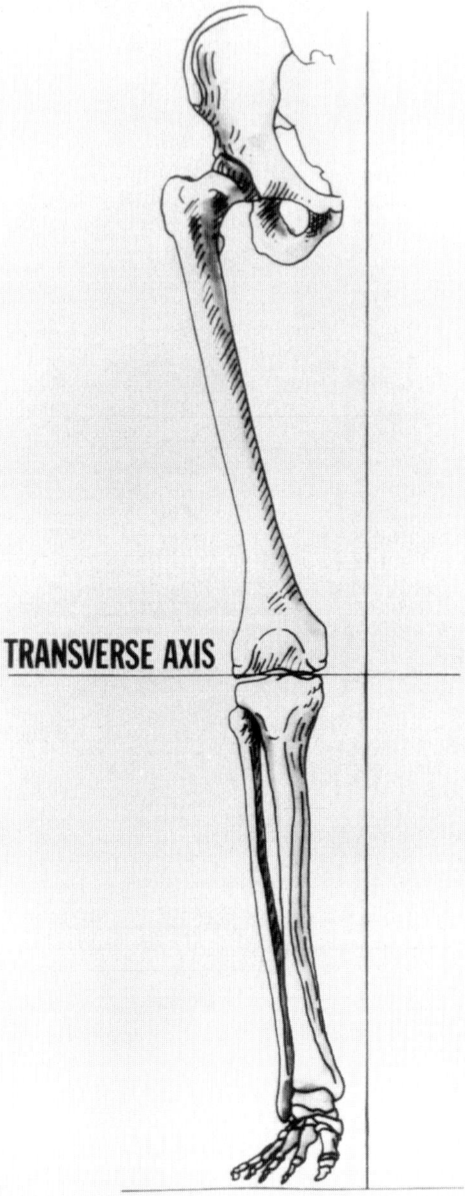


**Fig. 6-26C** The transverse axis is perpendicular to a vertical axis.

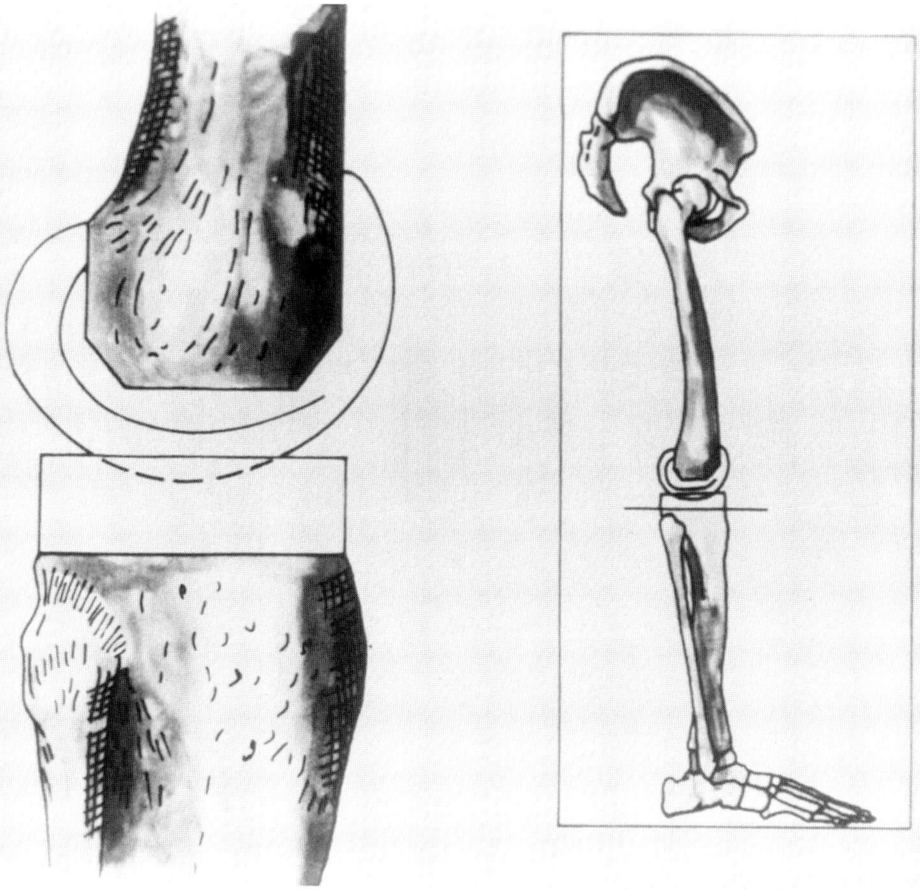

**Fig. 6-27A** In the sagittal plane, the tibial component should sit squarely on the resected tibia.

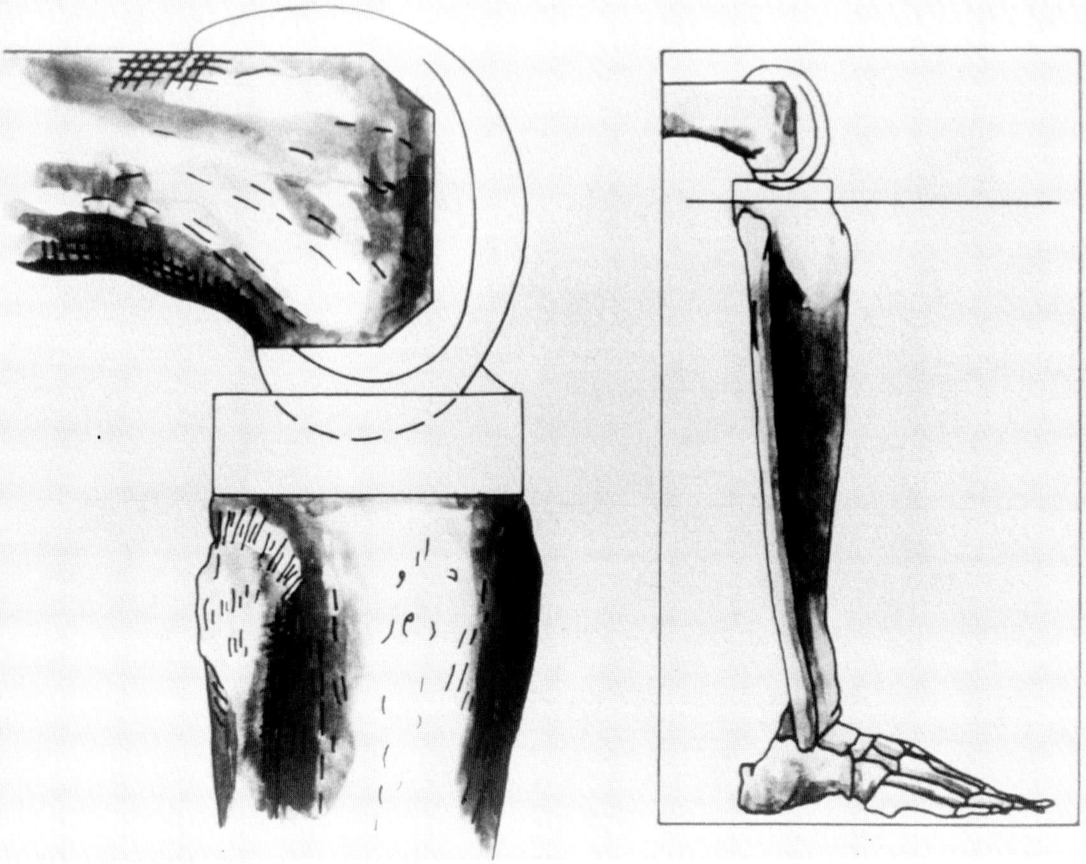

**Fig. 6-27B** The anterolateral bow of the femur results in an alignment of the component 5°–10° away from the perpendicular axis of the femur.

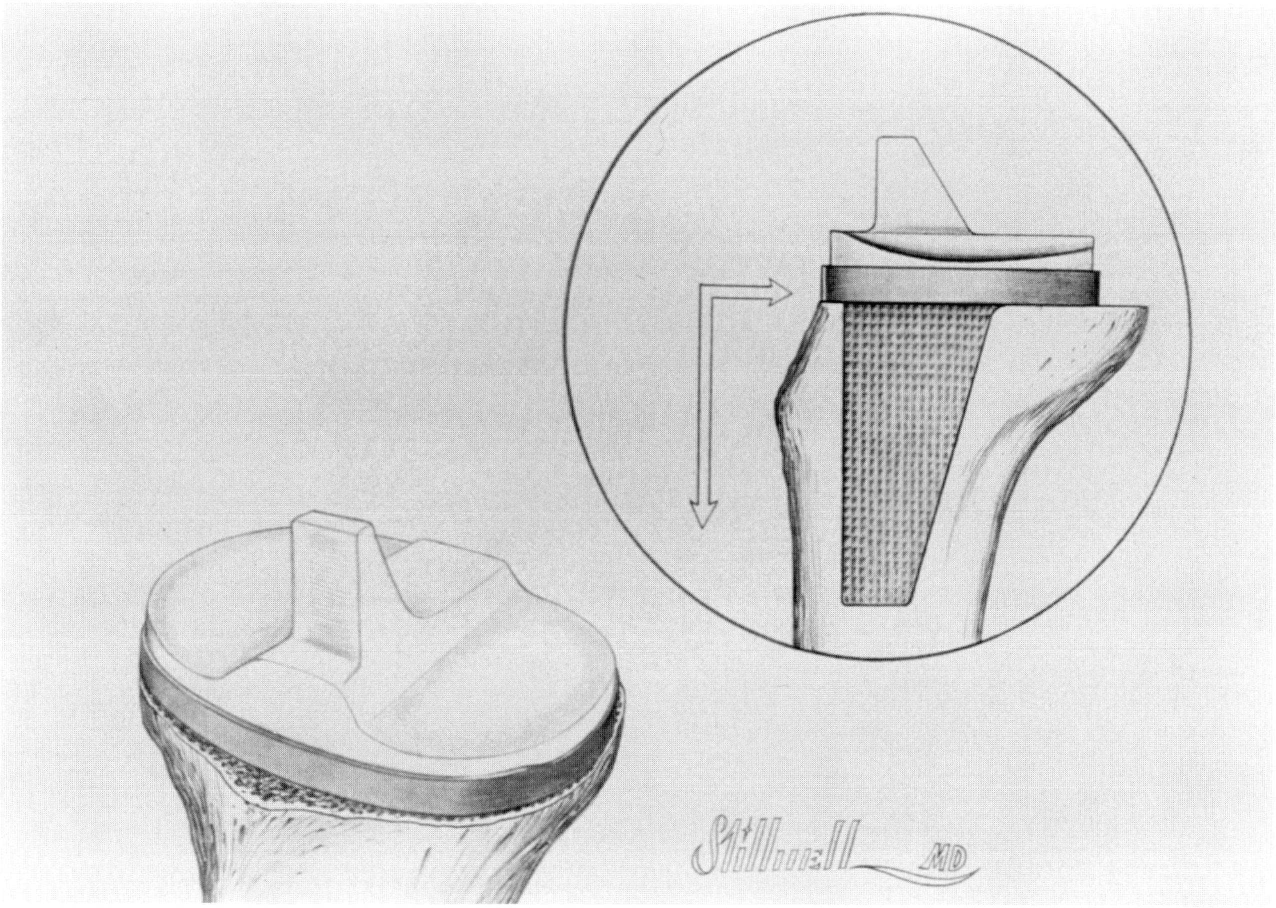

**Fig. 6-27C** The right angle relationship between the component and the tibia.

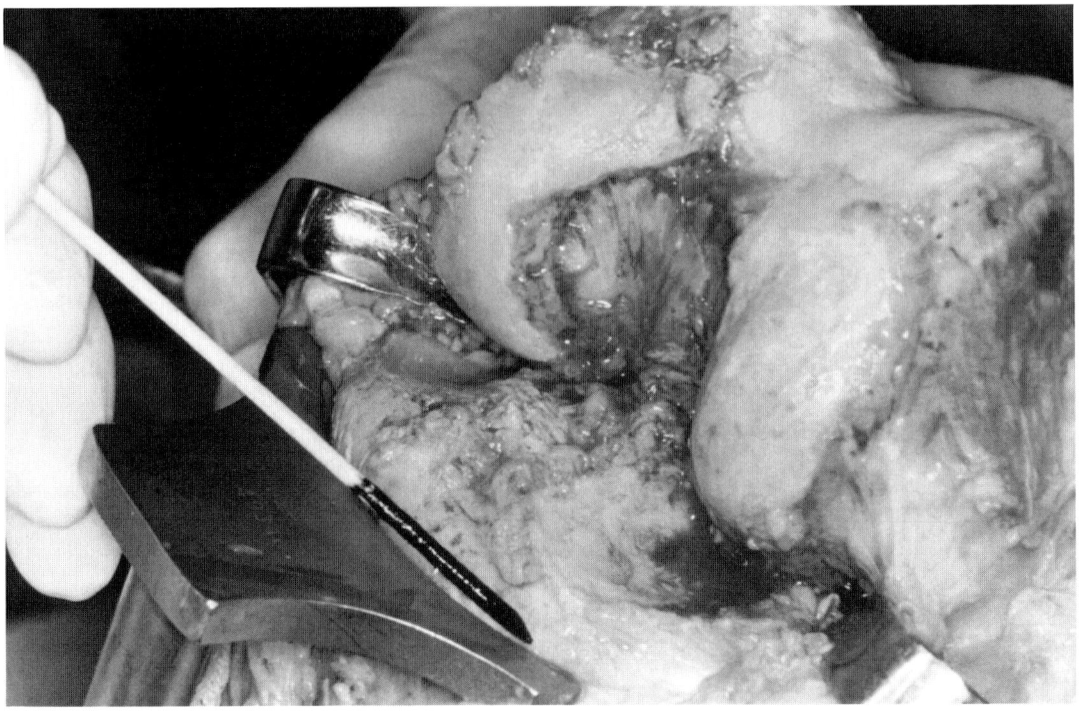

**Fig. 6-28A** The level of tibial resection can be marked with methylene blue.

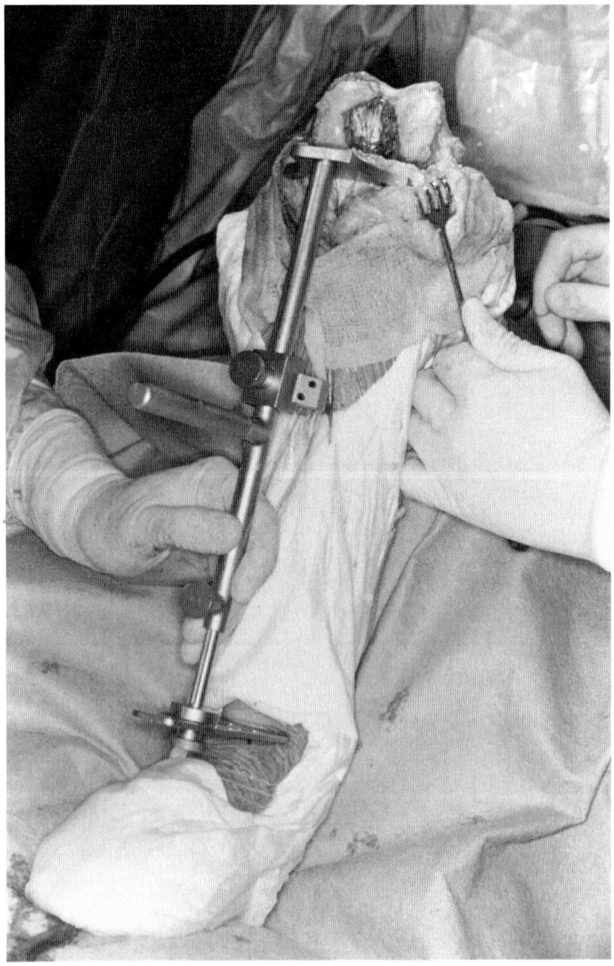

**Fig. 6-28B** In systems where the tibial cut is outlined by an aligning system that centers on the tibial shaft, one must beware too much tibial bowing.

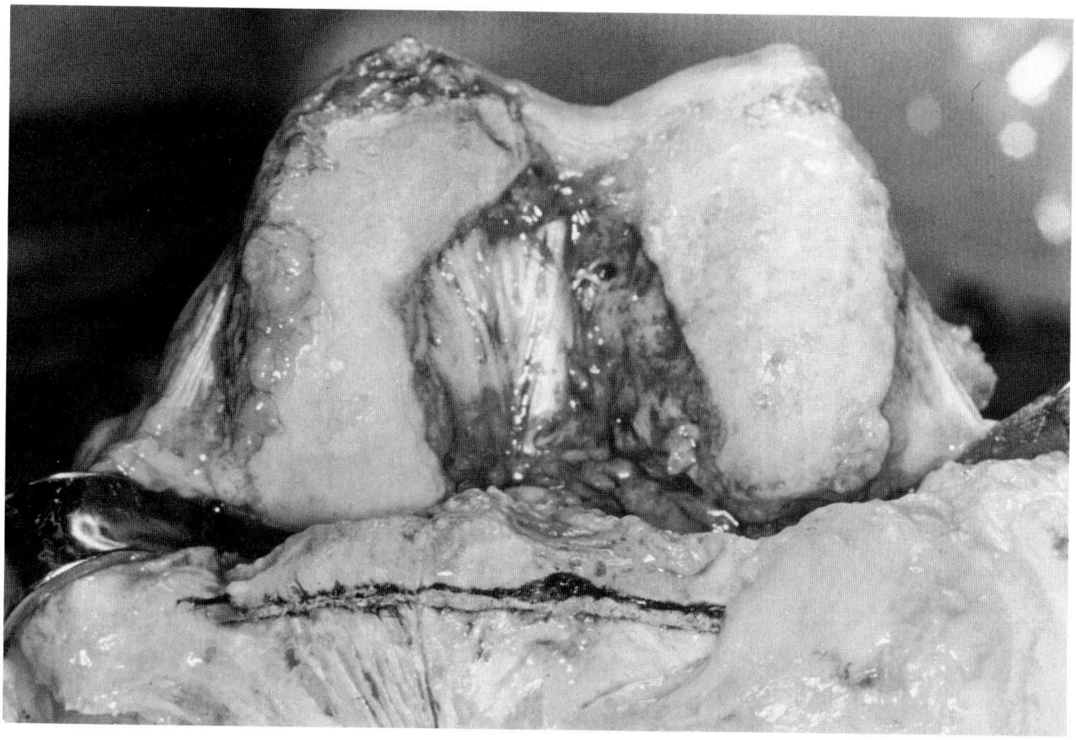

**Fig. 6-28C** Having indicated the level of resection, the tibia can be cut either by "eyeball" or with a "cutting guide."

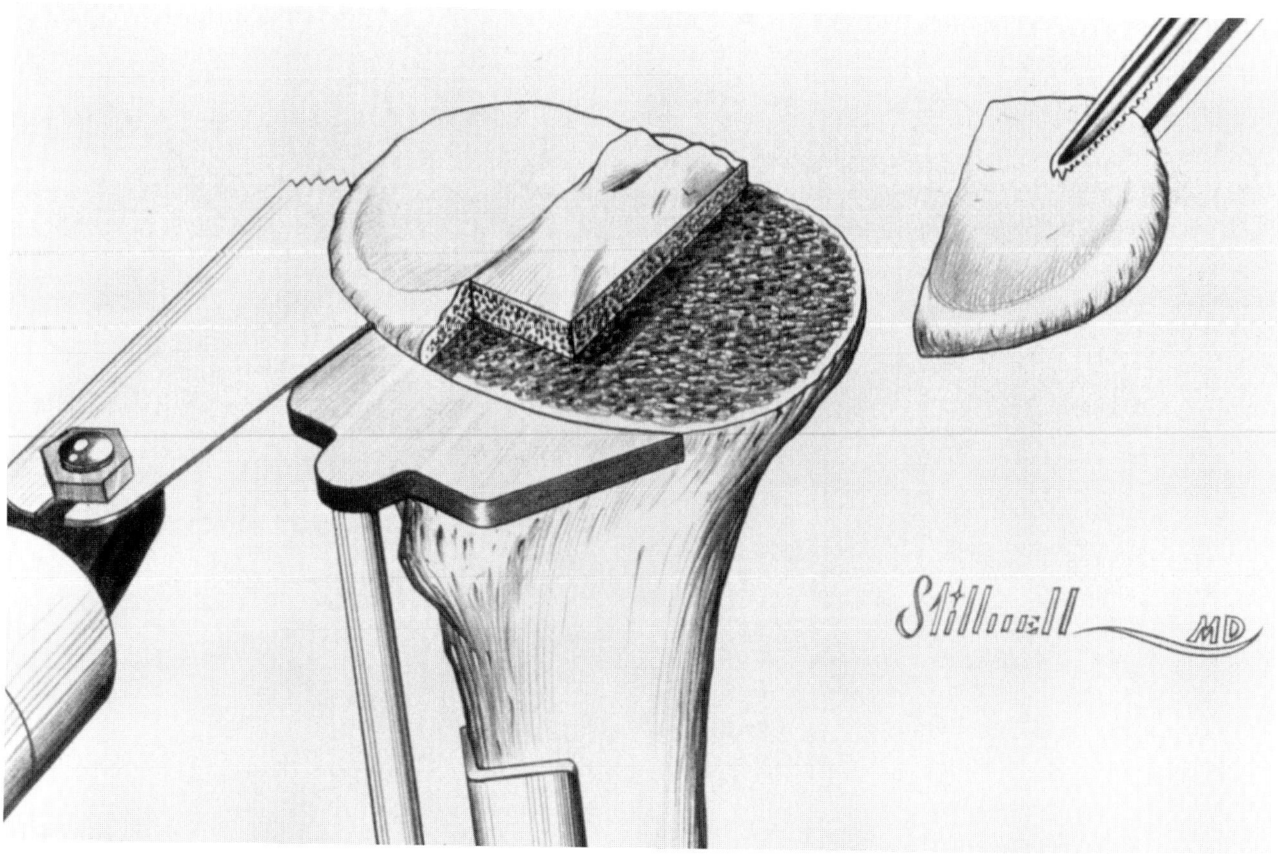

**Fig. 6-28D** If there is no bony deformity, equal amounts of bone are removed from both the medial and lateral plateau.

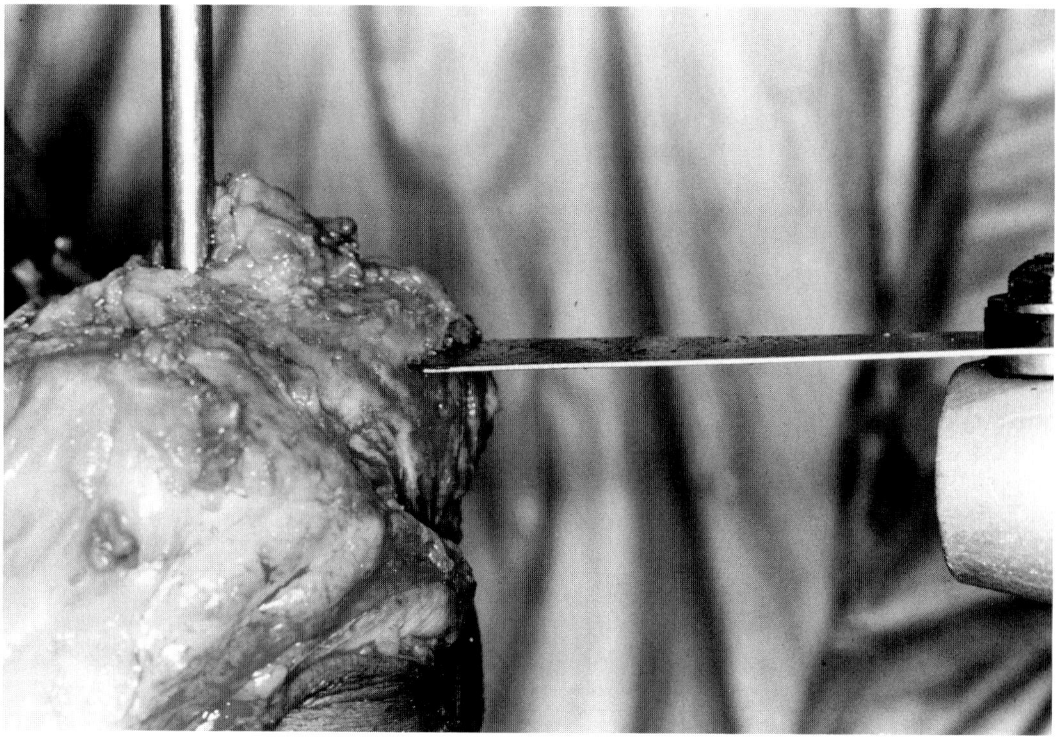

**Fig. 6-29A** Placing a rod in the tibial metaphysis and the saw blade at a right angle to the rod will ensure an even cut in both the coronal and sagittal plane.

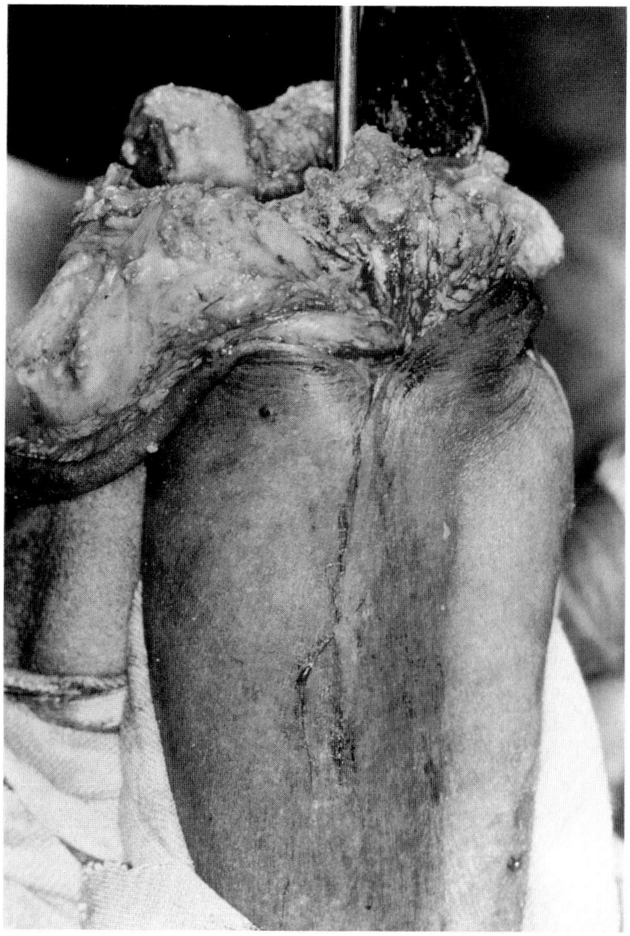

**Fig. 6-29B** The rod does not have to extend to the diaphyseal region, thus avoiding any anatomical deformity.

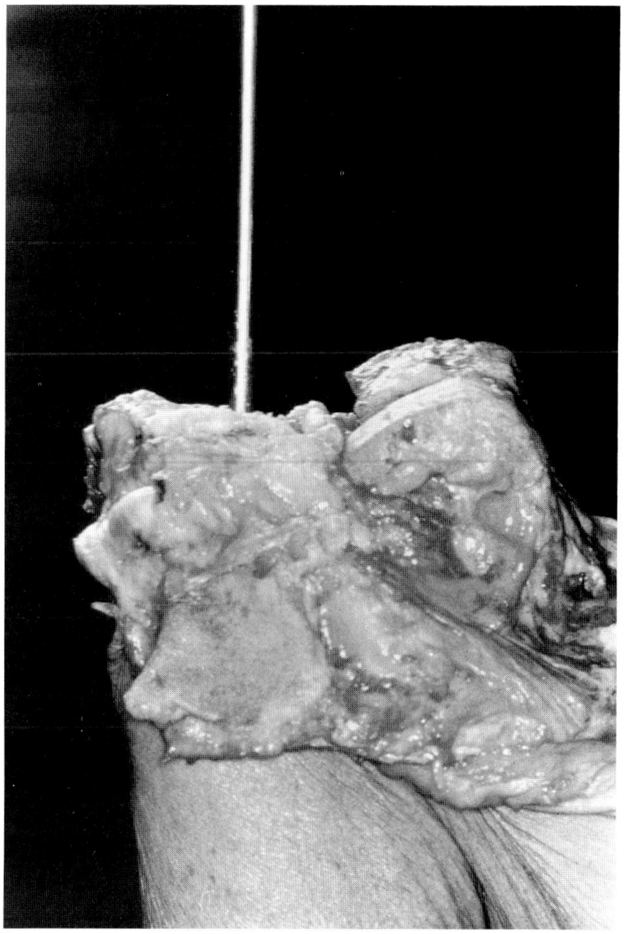

**Fig. 6-29C** A lateral view showing the posterior slope of the proximal tibia.

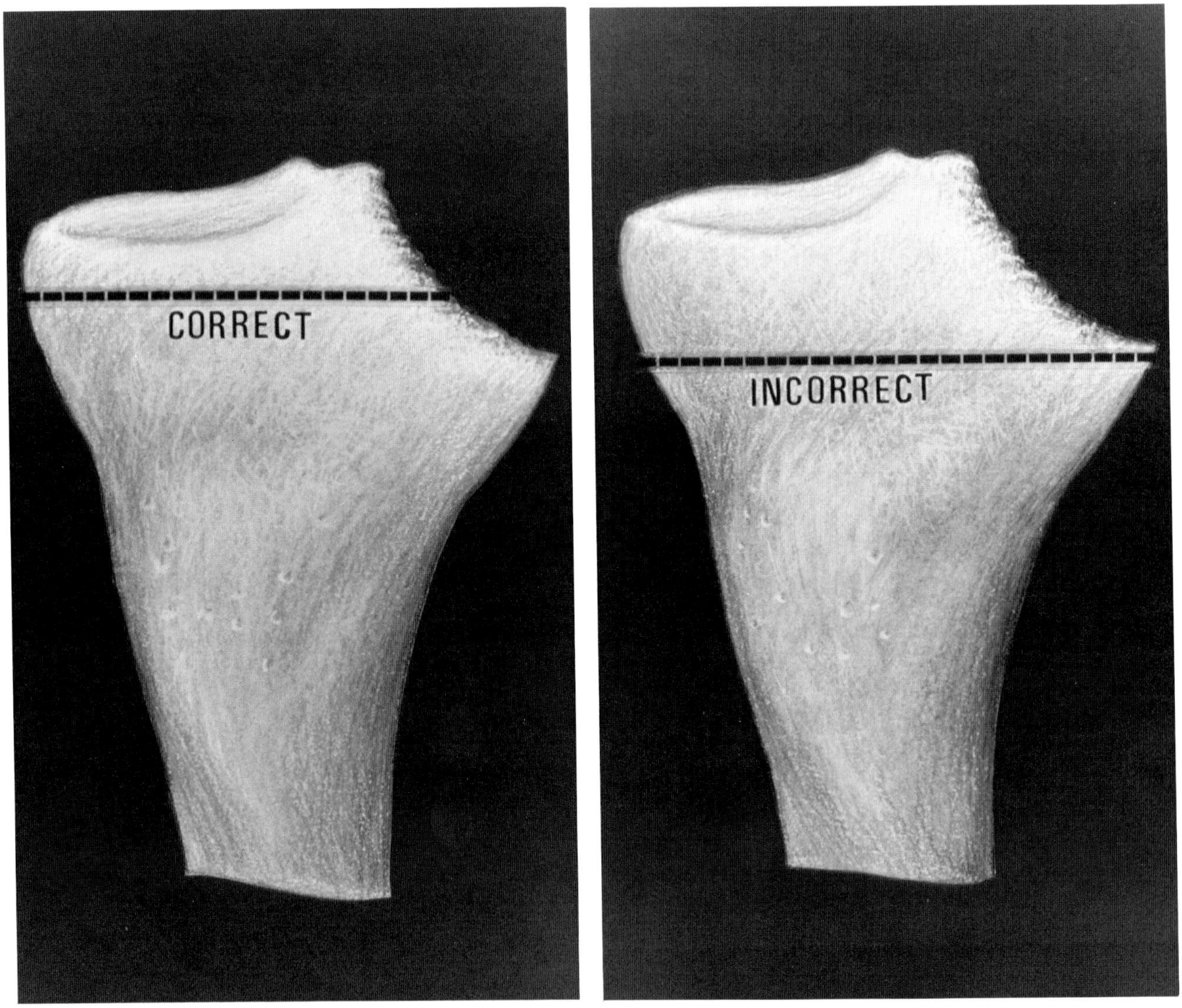


**Figs. 6-30A and B** With a bone deformity, it is important not to resect bone at the base of the deformity, but rather concentrate on augmenting the final depression.

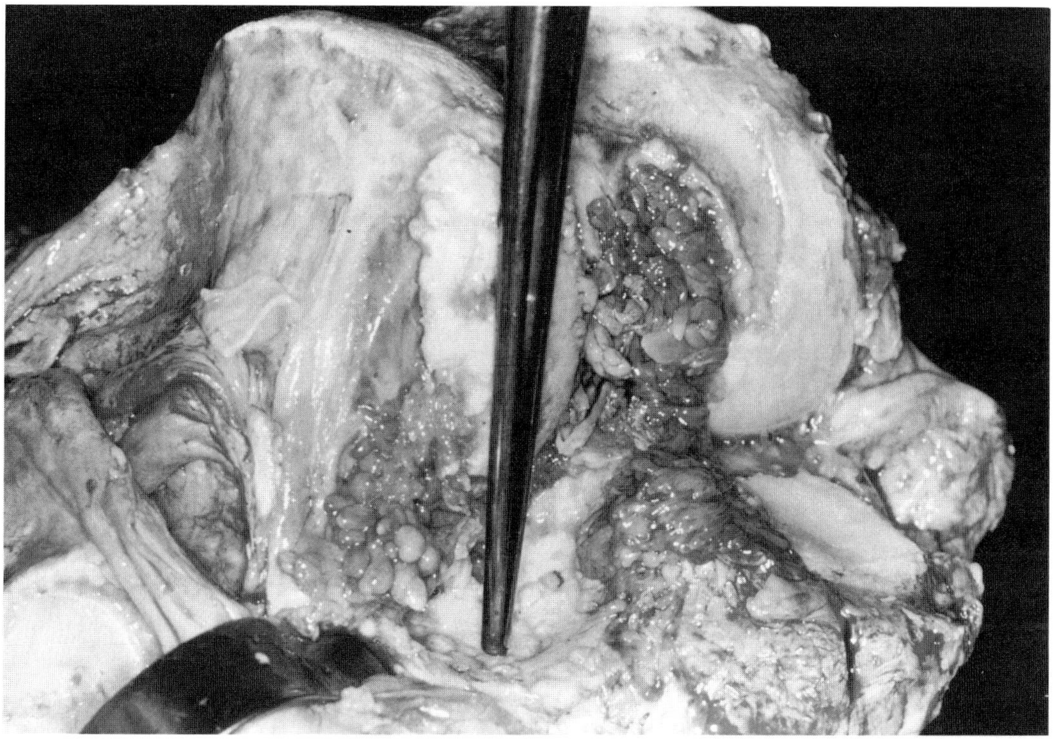

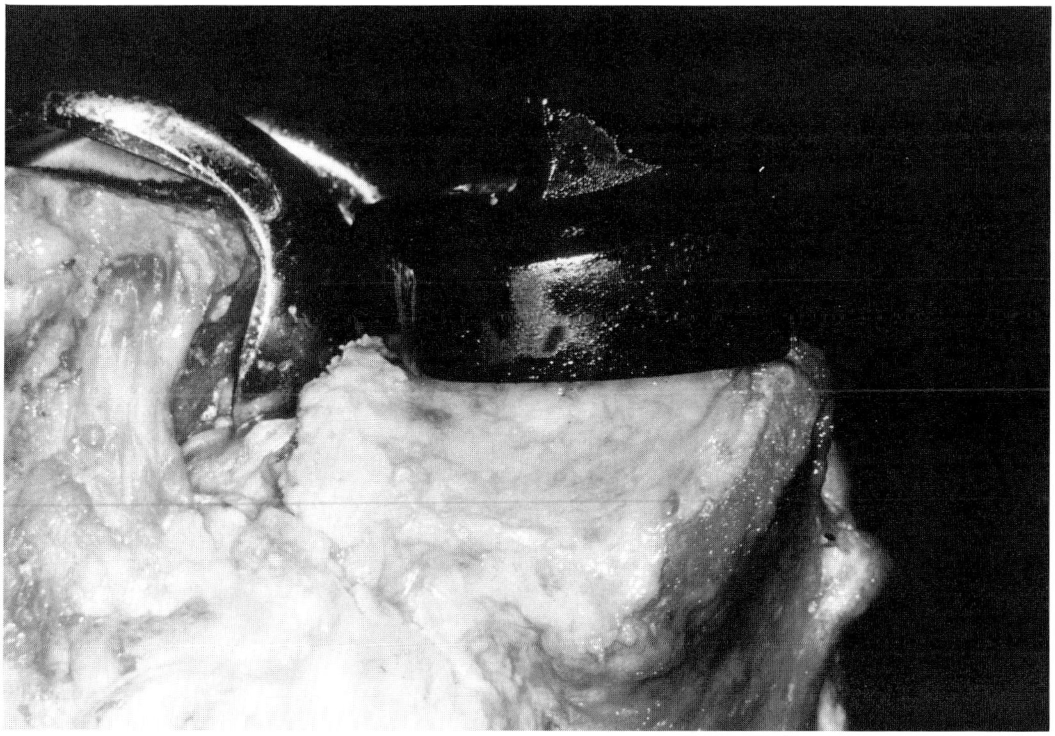

**Figs. 6-31A and B** A depression of the tibial plateau prior to and after bone resection.

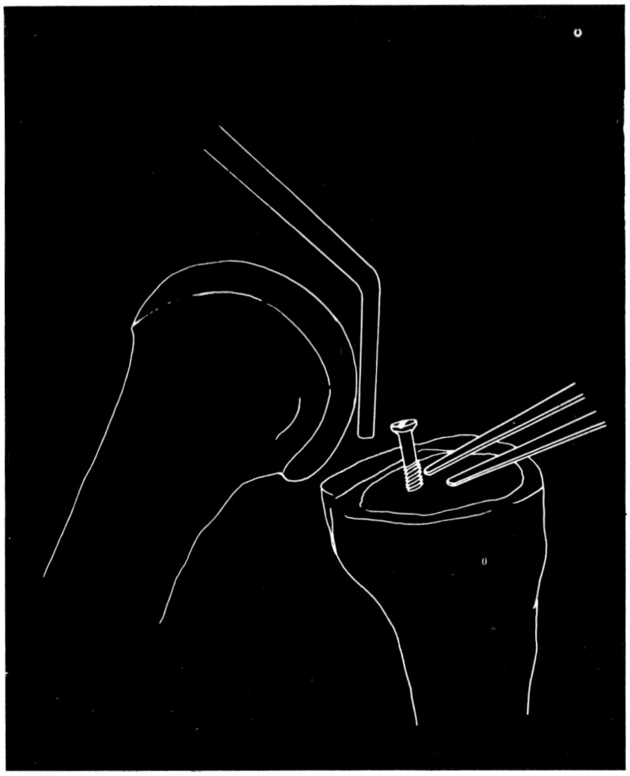

**Fig. 6-31C** Depressions can be augmented via screws alone, screws and cement, and bone grafts.

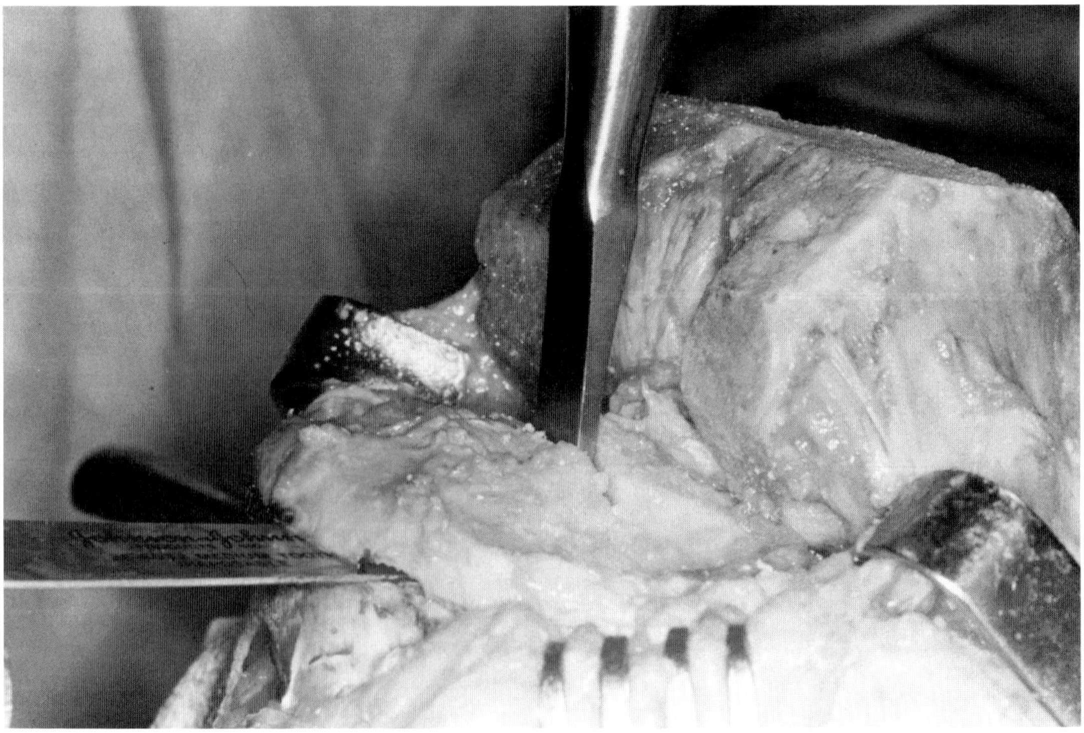

**Figs. 6-32A–C** Depending on the type of prosthesis, the tibial plateau must be resected either completely (cruciate sacrificing) or by preserving the posterior central island to ensure the integrity of the posterior cruciate ligament.

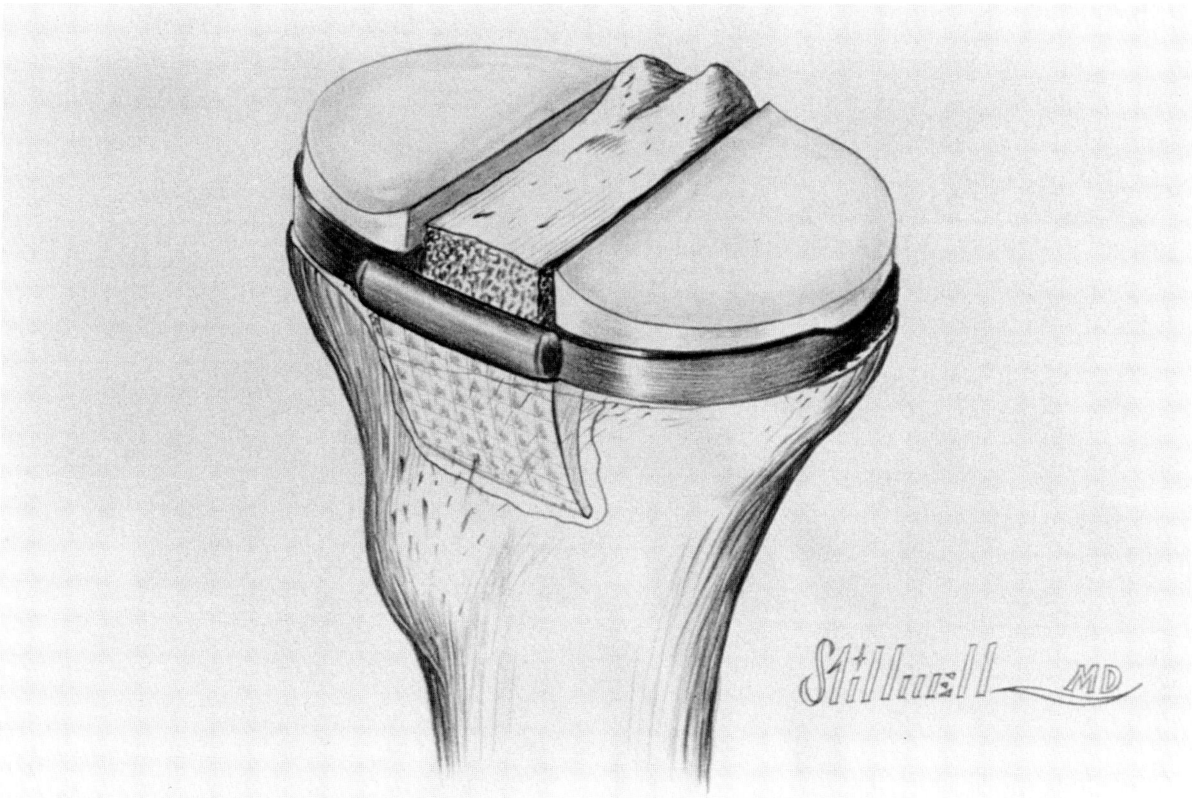

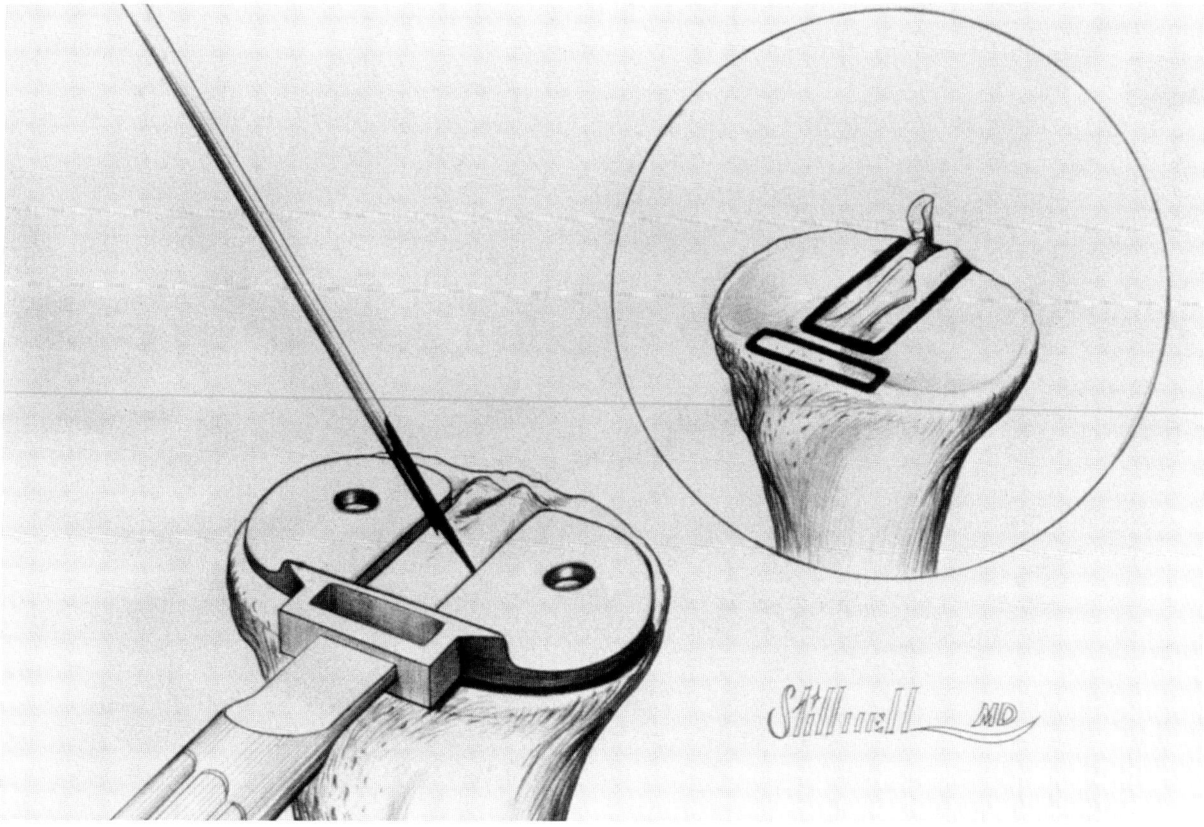

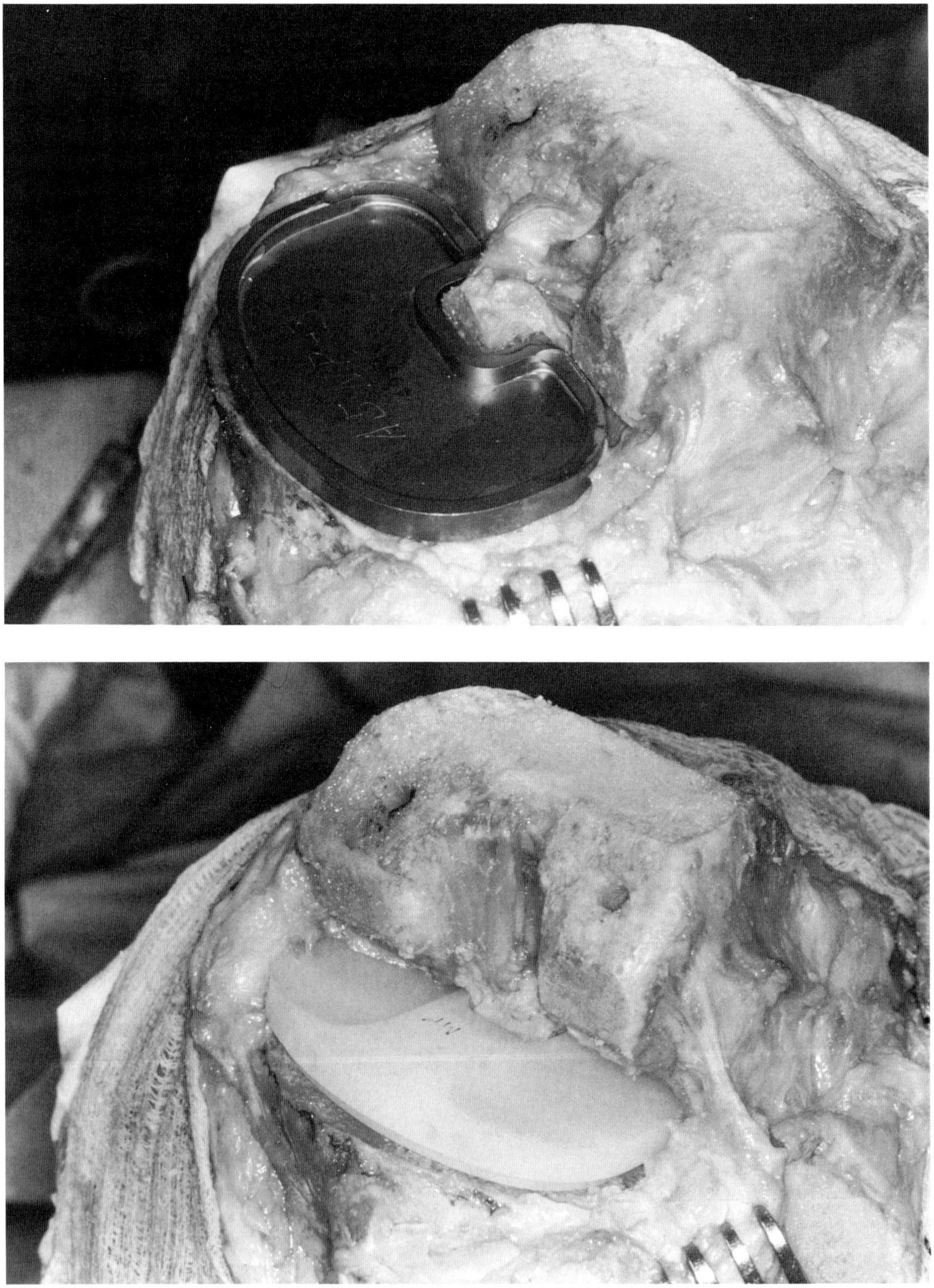

**Figs. 6-33A and B** Posterior cruciate retaining plateaus that preserve enough bone to ensure that the cruciate attachment on the posterior cortex is not disrupted.

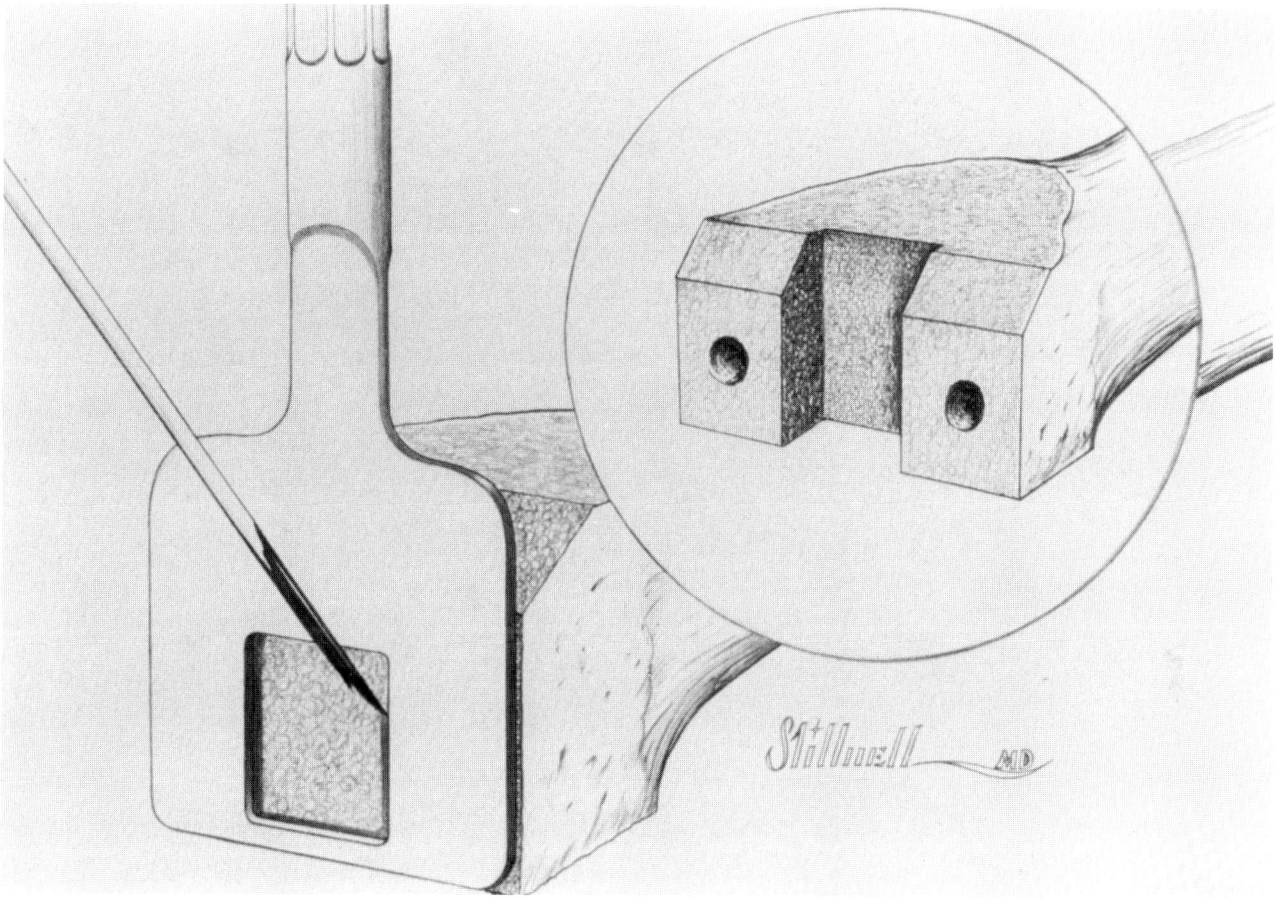


**Fig. 6-34A–C** In certain designs the central portion of the femoral housing will be aligned to the proximal tibia, otherwise, the rotation of this component can usually be aligned with the tibial tubercle.

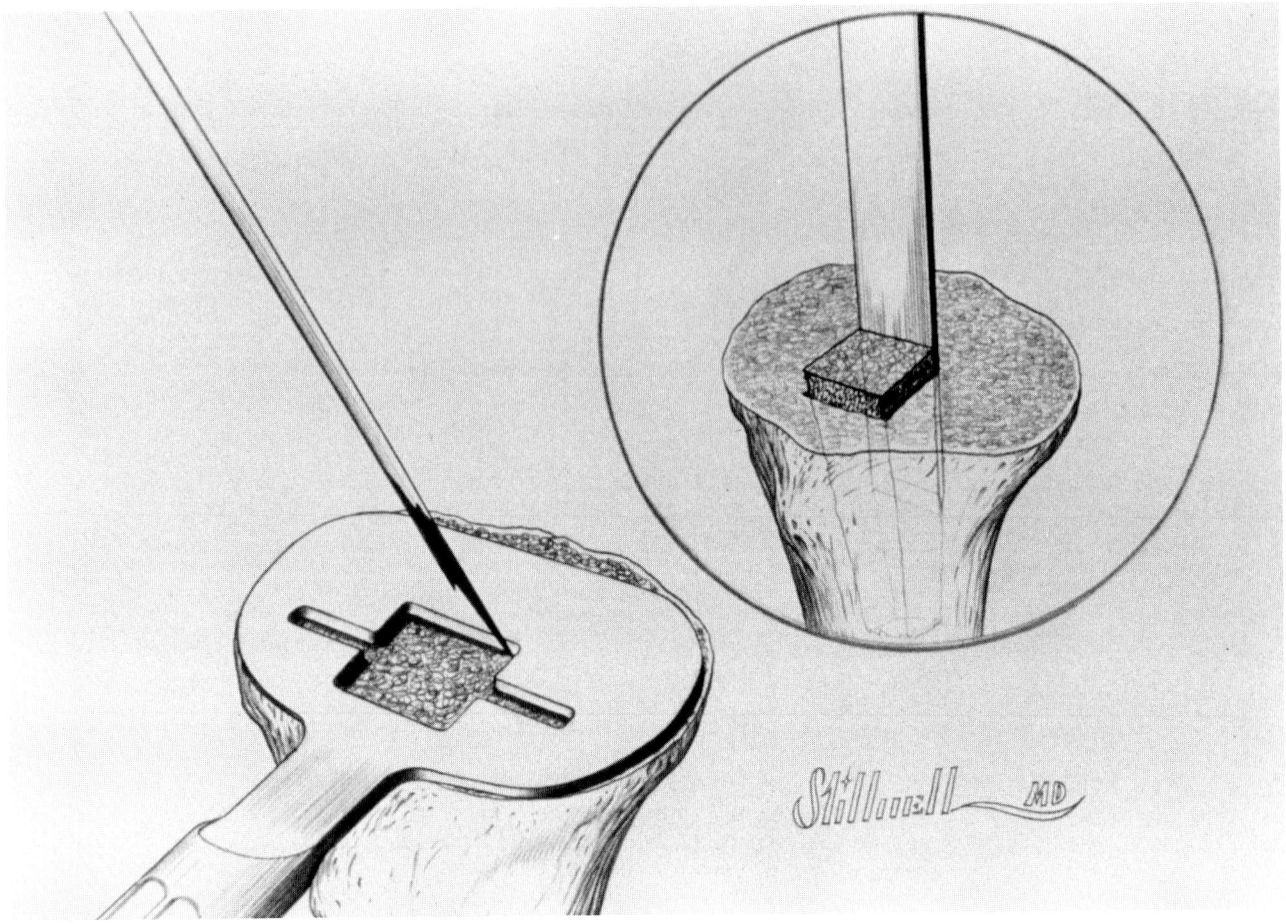

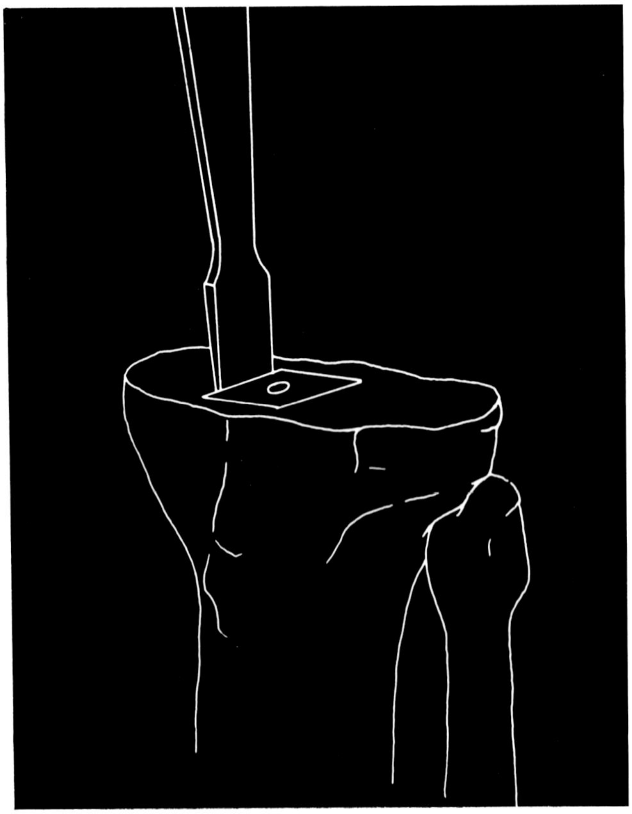

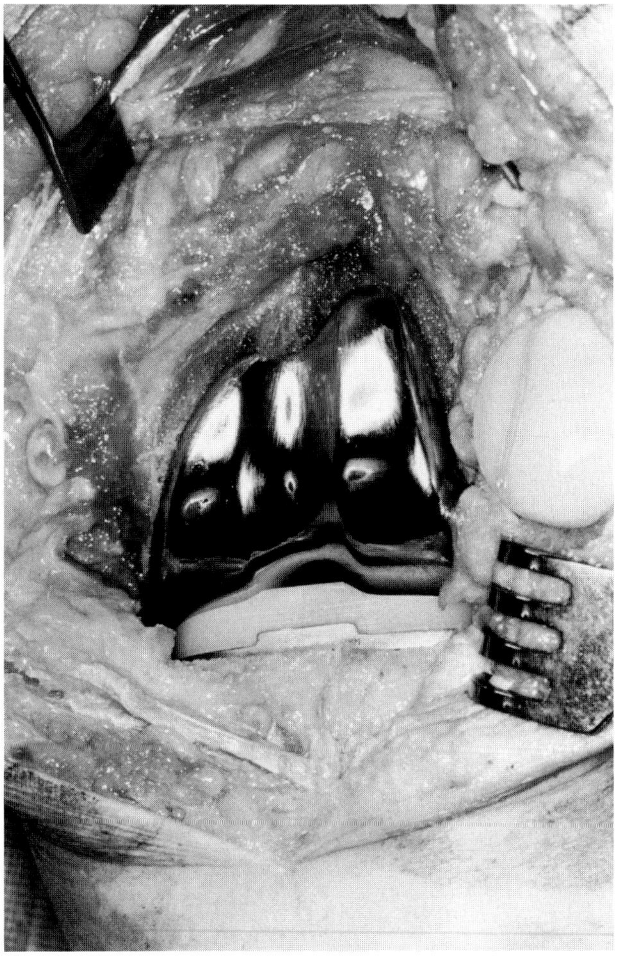

**Fig. 6-34D** The femoral and tibial components are centered, ensuring no malrotation.

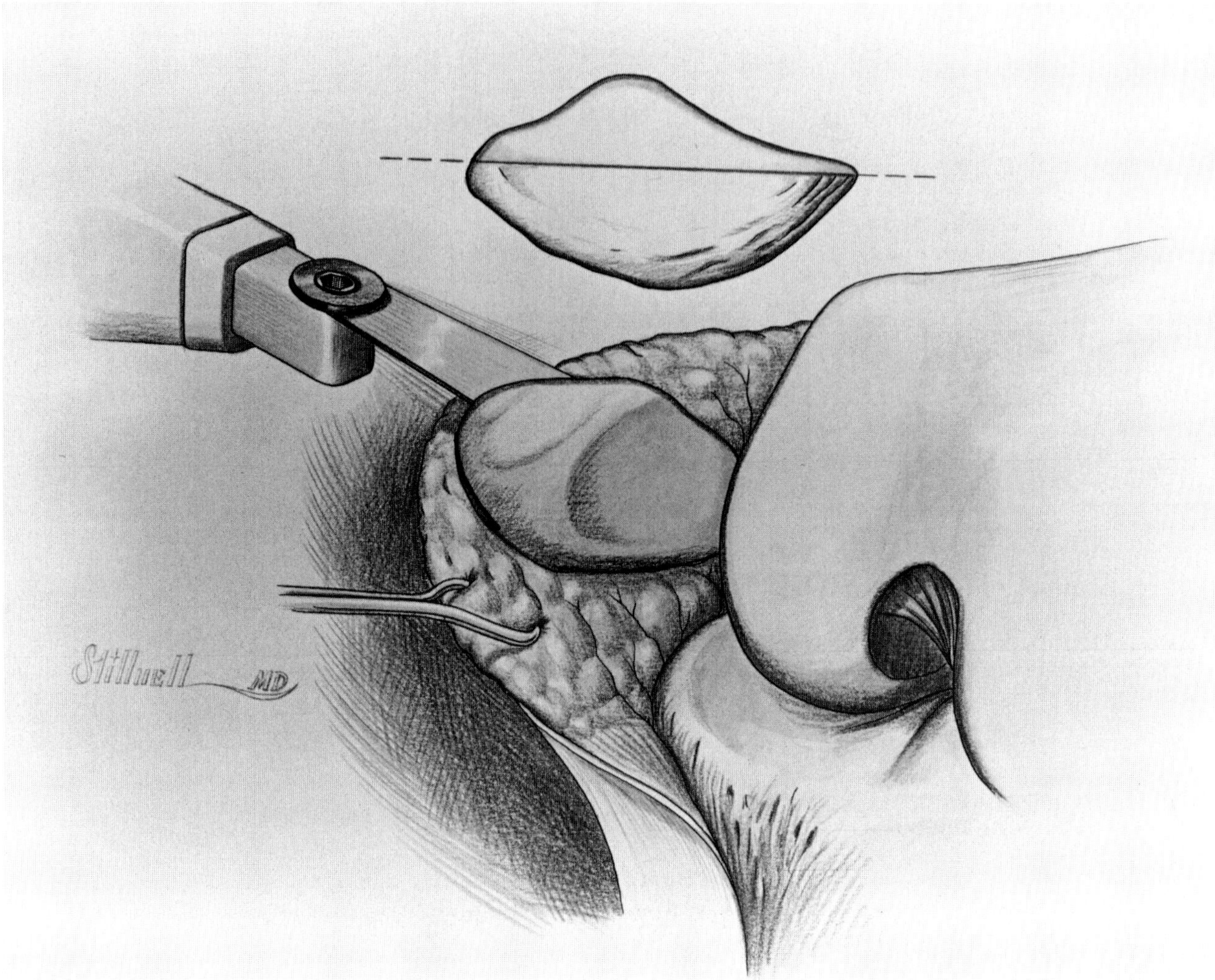


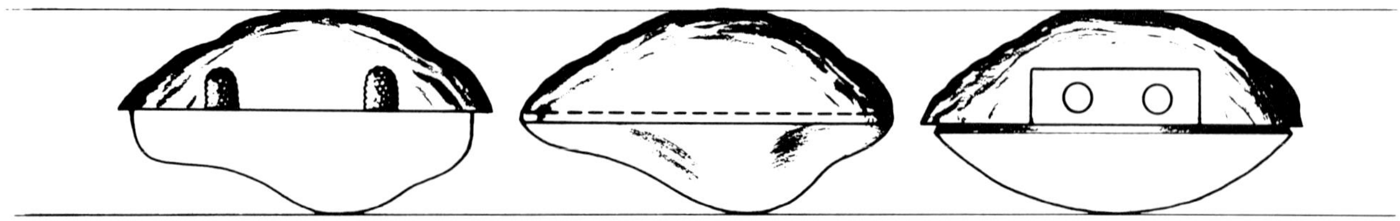

**Figs. 6-35A and B** Whether the patella prosthesis has one central peg or smaller fixation lugs, minimal bone is resected, less than one-third the surface, producing a totally flat area.

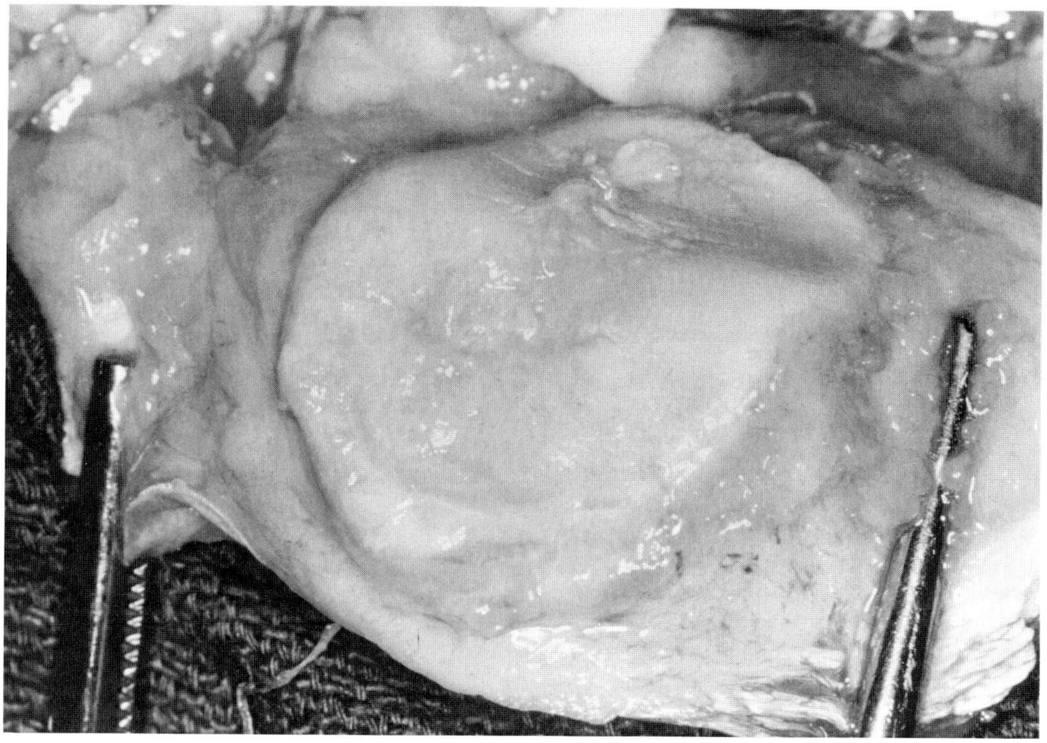

**Fig. 6-36A** The quadriceps and patella tendon are everted and clamped to facilitate exposure for resection.

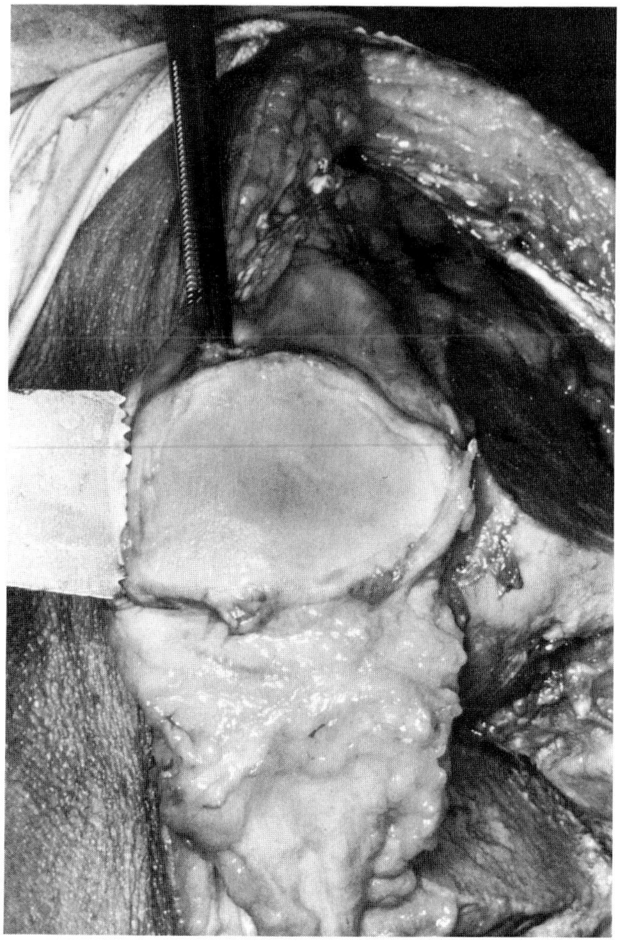

**Fig. 6-36B** Owing to the facets of the patella, the blade is usually placed just below the lowest facet that is dependent on the disease process.

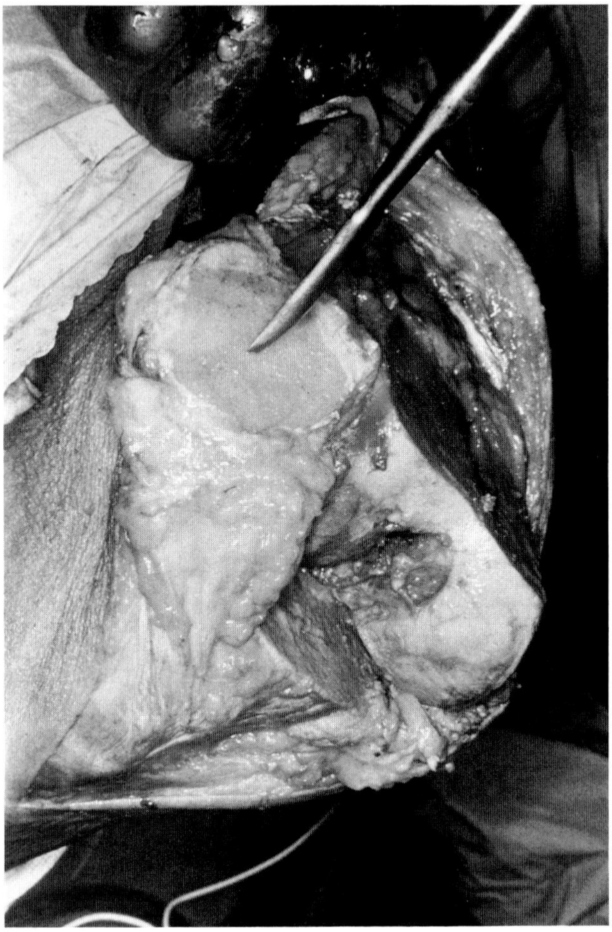

Figs. 6-37A and B Appropriate patella fixation hole(s) is made in the cancellous surface.

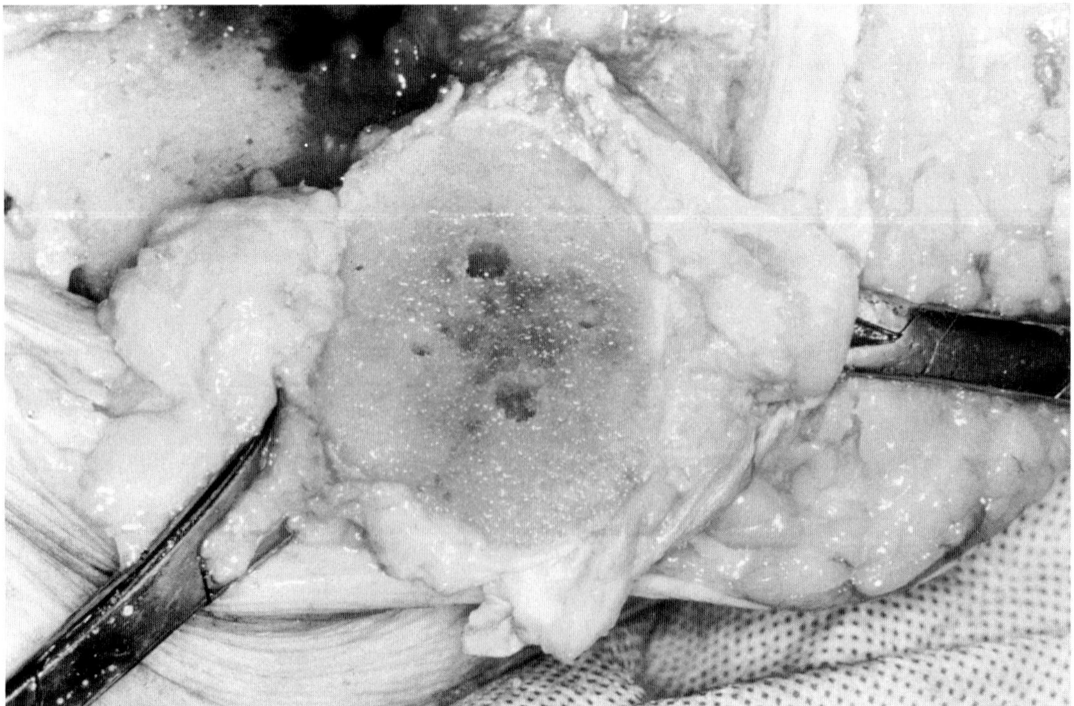

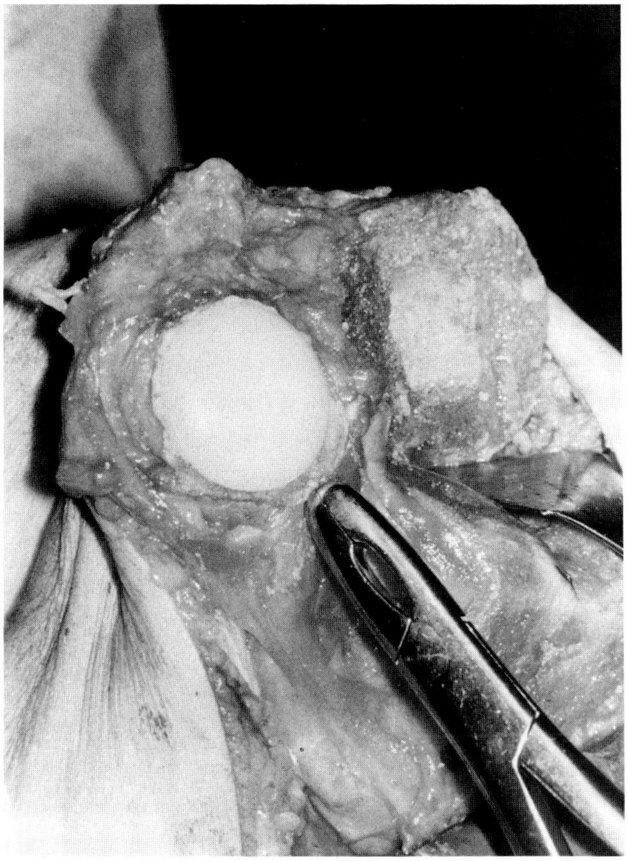

**Fig. 6-38A** Overhanging osteophytes should be removed from the surface of the patella.

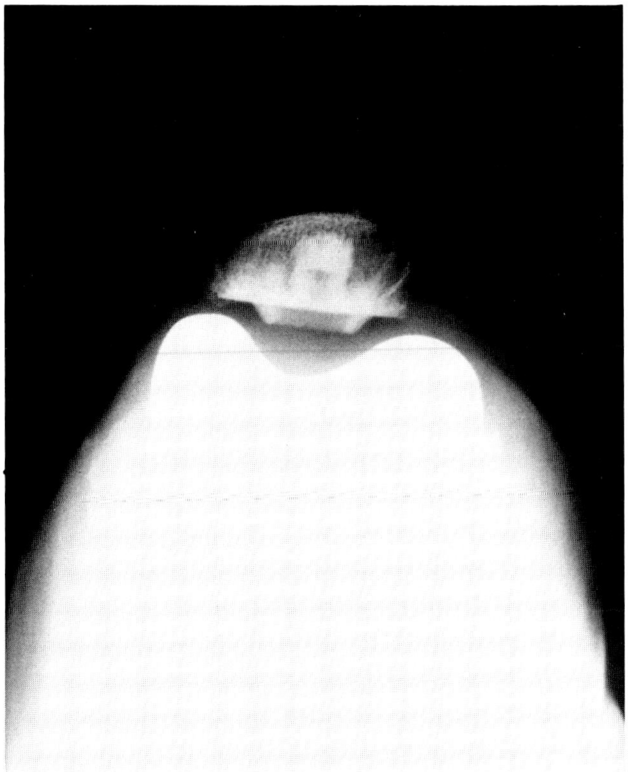

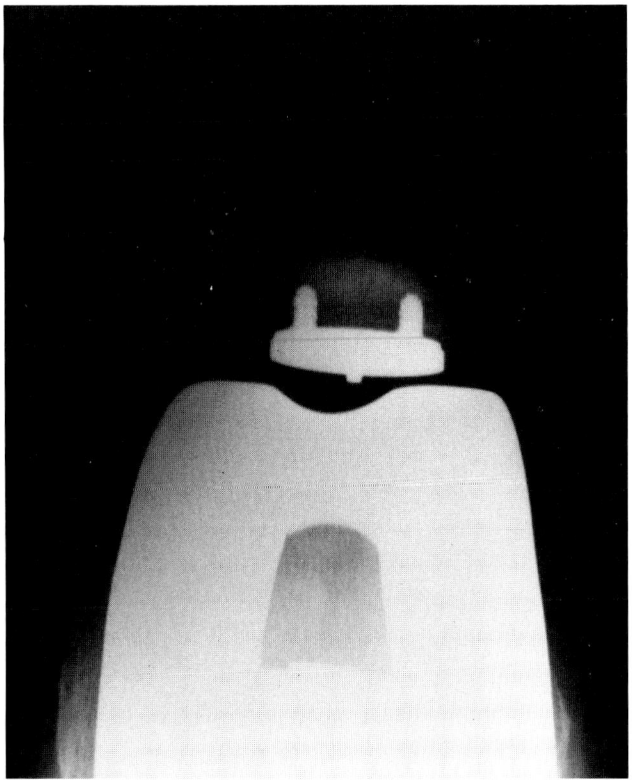

**Figs. 6-38B and C** Cemented and noncemented patella replacements.

## References

1. Scott, W.N. (Ed.). *Total Knee Arthroplasty, Five and Ten Year Statistics,* 204:36–39, 1986.
2. Scott, W.N., Tria, A., Insall, J. Total knee arthroplasty: Past, present & future. *Orthop. Surv.* 3(2),1979.
3. Walldius, B. Knaledsplastik Med Plastprotes. *Tidskrift, Militzis Halsovard* 78:77, 1953.
4. d'Aubique, M.R., Lacheretz, C.M. Traitement des ankylosis. *Rev. Chir. Orthop.* 39:495, 1953.
5. Thornhill, T. Unicompartmental knee arthroplasty. *Clin. Orthop. Rel. Res.* 205:121–130.
6. Insall, J. The Total Condylar Prosthesis. *Clin. Orthop. Rel. Res.* 205:43–49.

# Index